CATALINA ALEGRE D

HEMATOLOGIC PROBLEMS IN THE NEWBORN

Second Edition

By

Frank A. Oski, M.D.

Associate Professor of Pediatrics, Department of
Pediatrics, University of Pennsylvania School of
Medicine; Hematologist, Children's Hospital
of Philadelphia

and

J. Lawrence Naiman, M.D.

Associate Professor of Pediatrics, Temple
University School of Medicine; Director of
Hematology, St. Christopher's Hospital for
Children, Philadelphia

Volume IV in the Series

MAJOR PROBLEMS IN CLINICAL PEDIATRICS

ALEXANDER J. SCHAFFER
Consulting Editor

W. B. Saunders Company, Philadelphia, London, Toronto   1972

W. B. Saunders Company: West Washington Square
                           Philadelphia, Pa. 19105

                           12 Dyott Street
                           London, WC1A   1DB

                           1835 Yonge Street
                           Toronto 7, Ontario

Hematologic Problems in the Newborn   ISBN 0-7216-7021-0

Print No.:   9   8   7   6   5   4   3   2   1

TO
Our children
Jonathan, Jane, Jessica, Matthew, Jonathan, and Michael
and
to all of those who care for
or care about the newborn infant

Foreword

The first edition of this volume met with the enthusiasm it merited. It fulfilled precisely the conditions we envisaged as requisite for a succession of books of this nature. These were, first, that they describe exhaustively all the information with respect to one circumscribed segment of pediatrics, including the pertinent embryology, anatomy, physiology, and pathology; second, that they present all the clinical and laboratory data needed to aid one in arriving at proper diagnoses; third, that they indicate clearly the available and preferable modes of treatment; and, finally, that they be written by one or more authors who had devoted an appreciable number of years to work in the field under question.

In the six years which have intervened since the publication of their first edition neonatal hematology has almost literally leaped forward. Drs. Oski and Naiman have not only gathered together all of this material; they have themselves continued to contribute much to the advance. As a result, this edition contains one hundred pages more than the first, with almost every chapter covering ten to twenty more pages. All of this added matter brings each subtopic absolutely up to date.

The writing is superb, therefore the reading is easy. I myself read the book in page proof as though I were immersed in a novel, and I suspect that you will do the same.

ALEXANDER J. SCHAFFER, M.D.

Preface
to the Second Edition

In the space of six years, much to our gratification and embarrassment, our monograph has become obsolete. We are gratified because new knowledge in such areas as neonatal coagulation disturbances, the management of the fetus and newborn with erythroblastosis, and the problems of polycythemia, to cite only a few examples, enables the physician to better care for the infant. We are embarrassed because our students and house officers constantly remind us that our book is now either incorrect or inadequate. We hope the revisions in this second edition will ensure that the book will continue to be useful to those daily confronted with the hematologic problems of the newborn infant.

We have appreciated the wide usage of the first edition and are equally appreciative of those, who by their comments or by their efforts, are responsible for this second edition. The help of Dr. Michael E. Miller in revising the chapter on Disorders of the Leukocytes deserves special mention. We are particularly grateful for the secretarial assistance of Mrs. Judy Clark, Miss Ilene Levinson, Miss Ellen Rensel and Miss Rhonda Premit, for the artistic help of Dr. Thomas Tedesco, and for the editorial guidance of Mr. Robert Rowan, of W. B. Saunders Company.

FRANK A. OSKI
J. LAWRENCE NAIMAN

Preface
to the First Edition

During the first few weeks of life, there are more diagnostic problems with hematologic aspects than at any time thereafter. The pediatrician is asked to distinguish inherited disorders from acquired disease and the consequences of maternal-fetal interaction, all at a time when normal physiologic processes are in a state of rapid change. As Dr. Clement Smith has stated, "This is a time during which life is more dynamic than static, for in no other equally brief span of existence do such profound alterations and adjustments occur as in the weeks, or even the days or hours following birth."

It is the purpose of this book to provide in a single source much of what is known concerning both the normal and abnormal hematologic processes of the first month of life and the effects of prenatal factors on them. We hope this book will provide a useful guide to all who care for, or are interested in, the newborn infant—those who are continually confronted with infants who are bleeding, anemic, jaundiced, or purpuric. We also hope that this discussion of what is known regarding the normal, the hematologic manifestations of the maternal-infant relationship, the disorders of the formed elements of the blood, and the coagulation process will serve as a stimulus to others to explore the areas in which little is as yet known.

It should not be forgotten in this era of mass screening tests for the unusual diseases that a well taken history, a careful physical exam, and a few well chosen laboratory tests can still disclose many common yet serious disturbances. In this book we have indicated how important information can be obtained in an easy manner to aid in the diagnosis and treatment of infants with hematologic disorders.

We regret that all who have made observations relevent to the topics included in this book could not be cited in the text; their numbers are legion and to all we are grateful. In each chapter an attempt has been made to cite the work of the original observer and to bring these observations into focus, based on the most recent work. The chapter on erythroblastosis fetalis clearly illustrates the shortcomings of this approach. So much has been done and is being done that only a summary could be made within the confines of this book.

To Dr. Louis K. Diamond goes much of the credit for nurturing our interest in the field of pediatric hematology. We have benefited from his many years of experience. His own work in these areas has been a beacon, facilitating the studies of others. We are also indebted to Dr. Lewis A. Barness for stimulating our curiosity and providing the necessary encouragement and wisdom for the completion of this task.

We wish to thank Dr. Alexander Schaffer for providing us with an opportunity to assemble this information and for his helpful criticism at each step along the way.

As in all endeavors of this nature, we wish to express special thanks to those who only sit and work — our typists, Miss Loretta Plunkett and Mrs. George Seeley; our artist, Mrs. Libby Rudnick; and our photographer, Mr. Edward Glifort.

F.A.O.
J.L.N.

Contents

Chapter One

NORMAL BLOOD
VALUES IN THE
NEWBORN PERIOD

Because birth is merely a transient event in the development of the infant, the interpretation of the blood picture in the newborn requires an understanding of the maturational processes that precede it.

HEMATOPOIESIS IN UTERO

Hematopoiesis in the embryo and fetus can be conveniently divided into three periods: mesoblastic, hepatic, and myeloid (Wintrobe, 1961). All blood cells are derived from the embryonic connective tissue—the mesenchyme—and blood formation can first be detected about the nineteenth day of gestation. At this time, blood islands in the yolk sac can be observed to differentiate in two directions. Peripheral cells in the islands form the walls of the first blood vessels, and centrally located cells become the primitive blood cells or hemocytoblasts (Maximow, 1924; Bloom and Bartelmez, 1940). By the twenty-second day of gestation, similar blood islands may be observed scattered throughout the mesodermal tissues of the body stalk. By the sixth week of gestation, the activity of this intravascular, mesoblastic stage of erythropoiesis begins to decline, and by the end of the third fetal month it can no longer be observed (Gilmour, 1941).

About the thirty-fifth gestational day, blood formation begins in the liver. The fetal liver appears to be a site of pure erythropoiesis

1

and, during the third to fifth months of gestation, erythroid precursors represent approximately 50 per cent of the total nucleated cells of this organ (Thomas and Yoffey, 1964). The liver is the chief organ of hematopoiesis from the third to the sixth fetal month and continues to produce formed elements into the first postnatal week (Fig. 1–1). During the third fetal month, hematopoiesis also can be detected in the spleen and thymus, and shortly afterward in the lymph nodes. Blood cell formation can still be observed in the spleen during the first week of postnatal life.

The myeloid period of hematopoiesis commences during the fourth to fifth fetal months and becomes quantitatively important by the sixth fetal month. During the last three months of gestation, the bone marrow is the chief site of blood cell formation. Marrow cellularity becomes maximal at about the thirtieth gestational week, although the volume of marrow occupied by hematopoietic tissue continues to increase until term (Kalpaktsoglu and Emery, 1965). Following birth, the amount of marrow tissue continues to grow with no apparent increase in cellular concentration. The only way for an infant to increase cell production is to effect a more rapid turnover

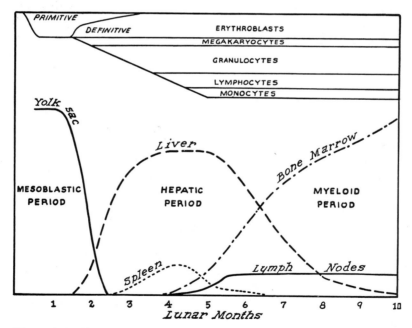

Figure 1–1 The stages of hematopoiesis in the developing embryo and fetus indicating the time of appearance and the comparative participation of the chief centers of hematopoiesis. (From Wintrobe, M.: *Clinical Hematology.* 5th Ed., Philadelphia, Lea & Febiger, 1961.)

of cells or to increase the volume of hematopoietic tissue. This increase in tissue produces the marrow expansion that is most readily observed in the calvarium.

Erythropoiesis

The first blood cells produced by the embryo belong to the red cell series. Two distinct generations of erythrocytes can be observed in the developing embryo. Red cells arise as a result of either primitive, megaloblastic erythropoiesis or definitive normoblastic erythropoiesis. Both types of cells apparently derive from similar-appearing hemocytoblasts and develop through roughly similar but morphologically distinct series of erythroblasts. In the very early embryo, the red cells arise from the primitive erythroblasts. These cells were termed megaloblasts by Ehrlich (1880) because of their resemblance to the erythroid precursors found in patients with pernicious anemia. Megaloblasts are large cells with abundant polychromatophilic cytoplasm, and they possess a nucleus in which the chromatin is fine and widely dispersed. Megaloblasts give rise to large, irregularly shaped, somewhat hypochromic erythrocytes. The primitive erythroblasts arise primarily from intravascular sites; as development continues, these cells gradually are replaced by smaller cells of the definitive or normoblastic series.

Normoblastic erythropoiesis begins about the sixth gestational week and by the tenth week of development accounts for more than 90 per cent of the circulating erythrocytic cells. Maturation of normoblastic erythroid cells resembles that seen in postnatal life and is primarily extravascular.

From the studies of numerous investigators (Wintrobe and Shumacker, 1935; Mugrage and Andresen, 1936; Javert, 1939; Walker and Turnbull, 1953; and Thomas and Yoffey, 1962), a general pattern of red cell changes is evident. In the early embryo, the red cell count, hemoglobin concentration, and packed cell volume are very low in comparison to those of the term infant or adult. However, the red cells are very large. Most of them are nucleated, and they contain large amounts of hemoglobin. As the fetus develops, the number of red cells, the hemoglobin concentration and the volume of packed cells increase, and the mean size of the cells, their mean corpuscular hemoglobin, and the proportion of circulating immature erythrocytes decrease. The mean cell thickness, which is determined from the mean cell volume and the mean cell diameter, also undergoes a progressive decrease throughout gestation. In the first trimester it averages 2.36 μ, in the second trimester 2.29, and at term 2.14, as contrasted with the normal adult value of 1.98 μ (Schulman, 1959). Despite these changes the mean corpuscular hemoglobin concentration remains relatively constant.

By the tenth gestational week, the red cell count ranges from 500,000 to 1,500,000 per cu. mm. At this time, 5 to 10 per cent of all the circulating erythrocytes are nucleated and the reticulocyte count is approximately 80 per cent. The reticulocytes have a mean diameter of 10.5 μ and a mean cell volume of 250 cu. μ. The hemoglobin concentration ranges from 6 to 9 gm./100 ml., and the hematocrit ranges from 20 to 30 per cent.

By the twenty-fourth week of gestation, the hemoglobin has risen to approximately 14 gm./100 ml., the hematocrit is 40 per cent, and the red blood cell count is 3,500,000. From this period until the termination of gestation at the fortieth week, there is a slow rise in hemoglobin, hematocrit, and red blood cell count. At the twenty-fourth week only 0.3 to 0.5 per cent of the circulating erythrocytes are nucleated, and the reticulocyte count has decreased to 10 per cent or less. Table 1–1 summarizes the changes observed during gestation.

Myelopoiesis

The production of leukocytes in the parenchyma of the liver and in various connective tissues such as the meninges, mesentery, and stroma of the lymph plexuses has been observed in the seven week embryo, but significant leukocyte production does not take place until the myeloid period of hematopoiesis. Marrow in the clavicle is the first to produce leukocytes (Gilmour, 1941).

The observations of Thomas and Yoffey (1962) and Playfair et al. (1963) indicate that there are very few circulating granulocytes during the first half of gestation. Granulocyte counts in excess of 1000 per cu. mm. were not observed during this period. During the last trimester of pregnancy, the granulocyte count seems to rise rapidly, and at birth the count is greater than in the adult.

Lymphopoiesis

Lymphopoiesis begins during the eighth week of development in the lymph plexuses; during the ninth week it can be observed in the thymus, and during the third fetal month in the lymph glands. After the appearance of circulating lymphocytes, their number increases rapidly, and by the twentieth week of gestation it may reach a gestational high of 10,000 per cu. mm. During the second half of intrauterine life, the number of lymphocytes decreases slowly to approximately 3000 per cu. mm. at term (Playfair et al., 1963).

The time of appearance of monocytes is variable. Monocytes were seen for the first time during the fifth fetal month by Knoll (1949), while Playfair and associates (1963) observed them as early as the fourth gestational week.

Table 1–1 Mean Red Cell Values During Gestation

Age (in weeks)	Hb (gm./100 ml.)	Hemato-crit (%)	RBC (10⁶/cu.mm.)	Mean Corpusc. Vol. (μ^3)	Mean Corpusc. Hb ($\gamma\gamma$)	Mean Corpusc. Hb Conc. (%)	Nuc. RBC (% of RBC's)	Retic. (%)	Diam. (μ)
12	8.0–10.0	33	1.5	180	60	34	5.0–8.0	40	10.5
16	10.0	35	2.0	140	45	33	2.0–4.0	10–25	9.5
20	11.0	37	2.5	135	44	33	1.0	10–20	9.0
24	14.0	40	3.5	123	38	31	1.0	5–10	8.8
28	14.5	45	4.0	120	40	31	0.5	5–10	8.7
34	15.0	47	4.4	118	38	32	0.2	3–10	8.5

Megakaryocytes

Between the fifth and sixth weeks of gestation, megakaryocytes can be observed in the yolk sac, and from this time until the conclusion of gestation they also can be seen in the liver. Gilmour (1941) noted that after the third fetal month megakaryocytes were consistently present in the bone marrow. Platelets can be observed in the blood by the eleventh gestational week (Bleyer et al., 1971). By the thirtieth gestational week, megakaryocytic activity and the platelet count are similar to those of the adult (Kalpaktsoglou and Emery, 1965).

THE HEMATOLOGIC PICTURE AT BIRTH

Several important factors influence what is described as the normal blood picture in the newborn infant. The site of sampling, the time of sampling, the treatment of the umbilical vessels at the time of delivery, and the possibility of previous fetal-to-maternal or maternal-to-fetal transfusions all influence the so-called normal blood picture. These factors primarily affect hemoglobin and hematocrit values and the red cell count.

Site of Sampling

Capillary samples obtained by skin prick, generally from the heel or toe, have a higher hemoglobin concentration than simultaneously collected venous samples. Oettinger and Mills (1949) found that during the first hour of life the hemoglobin concentration of capillary blood averaged 20.3 gm./100 ml., while blood obtained from the jugular vein averaged 16.7 gm./100 ml. In some infants the difference in hemoglobin concentration amounted to 8 gm./100 ml. Vahlquist (1941) observed that immediately after birth the hemoglobin concentration of heelprick samples was ·about 10 per cent greater than that taken at the same time from the femoral vein; Mollison (1961) observed only a 5 per cent difference in capillary and venous samples obtained a few hours after birth. Oh and Lind (1966) demonstrated that the capillary-venous hematocrit differences were greater in infants whose umbilical cord was clamped after all arterial pulsations had ceased. During the first five days of life, those infants who received a large placental transfusion maintained a greater capillary-venous hematocrit difference than the infants in whom the cord was clamped immediately after birth. Stasis of blood in the peripheral vessels, because of sluggish circulation with resultant transudation of plasma, is believed to be responsible for the discrepancy in the samples obtained from the different sites, which results in the higher capillary hemoglobin.

Even on the fifth day of life, Oettinger and Mills (1949) found that capillary samples had hemoglobin concentrations 12 per cent higher than those of venous blood, although Vahlquist (1941) could only demonstrate a 2.5 per cent difference on the sixth day of life.

The clinical importance of the site of sampling was illustrated by Moe (1967). In his study of 54 infants with erythroblastosis fetalis, cord blood and capillary blood specimens were obtained for hemoglobin and hematocrit determinations. Forty-one infants eventually required exchange transfusions for hyperbilirubinemia. Of these 41 infants, 25 were found to be anemic based on determinations performed on cord blood samples, while only 14 could be considered anemic according to values obtained from capillary samples. The discordant results from the two sampling sites are illustrated in Figure 1–2.

Differences in hemoglobin concentration between venous and capillary blood can be minimized by first warming the extremity before skin prick, obtaining good spontaneous blood flow, and discard-

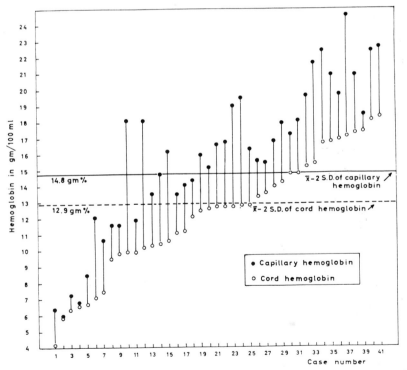

Figure 1–2 Umbilical cord and capillary hemoglobin values in 41 patients who required exchange transfusion. (Moe, P., Acta Paediat. Scand. 56:391, 1967.)

ing the first few drops before obtaining the samples. Capillary values should not be compared to previously obtained cord venous blood values when one is looking for changes in hemoglobin concentration during the first week of life. For this purpose venous blood should be obtained whenever possible. The selection of the vein is unimportant, for blood drawn from the external jugular, internal jugular, femoral, and scalp vein gave similar results (Gairdner et al., 1953; Oh and Lind, 1966).

Time of Sampling

During the first few hours after birth, an increase in hemoglobin concentration takes place. In some infants this rise may be as great as 6 gm./100 ml. This increase is partially a result of the placental transfusion that occurs at the time of delivery. The total blood volume of the infant rapidly adjusts after birth, decreasing in plasma volume while red cell volume remains essentially unchanged (Usher et al., 1963). This results in an increase in red cell count, hematocrit, and hemoglobin concentration. Gairdner et al. (1958) have shown that an increase in hemoglobin concentration occurs shortly after birth even when the cord was clamped "as soon as conveniently possible." They noted that the hemoglobin increased from 16.6 to 19.1 gm./100 ml. during a period of eight hours. At the same time, the plasma protein concentration increased from 6.5 to 7.0 gm./100 ml. Although this increase in hemoglobin concentration after birth appears to be a relatively uniform phenomenon, the magnitude of the increase depends on the amount of the placental transfusion (Oh and Lind, 1966).

Treatment of the Umbilical Vessels

The manner in which the umbilical vessels are treated influences the hematologic values obtained during the first week of life and may even exert an effect throughout the first year of life.

At birth the blood volume of the infant may be increased by as much as 61 per cent by allowing complete emptying of the placental vessels before the cord is clamped (Usher et al., 1963; Yao et al., 1969). It has been estimated that the placental vessels contain 75 to 125 ml. of blood at birth — or one-quarter to one-third the fetal blood volume (Haselhorst and Allmeling, 1930; Goodall et al., 1938; Demarsh et al., 1942; and Colozzi, 1954). Under normal circumstances, about one-quarter of the placental transfusion takes place within 15 seconds of birth and one-half by the end of the first minute (Usher et al., 1963; Yao et al., 1969). The percentage ratio of blood between the infant's and placenta's circulation has been found to average 67:33 at birth, 80:20 at one minute, and 87:13 at the end of the placental transfusion

(Yao et al., 1969). The placental transfusion occurs more rapidly in women who receive ergotamine derivatives at the onset of the third stage of labor (Yao et al., 1968).

The umbilical arteries generally constrict shortly after birth, so that no blood flows from the infant to the mother, although the umbilical vein remains dilated, permitting blood to flow in the direction of gravity. Infants held below the level of the placenta will continue to gain blood; infants held above the placenta may bleed into it (Gunther, 1957). Yao and Lind (1969) demonstrated that hydrostatic pressure, produced by placing the infant 40 cm. below the mother's introitus, hastened placental transfusion to virtual completion in 30 seconds. When the infant was held above the introitus the placental transfusion was either markedly reduced or completely prevented. In infants born by cesarean section, it would appear advisable to keep the baby at least 20 cm. below the placenta for approximately 30 seconds before clamping the cord, in order to insure a partial placental transfusion. This recommendation does not apply when dealing with infants suspected of having erythroblastosis fetalis. In this situation the cord should be clamped promptly in order to minimize the transfer of sensitized cells. Although Redmond et al. (1965) have presented evidence to indicate that the time of cord clamping in relation to the onset of respiration determines the amount of placental transfusions, the studies of Usher and associates (1963) and those of Yao et al. (1969) have failed to confirm their findings.

Results from reports on the effects of placental transfusion on the total blood volume of the infant show wide variability. This is partially because of the techniques employed and partially because of the time at which the samples were taken. During the first hours after birth, plasma apparently leaves the circulation (Gairdner et al., 1958; Usher et al., 1963). It seems that the greater the placental transfusion, the greater the plasma loss. Thus, by the third day of life there are only small differences in total blood volume, regardless of the method of cord clamping. Usher found that infants with delayed cord clamping had an average blood volume of 93 ml./kg. at an age of 72 hours; infants with immediate cord clamping had a blood volume of 82 ml./kg. Although the total blood volume may be only slightly altered by the timing of the cord clamping, more significant differences can be observed in the red cell mass or hemoglobin concentration. In the study of Usher and associates, infants with delayed cord clamping had an average red cell mass of 49 ml./kg. at 72 hours of age as compared with a red cell mass of only 31 ml./kg. in infants with immediate cord clamping. Similar results were later obtained by Yao and co-workers (1969). In Table 1-2 are listed the results of other investigators, which indicate that infants with delayed cord

Table 1–2   Effect of Cord Clamping on Hemoglobin Concentration

AUTHOR	EARLY CLAMPING HB (GM./100 ML.)	DELAYED CLAMPING HB (GM./100 ML.)	TIME OF STUDY
Phillips (1941)	15.6	19.3	20–30 hours of age
DeMarsh et al. (1948)	17.4	20.8	3rd day
Colozzi (1954)	14.7	17.3	72 hours
Lanzkowsky (1960)	18.1	19.7	72–96 hours
	11.1	11.1	3 months of age

clamping tend to have higher hemoglobin values during the first week of life.

Infants in whom cord clamping was delayed demonstrated a slower onset of respirations, a more rapid respiratory rate during the first few hours of life, and a higher systolic blood pressure (Oh et al., 1966). In addition, their pulmonary artery pressure (Arcilla et al., 1966), their central venous pressure (Jegier et al., 1963), and their right atrial pressure were higher than those of early clamped infants (Arcilla et al., 1966). Urine flow, glomerular filtration rate, PAH clearance, and effective renal blood flow were also higher during the first 12 hours of life (Oh et al., 1966) in infants with delayed cord clamping. Bound et al. (1962) and Moss et al. (1963) found a decreased incidence of the respiratory distress syndrome in infants in whom cord ligation was delayed; neither Taylor and associates (1963) nor Yao et al. (1969) could demonstrate any benefit from this procedure. Premature infants with increased red cell volumes as a consequence of delayed cord clamping have been found to have higher serum bilirubin levels (Taylor et al., 1963; Usher and Lind, 1965).

Fetal-Maternal and Maternal-Fetal Transfusions

In tabulating normal hematologic data for the newborn, most investigators encounter a great range of variability. Cord blood hemoglobin values in apparently normal infants have ranged from 13 to 22 gm./100 ml. (Guest et al., 1938). It is now recognized that in as many as 50 per cent of pregnancies some fetal cells pass into the maternal circulation at some time during gestation or during the birth process. In 10 per cent of pregnancies, these transplacental losses range from 0.5 to 40.0 ml. of blood; in about 1 per cent, the losses are even greater and may approximate 100 ml. (Cohen et al., 1964).

In addition to this high incidence of fetal-maternal transfusion, which may explain some of the low hemoglobin values recorded in cord samples from apparently normal infants, is the observation that on occasion the infant may receive a transfusion from the mother resulting in plethora with hemoglobin values in the 21.0 to 26.0 gm./100 ml. range (Michael and Mauer, 1961). Andrews and Thompson (1962) recognized this phenomenon in 2 of 207 consecutive deliveries.

As yet no systematic attempt has been made to determine normal hematologic values in the newborn period while eliminating the erroneous results caused by transplacental transfusions.

NORMAL VALUES IN THE NEWBORN PERIOD

With the realization that many factors influence what is considered as normal, an attempt is made to present a consensus based on the observations of many investigators.

Hemoglobin Concentration

Within the last decade, techniques for obtaining hemoglobin standardization have improved and with it has come closer agreement as to what constitutes the normal value. Values for the normal mean hemoglobin concentration of cord blood have ranged from 15.7 (Sturgeon, 1956) to 17.9 gm./100 ml. (Dochain et al., 1952). The bulk of recent studies has placed the normal value in the range of 16.6 to 17.1 gm./100 ml. (Table 1–3). When these results are corrected according to the number of observations in the series, the value for the mean cord hemoglobin concentration is 16.8 gm./100 ml. Approximately 95 per cent of all values fall between 13.7 and 20.1 gm./100 ml. Sisson (1958) has suggested that 13.5 gm./100 ml. be considered the lowest normal value, which agrees well with Mollison's (1961) figure of 13.6 gm./100 ml. These values may prove to be too low when infants with recognized transplacental hemorrhages are separated from the group. Hemoglobin values in this low range of normal can best be interpreted when a reticulocyte count and a nucleated red cell

Table 1–3   The Normal Cord Blood Hemoglobin

AUTHORS	MEAN HEMOGLOBIN (GM./100 ML.)	RANGE (GM./100 ML.)	NUMBER OF OBSERVATIONS
Mollison (1951)	16.6		134
Dochain et al. (1952)	17.9	14.4–21.6	40
Walker et al. (1953)	16.5		145
Marks et al. (1955)	16.9	12.3–22.0	221
Guest et al. (1957)	17.1	13.0–25.0	59
McKay (1957)	17.4		60
Rooth et al. (1957)	16.7	11.2–26.6	414
Mean	16.8		

count are also taken into account. If either or both of these last two values are elevated, it suggests that the body of the infant is attempting to compensate for a lower than normal hemoglobin and that the observed value represents anemia for the child under study.

Hemoglobin values for umbilical artery blood tend to be about 0.5 gm./100 ml. higher than samples obtained from the umbilical vein (Chaplin, 1961).

Few studies are available that document the normal hemoglobin of capillary blood at the time of birth. Results of older studies, performed at various times during the first day of life, show average values that range from 16.6 to 23.4 gm./100 ml., the mean value being 19.8 gm./100 ml. (Smith, 1959).

Walker and Turnbull (1953) concluded that the mean hemoglobin concentration of cord blood increases during the last two weeks of gestation and continues to increase in infants born after the fortieth week of pregnancy as a result of progressive oxygen lack. They found the mean hemoglobin concentration at 38 weeks to be 15.2 gm./100 ml.; at 40 weeks, 16.5 gm./100 ml.; and at 42 weeks, 18.0 gm./100 ml. Neither Marks et al. (1955) nor Rooth and Sjöstedt (1957) could demonstrate any upward trend in hemoglobin concentration in the postmature infant. The data of Rooth and Sjöstedt, as well as Mollison (1961), do suggest, however, that the hemoglobin value does increase by approximately 1.3 gm./100 ml. between the thirty-eighth and fortieth week of pregnancy. Previously stated values for normal cord hemoglobin do not take this factor into consideration.

Hemoglobin Values During the First Week of Life. In most normal infants the hemoglobin concentration at the end of the first week of life is as high as, if not higher than, it was in the cord blood. In the first several hours after birth, there is an increase in hemoglobin concentration. Wegelius (1948) performed a detailed study of the blood changes that occur during the first few hours of life and noted that the hemoglobin value increases by 17 to 20 per cent of the initial value during the first two hours of life, but then falls slightly during the next two hours. Usher et al. (1963) observed that the increase in hematocrit that occurs during the first four hours of life is confined to infants whose cords were not clamped immediately. In Table 1–4 are listed the results of serial hemoglobin determinations performed during the first two weeks of life. It is apparent that there is no real decrease in hemoglobin concentration until some time between the first and third week of life. A decreasing hemoglobin during the first week of life indicates either increased red cell destruction or blood loss. Mollison has suggested that any venous hemoglobin value below 13.0 gm./100 ml. in the first two weeks should be regarded as evidence of anemia. A capillary hemoglobin below 14.5 gm./100 ml. is regarded as evidence of anemia in our laboratory.

Table 1–4 Normal Hematologic Values During the First Two
Weeks of Life in the Term Infant

Value	Cord Blood	Day 1	Day 3	Day 7	Day 14
Hb (gm./100 ml.)	16.8	18.4	17.8	17.0	16.8
Hematocrit (%)	53.0	58.0	55.0	54.0	52.0
Red cells (cu. mm. × 10⁶)	5.25	5.8	5.6	5.2	5.1
MCV (μ^3)	107	108	99.0	98.0	96.0
MCH ($\gamma\gamma$)	34	35	33	32.5	31.5
MCHC (%)	31.7	32.5	33	33	33
Reticulocytes (%)	3–7	3–7	1–3	0–1	0–1
Nuc. RBC/(cu. mm.)	500	200	0–5	0	0
Platelets (1000's/cu. mm.)	290	192	213	248	252

MCV = mean corpuscular volume
MCH = mean corpuscular hemoglobin
MCHC = mean corpuscular hemoglobin concentration

The Hematocrit

Studies of cord blood hematocrit values have not been reported as frequently as hemoglobin concentrations. Reports of normal values have ranged from a mean of 51.3 per cent (Wauth et al., 1939) to 56.0 per cent (Gairdner et al., 1956). Hematocrit value, just as the hemoglobin value, shows an abrupt increase during the first few hours of life and then slowly declines, so that by the end of the first week of life it is very near the original cord blood value. Guest and Brown (1957) recorded a mean cord blood hematocrit of 52.3 per cent; on the first day of life the hematocrit was 58.2 per cent, at three days of age the hematocrit was 54.5 per cent, and at the end of seven days the hematocrit value was 54.9 per cent (Table 1–4). Gatti (1967) measured the hematocrit levels of the capillary blood of 629 healthy newborn infants during the first ten days of life. The mean level on the first day of life was 62.9 ± 3.2 per cent; it then decreased to 56.6 ± 2.6 per cent by day seven, and was 53.7 ± 2.5 per cent on day ten. At one week of age the mean capillary hematocrit value was two percentage points higher than the mean venous hematocrit value.

The Red Cell Count and Red Cell Indices

The red cell count, just as the hemoglobin and hematocrit values, shows great variability at the time of birth. Wegelius (1948) and Guest and Brown (1957) reported the mean red cell count to be approximately 4,600,000/cu. mm. Marks and associates (1955) found the mean value to be 5,100,000/cu. mm., while Lippman (1924) reported a value of 5,200,000/cu. mm. The red cell count also rises rapidly during the first hours of life to a level that is approximately 500,000/cu. mm. more than the cord blood value. By the end of the first week of life, the red cell count is near 5,200,000/cu. mm. (Table 1–4).

The red cells of the newborn infant are in general much larger than the cells of the normal adult, although much variation in size can be observed in any child. Saragea (1922) found the average diameter of the erythrocytes to be 8.5 μ at birth. By the time the infant is six months of age, the diameter of the red cells has decreased to the normal adult size of 7.5 μ. Heissen and Schalloer (1928) found the average diameter of the cells to lie between 8.5 and 9.3 μ as compared with 7.5 μ in adult red blood cells. Marked anisocytosis was evidenced because there was a difference of 8.2 μ between the diameters of the smallest and largest cells in the population. In the adult, there was only a 2.5 μ difference between cells of maximum and minimum diameter. More recent studies of red cell diameter (Katō, 1933; Faxen, 1937; Walker et al., 1953) all confirm the presence of a relative macrocytosis in the newborn, and these studies place the mean red cell diameter between 8.0 and 8.3 μ compared to the normal adult mean of 7.5 μ.

By special staining techniques, Breatnach (1962) demonstrated that the macrocytes, cells with a diameter greater than 9 μ, seldom contained fetal hemoglobin, while the microcytes, cells with a diameter of less than 6 μ, invariably did.

The mean diameter of the red cell population, as well as the mean corpuscular volume, rapidly decreases during the first weeks of life (Table 1–4), suggesting either that many of the macrocytes are quickly eliminated from the circulation or that the cells rapidly decrease in size. In the term infant, by the end of the second month of life, cell size values comparable to those in adult cells are reached.

The mean corpuscular volume of erythrocytes, at birth, has been estimated to range from 104 to 118 cu. μ (Marks et al., 1955; Walker et al., 1953), compared to the normal adult value of 82 to 92 cu. μ. The mean corpuscular hemoglobin is also increased with reported values ranging from 33.5 to 41.4 $\mu\mu$g. as contrasted with the normal adult value of 27 to 31 $\mu\mu$g. Although both the mean corpuscular volume and the mean corpuscular hemoglobin are elevated, the value of the mean corpuscular hemoglobin concentration in the newborn is quite similar to that in the normal adult. The mean corpuscular hemoglobin concentration has been estimated to range from 30 to 35 per cent in the newborn and 32 to 36 per cent in the adult (Table 1–4).

Matoth and co-workers (1971), employing an electronic cell sizer and counter, and using capillary blood samples, recorded sequential values in a group of healthy term infants during the first 12 weeks of life. Their results (Table 1–5) differ slightly from those

Table 1–5   Normal Hematologic Values During the First Twelve Weeks of Life in the Term Infant as Determined by an Electronic Cell Counter*

AGE	NO. OF CASES	HB GM. % ± S.D.	RBC × 10⁶ ± S.D.	HCT % ± S.D.	MCV CU.μ ± S.D.	MCHC % ± S.D.	RETIC % ± S.D.
Days							
1	19	19.0 ± 2.2	5.14 ± 0.7	61 ± 7.4	119 ± 9.4	31.6 ± 1.9	3.2 ± 1.4
2	19	19.0 ± 1.9	5.15 ± 0.8	60 ± 6.4	115 ± 7.0	31.6 ± 1.4	3.2 ± 1.3
3	19	18.7 ± 3.4	5.11 ± 0.7	62 ± 9.3	116 ± 5.3	31.1 ± 2.8	2.8 ± 1.7
4	10	18.6 ± 2.1	5.00 ± 0.6	57 ± 8.1	114 ± 7.5	32.6 ± 1.5	1.8 ± 1.1
5	12	17.6 ± 1.1	4.97 ± 0.4	57 ± 7.3	114 ± 8.9	30.9 ± 2.2	1.2 ± 0.2
6	15	17.4 ± 2.2	5.00 ± 0.7	54 ± 7.2	113 ± 10.0	32.2 ± 1.6	0.6 ± 0.2
7	12	17.9 ± 2.5	4.86 ± 0.6	56 ± 9.4	118 ± 11.2	32.0 ± 1.6	0.5 ± 0.4
Weeks							
1–2	32	17.3 ± 2.3	4.80 ± 0.8	54 ± 8.3	112 ± 19.0	32.1 ± 2.9	0.5 ± 0.3
2–3	11	15.6 ± 2.6	4.20 ± 0.6	46 ± 7.3	111 ± 8.2	33.9 ± 1.9	0.8 ± 0.6
3–4	17	14.2 ± 2.1	4.00 ± 0.6	43 ± 5.7	105 ± 7.5	33.5 ± 1.6	0.6 ± 0.3
4–5	15	12.7 ± 1.6	3.60 ± 0.4	36 ± 4.8	101 ± 8.1	34.9 ± 1.6	0.9 ± 0.8
5–6	10	11.9 ± 1.5	3.55 ± 0.2	36 ± 6.2	102 ± 10.2	34.1 ± 2.9	1.0 ± 0.7
6–7	10	12.0 ± 1.5	3.40 ± 0.4	36 ± 4.8	105 ± 12.0	33.8 ± 2.3	1.2 ± 0.7
7–8	17	11.1 ± 1.1	3.40 ± 0.4	33 ± 3.7	100 ± 13.0	33.7 ± 2.6	1.5 ± 0.7
8–9	13	10.7 ± 0.9	3.40 ± 0.5	31 ± 2.5	93 ± 12.0	34.1 ± 2.2	1.8 ± 1.0
9–10	12	11.2 ± 0.9	3.60 ± 0.3	32 ± 2.7	91 ± 9.3	34.3 ± 2.9	1.2 ± 0.6
10–11	11	11.4 ± 0.9	3.70 ± 0.4	34 ± 2.1	91 ± 7.7	33.2 ± 2.4	1.2 ± 0.7
11–12	13	11.3 ± 0.9	3.70 ± 0.3	33 ± 3.3	88 ± 7.9	34.8 ± 2.2	0.7 ± 0.3

MCV   = mean corpuscular volume.
MCH   = mean corpuscular hemoglobin.
MCHC = mean corpuscular hemoglobin concentration.
*From Matoth et al., Acta Paediat. Scand. 60:317, 1971.

previously obtained using manual methods, but provide a valuable reference for laboratories where this newer equipment is available.

Reticulocyte Count and Nucleated Red Cells

Most authors have reported considerable variation in the reticulocyte count from infant to infant, and there have been marked differences in what has been considered the normal mean. Values for the average percentage of reticulocytes at birth have ranged from 1.6 (Kato, 1932) to 6.2 per cent (Seyfarth and Jurgens, 1927). Differences in staining techniques and counting methods are responsible for much of this variation in the literature. Seip (1955), in a small but carefully controlled study, found the mean reticulocyte count to be 5.1 per cent on the first day of life in term infants. Normal values ranged from 4.1 to 6.3 per cent—approximately 300,000 reticulocytes/cu. mm. Zinkham's (1963) figure of 5.5 per cent with a range of 4.2 to 7.2 per cent is in close agreement with that of Seip. In our laboratory, the mean reticulocyte count for term infants on the first day of life is 4.7 ± 1.9 per cent. During gestation the reticulocyte count progressively decreases from a value of approximately 80 per cent in the third fetal month. Infants born prematurely have higher reticulocyte counts. Values between 6 and 10 per cent are frequently observed in infants born between the thirtieth and thirty-sixth week of gestation. The percentage of reticulocytes increases slightly during the first two to three days after birth (Wegelius, 1948; Seip, 1955; DeMarsh et al., 1948). DeMarsh et al. observed that the increase is greatest in infants whose cords are clamped immediately after birth.

Evidence of very active erythropoiesis, as reflected in the elevated reticulocyte count, persists for the first three days of life. Then the reticulocyte count drops abruptly to values of about 1 per cent by the seventh day of life (Table 1–4). More rapid falls are seen in infants who are small for gestational age (Humbert et al., 1969). Persistent reticulocytosis suggests the presence of a hemolytic process, blood loss, or hypoxia.

Nucleated red blood cells may be observed in the blood of almost all infants at the time of birth and during the first day of life (Lippman, 1924). Unfortunately, most authors have expressed the number of nucleated red cells as a percentage of the white cells. Because of the marked variability in the number of white cells normally present at birth, it is more meaningful to express the nucleated red cells in absolute numbers or as a percentage of the red cells as is done for the reticulocytes. The term infant has approximately 500 nucleated red cells/cu. mm. of blood at birth, or 0.1 per cent of his red cell population. By the time the newborn is 12 hours old this number has decreased by about 50 per cent. By the end of 48 hours, 20 to 30 nucleated red cells/cu. mm. may be observed, and by the fourth day of life it is unusual to see any nucleated red cells in the peripheral blood of the term infant.

In the premature infant, 1000 to 1500 nucleated red cells/cu. mm. may be present at the time of birth. The younger the infant is, the greater the number. These values also decrease rapidly during the first week of life, although it is not unusual to see an occasional nucleated red cell in the peripheral blood smear of a small infant seven days old.

When expressed in terms of white cells, as is the common practice, the term infant has an average of 7.3 nucleated red cells per 100 leukocytes at birth with a range of 0 to 24 (Anderson, 1941). In the premature infant, the average figure is 21 nucleated erythrocytes per 100 white blood cells. Javert concluded from his studies of cord blood that prematurity should be considered likely when there are more than ten nucleated red cells per 100 white cells present in the peripheral blood at the time of birth. Both twins and Blacks tended to have lower counts in proportion to their weight, suggesting advanced gestational age despite low birth weight. Increased numbers of nucleated red cells are observed in hemolytic disease, after hemorrhage, during hypoxia (Merenstein et al., 1970), in Down's syndrome, and in infants with congenital anomalies.

Red Cell Surface Alterations and Inclusions

Interference–contrast microscopy studies of the red cell membrane have revealed morphologic differences between the red cells of the newborn infant and those of the adult (Holroyde et al., 1969).

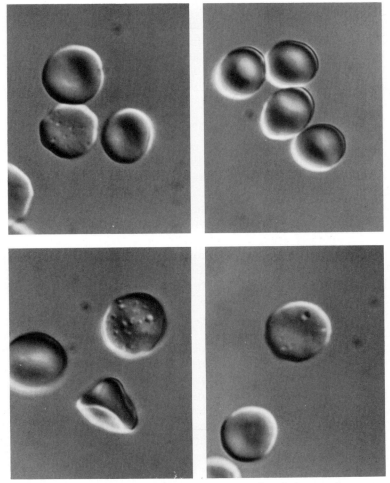

Figure 1–3   Red cell surface morphology as viewed with the interference-contrast microscope. (Wet preparation, original magnification × 1000.) *Upper left*, normal adult cells; *upper right* and *lower left*, cells from term infants; *lower right*, cells from an infant of 32 weeks' gestation. Note surface pits on infant's cells. Supplied by courtesy of Dr. Christopher P. Holroyde.

In normal adults 2.6 per cent of erythrocytes appear to have pits or craters 0.2 to 0.5 μ in diameter on their surface (Fig. 1–3). By contrast, premature and term infants have a mean of 47.2 per cent and 24.3 per cent, respectively. By approximately two months of age, the cells of the term infant resemble those of the adult, while it takes several weeks longer for the cells of the premature infant to reach this appearance. These defects, which appear as pits by interference-contrast microscopy, are probably cytoplasmic vacuoles. It is believed that the finding of increased numbers of these cells in the newborn infant reflects the presence of splenic or reticuloendothelial hypofunction since this type of cell has only been observed with such high frequency in patients without spleens.

The number of red cells containing siderotic (iron-containing) granules is also increased in the normal newborn, averaging 3.16 per cent as compared with a mean of 0.09 per cent in adult males (Kurth et al., 1969). The presence of increased numbers of these cells is believed to be another reflection of decreased splenic function.

The White Cell Count and Differential

The white cell count at birth may range from 9000 to 30,000/cu. mm. with the mean count generally in the range of 15,000 to 20,000/ cu. mm. for the term infant. The premature infant has a slightly lower total white cell count (Lichtenstein, 1917; Burrell, 1952). During the first hours of life, a small increase in the white count is frequently observed. After this initial peak, the total white count gradually falls to a mean level of approximately 12,000/cu. mm. by the end of the first week of life (Lucas, 1921; Bakwin and Morris, 1923; Lippman, 1924; Washburn, 1935; and Wegelius, 1948).

During the first days of life, the differential count reveals a preponderance of polymorphonuclear neutrophils. Neutrophils average about 61 per cent of the total cells, and they generally demonstrate a "shift to the left" with 20 to 40 per cent of the neutrophils being band forms. Promyelocytes and myelocytes may occasionally be seen (Agress and Downey, 1936) and metamyelocytes may comprise 5 per cent of the total white cells during the first 24 hours of life (Lippman, 1924). During the first three days of life myelocytes may number from 100 to 750/cu. mm., while occasional promyelocytes and blast cells may also be observed. These immature forms are more frequently observed in premature infants (Xanthou, 1970). Blast forms may also be observed with infections.

Some time between the fourth and seventh day of life, in the term infant, the lymphocyte becomes the predominant cell, and it remains so until the fourth year of life. A monocytosis may be observed toward the end of the first week of life, with monocyte counts of 10 per cent being common.

Table 1-6 The White Blood Cell Count and the Differential Count During the First Two Weeks of Life*

AGE	LEUKOCYTES	NEUTROPHILS			EOSINOPHILS	BASOPHILS	LYMPHOCYTES	MONOCYTES
		Total	Seg	Band				
Birth								
Mean	18,100	11,000	9400	1600	400	100	5500	1050
Range	9.0–30.0	6.0–26			20–850	0–640	2.0–11.0	0.4–3.1
Mean %	–	61	52	9	2.2	0.6	31	5.8
7 Days								
Mean	12,200	5500	4700	830	500	50	5000	1100
Range	5.0–21.0	1.5–10.0			70–1100	0–250	2.0–17.0	0.3–2.7
Mean %	–	45	39	6	4.1	0.4	41	9.1
14 Days								
Mean	11,400	4500	3900	630	350	50	5500	1000
Range	5.0–20.0	1.0–9.5			70–1000	0–230	2.0–17.0	0.2–2.4
Mean %	–	40	34	5.5	3.1	0.4	48	8.8

*From Altman, P. L., and Dittmer, D. S.: *Blood and Other Body Fluids.* Federation of American Societies for Experimental Biology, Washington, D.C., 1961.

Table 1–6 illustrates the white cell findings during the first two weeks of life.

Neither premature rupture of the membranes nor duration of labor appears to affect the total white count of the cord blood (Dorros et al., 1969). Total white cell counts show wide variation from infant to infant. Washburn (1935) found that leukocyte fluctuations were extremely irregular and showed considerable variability for the same baby at the same hour on different days and for any two babies of the same age and weight. The smallest variation observed for any one baby was from 5900/cu. mm. to 13,300/cu. mm. The greatest was from 8800/cu. mm. to 23,150/cu. mm. Washburn could find no evidence of an orderly rhythm in the leukocyte fluctuations or any evidence of correlation between the variations in white cell count and such factors as feeding, sleep, or increased activity. In contrast, Xanthou (1970) has observed that the neutrophil count in any given infant remains relatively constant from the third to the tenth day of life. In term infants the mean neutrophil count was 8000/cu. mm. at birth, rose to 13,000/cu. mm. at 12 hours, and then fell to 4000/cu. mm. by 72 hours of age, after which it remained unchanged. In the premature infants the mean value at birth was 5000/cu. mm., 8000/cu. mm. at 12 hours, 4000/cu. mm. at 72 hours, and then gradually fell to a mean of 2500/cu. mm. by the twenty-eighth day of life. The other formed elements also appeared to show consistent quantitative changes.

Eosinophils.   In the term infant, the eosinophil count ranges from 19 to 851 cells/cu. mm., with a mean of 267/cu. mm. (2.2 per cent) during the first 12 hours of life (Medoff and Barbero, 1950). In most infants the eosinophil count is higher by the fifth day of life and averages 483/cu. mm. by the end of the first month.

Premature infants have very low levels of circulating eosinophils at birth. Burrell (1952) could find no eosinophils on the first day of life in infants weighing less than 4.5 pounds. Following the first day of life, a progressive increase in eosinophils took place so that values of 900 to 1650/cu. mm. were reached in three to five weeks. Burrell noted that infants whose progress was unsatisfactory and who later died had marked eosinopenia. In all cases, on the day of death there was a complete absence of eosinophils.

The eosinophil response to adrenocorticotrophic hormone (ACTH) appears quite variable. Farquhar (1955) noted that 10 mg. of ACTH is required to produce a 30 per cent decrease in the level of circulating eosinophils and that there is no significant difference in the response on the first, third, or tenth day of life. Klein and Hanson (1950) noted that the eosinophil response to ACTH is much less during the first week of life than after this period.

Platelets

With the introduction of phase microscopy for platelet enumeration by Brecher and Cronkite (1950), more precise platelet counting has been possible. Despite this improvement in technique, wide variation in the platelet counts of normal infants is still evident.

During the first four days of life, platelet counts of approximately 100,000 to 300,000/cu. mm. are considered normal for the term infant (Ablin et al., 1961). Platelet counts may range from 84,000 to 478,000. Platelet counts generally fall into the normal adult range of 150,000 to 450,000 with a mean of approximately 250,000/cu. mm. after the first week of life.

Conflicting data concerning the normal platelet count in the premature infant have appeared. Although the platelet count of healthy premature infants is essentially the same as that of term infants during the first week of life, it was observed by Medoff (1964) that, in infants weighing less than 1700 gm. at birth, the mean platelet count on the seventeenth day was 35,000/cu. mm. and reached 100,000/cu. mm. by the end of the fifth week. In premature infants weighing more than 1700 gm., Medoff recorded a mean platelet count of 118,000 during the first two weeks of life. The platelet count increased to 185,000/cu. mm. by day 21. No bleeding was observed in any infant despite the thrombocytopenia. In contrast, Fogel et al. (1968), performing serial platelet counts at four day intervals on 73 premature infants, found only four of 36 infants weighing less than 1700 gm. at birth whose platelet count fell below 100,000/cu. mm. All four infants reached platelet counts of 100,000/cu. mm. by one month of age and none bled. The results of this study appear in Table 1–7. Aballi and co-workers (1968) studied a large group of thriving premature infants in two separate institutions and noted that only 1.8 per cent of 692 determinations performed on 298 premature infants during the first

Table 1–7 Comparison of Serial Platelet Counts per cu. mm. Obtained from Premature Infants Weighing < 1700 Grams and > 1700 Grams at Birth[*]

				Age (days)			
	1	4	8	12	16	20	24
< 1700 grams							
Mean	201,000	243,000	235,000	217,000	191,000	242,000	214,000
Range	112,000–380,000	46,000–363,000	71,000–378,000	14,000–344,000	28,000–334,000	63,000–275,000	95,000–253,000
> 1700 grams							
Mean	206,000	219,000	234,000	238,000	263,000	203,000	222,000
Range	120,000–380,000	152,000–282,000	129,000–389,000	138,000–346,000	178,000–375,000	182,000–272,000	186,000–309,000

*From Fogel et al., 1968.

month of life were less than 100,000/cu. mm. It would appear that a platelet count of less than 100,000/cu. mm., and certainly one of less than 50,000/cu. mm., during the first month of life, regardless of the infant's initial birth weight, should initiate a search for some pathological process (Appleyard and Brinton, 1971).

The Bone Marrow

Bone marrow aspirates are frequently unsatisfactory and are often dilute in newborns. This may lead to misinterpretations as to cellularity and to the number of megakaryocytes (see page 301). We prefer to use the posterior superior spine of the iliac crest for marrow aspirations during infancy and childhood.

The bone marrow at birth is an actively proliferating organ. Most of the marrow space of the body is normally involved in hematopoiesis, and thus the infant is left with virtually no marrow reserve to call upon to meet the demands of increased red cell production that accompany a hemolytic process. To meet the needs for increased red cell production the marrow cavity will expand outward. This outward expansion is reflected by the prominent frontal bossing and the radiologic "hair on end" appearance of the skull that develops in infants with congenital hemolytic anemias. Extramedullary hematopoiesis in the liver and spleen also takes place more readily in infants because of their lack of marrow reserve.

The cellularity of the marrow decreases during the first week of life and then slowly attains normal adult levels between the first and third months of life (Gairdner et al., 1952). On the first day of life, erythroid precursors account for 32 to 40 per cent of all the nucleated cells in the marrow (Shapiro and Bassen, 1941; Gairdner et al., 1952). By the end of the first week, the erythroid elements account for only 8 to 12 per cent of the nucleated cells. Myeloid cells average 46 to 77 per cent of the nucleated elements at birth and 50 to 77 per cent at the end of the first week of life. Thus the myeloid:erythroid ratio changes from about 1.5:1 at birth to slightly greater than 6:1 by the eighth day of life. By the end of the second month of life, the normal adult ratio of 2.5:1 to 3.0:1 has been established. The number of stem cells remains relatively constant during the entire first year of life. Although their proliferative activity is low during the first week of life, it gradually rises during the second and third week to a level which remains essentially unchanged for the next eight years (Lundmark, 1966). Both the percentage and the absolute numbers of lymphocytes in the bone marrow increase during the first 60 days of life, so that by the third month of life they comprise almost 50 per cent of the marrow nucleated cells. Table 1–8 lists the normal values for the marrow elements during the first weeks of life.

Table 1-8 The Bone Marrow Differential During
the First Week of Life*

	0–24 HOURS (%)	7 DAYS (%)	ADULT (%)
Myeloblasts	0–2	0–3	0.3–50
Promyelocytes	0.5–6.0	0.5–7.0	1.0–8.0
Myelocytes	1.0–9.0	1.0–11.0	5.5–22.5
Metamyelocytes	4.5–25.0	7.0–35.0	13.0–32.0
Band forms	10.0–40.0	11.0–45.0	–
Erythroblasts	0–1.0	0–0.5	1.0–8.0
Proerythroblasts	0.5–9.0	0–0.5	2.0–10.0
Normoblasts	18.0–41.0	0–15.0	7.0–32.0
Myeloid: erythroid ratio	1.5:1.0	6.5:1.0	3.5:1.0

*Adapted from Shapiro and Bassen (1941) and Gairdner et al. (1952).

Megakaryocytes appear to increase in number gradually during the first week of life. Shapiro and Bassen found 58.7 megakaryocytes/ cu. mm. of marrow aspirate at birth and 82.9/cu. mm. on the eighth day of life.

Plasma cells number less than one per 5000 nucleated marrow elements in the newborn (Steiner and Pearson, 1966) and are generally not observed in the peripheral blood (Washburn, 1967).

ERYTHROPOIETIN IN THE NEWBORN PERIOD

The physiology of initiation and control of erythropoiesis in the fetus during the early stages of development is presently unknown. Finne (1968) has demonstrated that the fetus, at least from the thirty-second week of gestation, reacts to hypoxia with increased erythropoietin production. Erythropoietin, one of the humoral factors known to govern red cell production, has been shown to be transferred from the fetus to the amniotic fluid (Halvorsen and Finne, 1963; Finne, 1964), and across the placenta to the mother (Finne, 1967).

At birth, when the marrow shows marked erythropoietic activity, erythropoietin can be demonstrated in the plasma (Halvorsen, 1963; Mann et al., 1965). The level is higher in term infants than in those born prematurely (Finne, 1966; Stoutenborough et al., 1969). After the first day of life, erythropoietin cannot again be detected in the plasma of normal term infants until some time between the sixtieth and ninetieth day of life (Mann et al., 1965). The reappearance of erythropoietin coincides with the resumption of marked marrow activity noted at this time.

Elevated levels of erythropoietin have been found in the cord blood of infants with erythroblastosis fetalis when the hemoglobin has fallen below the range of 11 to 13 grams per 100 ml. (Finne, 1966). Infants born with signs of dysmaturity or born of mothers with diabetes or pre-eclampsia also have elevated levels (Finne, 1966), as do infants with Down's syndrome (Naveh, 1971).

Anemic infants, or infants with hypoxia secondary to cyanotic heart disease, show elevated levels of plasma erythropoietin after the first day of life (Althoff et al., 1957; Jones and Klingberg, 1960; and Halvorsen, 1963). This suggests that the mechanism for regulation of erythropoiesis by erythropoietin is present in the fetus during the late stages of gestation, and it also indicates that adequate oxygenation is in part responsible, through the erythropoietin mechanism, for the postnatal decline in erythropoiesis that can be observed midway through the first week of life.

THE BLOOD VOLUME

Great variations in blood volume during the newborn period have been reported by various investigators. Here, as in determinations of hemoglobin, multiple factors may produce variations. Factors of obvious importance are the method of cord clamping, the time of sampling, the techniques employed, and the previous history of maternal-fetal blood exchange. Shortly after birth, blood volumes may range from 50 to 100 ml./kg. of body weight in the term infant, with a mean of approximately 85 ml./kg. (Mollison et al., 1950; Low et al., 1963; Usher et al., 1963; and Jegier et al., 1964).

Usher and associates found that in infants whose cords were clamped early the mean blood volume at one-half hour of age was 78.0 ml./kg. as compared to 98.6 ml./kg. for infants in whom cord clamping was delayed. By 72 hours of age, the blood volume in the early-clamped group was 82.3 ml. and was 92.6 ml. in the late-clamped group. Infants with delayed cord clamping had much larger red cell volumes; thus, red cell volumes appear to be the chief determinants of total blood volume. Mollison and others (1950) demonstrated that, in newborn infants with hematocrits ranging from 20 to 75 per cent, the blood volume increased as the hematocrit rose. Bratteby (1968) found that the red cell volume could be predicted from a measurement of the venous hematocrit in early infants. The formula: Red cell volume in ml./kg. = $-12.3 + 1.02$ hematocrit (venous) was found to be useful with a standard error of only approximately 10 per cent.

Yao and associates (1967) observed that infants born by elective cesarean section, in whom the cord was clamped in utero, had decreased blood volumes, while those delivered by the same method because of fetal distress had increased blood volumes. These same investigators noted that the blood volume was decreased in infants born with tight nuchal cords.

The blood volume of the premature infant ranges from 89 ml./kg. (Usher et al., 1965) to approximately 105 ml./kg. during the first few days of life (Schulman et al., 1954; Sisson et al., 1959). This increased blood volume is primarily the result of an increased plasma volume, with the total red cell volume per kilogram of body weight being quite similar to that of the term infant. Cassady (1966) has observed that the plasma volume decreases with increasing gestational age. Infants with intrauterine growth retardation, however, were found to have greater plasma volumes than those expected for infants of comparable weight.

In both the premature and term infants, change of the blood volume relative to that of the normal adult occurs during the first month of life. Mean blood volumes of 73 to 77 ml./kg. have been recorded for infants after the first month of life (Russell, 1949; Brines et al., 1941), while the normal adult has been found to have a blood volume of approximately 77 ml./kg. (Gibson and Evans, 1937).

Erythrocyte Life Span

A variety of techniques have been employed in an attempt to determine the life span of the newborn's red cells. Most studies appear to indicate that the life span of the erythrocytes of the premature infant is unquestionably shorter than that of the erythrocytes of a normal adult, while those of the term infant are the same or only slightly shorter.

In addition to the technical difficulties involved in the performance of life span studies in the newborn period and the calculation of values in a patient with a changing blood volume, the problem of interpretation is also present. Should the normal adult mean survival of 120 days serve as the point of reference? It must be remembered that the placental blood contains a disproportionate number of young cells, because during the last three months of pregnancy weight of the fetus triples, and thus its blood volume triples with an accompanying increase in new red cells.

Theoretically, the infant's blood, with its younger mean cell age, should show a slower rate of initial red cell destruction in comparison to the adult. This difference has not been seen, indicating that the erythrocytes of the newborn, or a certain fraction of the total erythrocyte population, have a life span that is definitely shorter than that of the adult.

The life spans of red cells have been determined by the use of the differential agglutination technique of Ashby, by the method of chromium-51 labeling, by following the disappearance of fetal hemoglobin containing cells transfused into an adult, by estimates based on radioiron incorporation and disappearance, and by simple calculations based on the rate of fall of hemoglobin and red count during the first few months of life.

Mollison (1951) transfused placental and adult cells simultaneously into newborn infants, and he followed their removal by differential agglutination. During the first ten days of the study approximately 20 per cent of the placental cells disappeared, while only 10 per cent of the adult cells left the circulation; some placental cells could be observed up to day 90. Seeleman (1954), also employing the method of differential agglutination, estimated that the life span of placental cells taken from a term infant was 111 days, while Vest (1959), using the same technique to measure survival of placental cells from premature infants, concluded that the life span in these cases was markedly shortened.

Hollingsworth (1955) traced the disappearance of chromium-51 labeled red cells of the newborn transfused into adults and found that about 50 per cent of these cells had disappeared in 20 days, compared to the chromium half-life of about 27 days for normal adult cells. Foconi and Sjolin (1959) found that 50 per cent of the chromium tag disappeared in 22.8 days when the cells of term infants were injected into adults, compared to 27.5 days for adult cells treated similarly. Giblett (1955) also noted a chromium half-life of 20 days for cells from term infants injected into normal adults.

Kaplan and Hsu (1961) found the chromium half-life for term infants, 0 to 5 days of age, to range from 21 to 35 days with 9 of 11 of the infants studied having chromium half-lives in the normal adult range of 25 to 35 days. Gilardi and Miescher (1957) also concluded that the chromium half-life of the red cells of term infants was near normal. The red cells of five infants had a mean half-life of 24 days, compared to an average of 30 days for those of the adults.

In all six premature infants studied by Kaplan and Hsu, red cell chromium half-lives were less than 20 days with a range of 10 to 20 days. Gilardi and Miescher also noted that the red cells of the premature infant exhibited a shortened half-life. The mean survival in seven infants was 16 days with a range of 15 to 19 days.

Objections have been raised to the use of chromium-51 as a tag for the red cells of newborns because it may elute more rapidly from these cells than from adult cells. Suderman et al. (1957), Erlandson et al. (1958), and Kaplan and Hsu (1961) all demonstrated that chromium-51 did elute more rapidly from hemolysates of newborn cells, but Erlandson and associates and Kaplan and Hsu could not demonstrate this increased elution from intact cells of newborns studied in vitro. Pearson and Vertrees (1961) provided an explanation for this difference in elution rates by demonstrating that chromium-51 appears to bind predominantly to the beta chains of hemoglobin, one of the normal polypeptide pairs of adult hemoglobin. Cells of new-borns contain mostly fetal hemoglobin, consisting of alpha and gamma chains. This in part may explain the differences in elution rates observed in hemolysates (see also Chapter 5).

When red cells of newborns, which contain fetal hemoglobin, were injected into normal compatible adults and their survival was followed by the staining of adult blood smears by the acid elution technique of Kleihauer et al. (1957), the life span of cord erythrocytes was found to range from 56 to 105 days by Zipursky (1965). Kleihauer and Brandt (1964), using the same method, estimated the mean sur-vival to be 70 to 80 days. Pearson (1966) studied the disappearance of cells containing fetal hemoglobin and chromium-51 labeled cells simultaneously and observed that both methods gave similar results. He found the life span of red cells from newborn term infants to be only about two-thirds that of the normal adult.

Garby et al. (1964) estimated the life span of red cells of new-borns by using iron-59 red cell incorporation and iron excretion pat-terns and concluded that the mean life span of red cells containing fetal hemoglobin present at birth must be shorter than 83 days and that many cells formed in the newborn period survive for only 65 to 100 days. Using the in vitro label diisopropyl fluorophosphate (DF^{32}P) for the tagging of cord blood erythrocytes, Bratteby and associates (1968) noted that these cells disappeared in a curvilinear fashion when transfused into normal adults. Approximately 1.0 to 1.5 per cent disappeared per day during the first month after trans-fusion, and 0.7 to 1.0 per cent per day during the following month. This finding of an increased rate of red cell destruction agrees closely with estimates based on endogenous carbon monoxide formation in which 4 moles of carbon monoxide are released from the breakdown of one mole of hemoglobin. Wranne (1967), using the carbon monox-ide technique, found that 1.5 per cent of the term infant's red cell mass was broken down daily during the first week of life. He con-cluded that the life span of most erythrocytes formed during the late fetal and early neonatal period is only 90 days.

Equations derived from accumulated data led Bratteby and co-workers (1968) to the observation that the mean life span of cells produced during the last 60 days of fetal life was between 45 and 70 days and that the life span frequency function was skewed, with a majority of the cells dying before the mean life span. This increased rate of destruction, coupled with the need for increased red cell production to keep pace with growth, results in a relative rate of pro-duction of erythrocytes during the last two months of gestation that is three to five times that found in adults.

This mass of information gives basis to the inescapable conclusion that the life span of the newborn's erythrocytes is considerably shorter than that of the normal adult's erythrocytes. Unfortunately, the precise defect (or defects) responsible for this accelerated destruction remains to be defined.

RED CELL OSMOTIC AND MECHANICAL FRAGILITY

The red cells of the newborn infant demonstrate increased mechanical fragility (Goldbloom et al., 1953; Sjolin, 1954). Anyone who has ever drawn blood from a newborn infant can readily confirm this fact. This mechanical fragility is greatest during the first week of life and reaches adult values by approximately three months of age.

The osmotic fragility of red cells during the newborn period has been extensively studied and thoroughly reviewed by Sjolin (1954). It appears that at birth the infant has some red cells with increased osmotic fragility, but the majority of cells are slightly more resistant to osmotic hemolysis. During the first few days of life, the fragile cells disappear from the circulation, either by removal or by a change in their osmotic properties. Sjolin concluded that the mean osmotic fragility of cord blood and adult blood did not differ, but the span of hemolysis was greater in cord blood, with the osmotically resistant cells more numerous than in the adult blood. His work indicates that throughout childhood the resistant cells are more numerous than in adult blood but that this is especially true during the first few days of life. In the fetus, the red cells appear more osmotically fragile than normal, but they begin to increase in resistance during the fourth to fifth month of gestation.

Waigh et al. (1939) also concluded that the osmotic fragility of erythrocytes is normal at birth, but during the first four days of life these cells show greater osmotic resistance than do adult cells. Crawford et al. (1953) demonstrated that 50 per cent lysis of red cells from cord blood occurs at a saline concentration of 0.422 per cent. This concentration drops to 0.395 per cent at age 2 to 5 days. Normal adults demonstrated 50 per cent lysis in a saline concentration of 0.424 per cent. Although the bulk of the newborn's cells are more resistant than those of the adult, Crawford et al. also demonstrated that a minor population displayed more fragility. Employing the newest technique for the measurement of osmotic fragility, the "fragiligraph," Danon and co-workers (1970) and Luzzatto and associates (1970) both confirmed these earlier findings that on the average the newborn's erythrocytes tend to be osmotically more resistant than those of the adult, but that a population of abnormally fragile cells is also present. Luzzatto et al. (1970) observed a normalization of the osmotic fragility curve at four to six weeks of age.

PLASMA HEMOGLOBIN, HAPTOGLOBIN, AND HEMOPEXIN

Hemolysis is often observed in samples of blood obtained from newborn infants. These elevations in plasma hemoglobin concentration generally reflect the trauma of the sampling process and are not an accurate measure of the true in vivo levels of this pigment (Michaëlsson and Sjolin, 1965). Perona and Sartorelli (1966), employing very careful techniques, have found that the concentration of plasma hemoglobin in cord blood samples is quite similar to that of normal adults. In term infants the level of plasma hemoglobin rises after birth to reach peak values of approximately 3 mg. per 100 ml. on the third day of life, and then returns to near adult levels of 0.37 mg. per 100 ml. by five days of age. In the premature infant, the plasma hemoglobin tends to remain elevated for longer periods of time.

Haptoglobin, an alpha$_2$-glycoprotein, and hemopexin, a beta-glycoprotein, are plasma constituents that bind free hemoglobin. In older children and adults, the finding of low levels of these proteins points to an accelerated rate of red cell destruction. However, in the newborn period, measurement of the concentration of these proteins is of no apparent diagnostic usefulness because during this period of life the low values reflect impaired synthesis of the proteins rather than accelerated consumption. Many infants have no measurable haptoglobin at birth and may not reach normal adult values for four to seven months (Bergstrand et al., 1962; Khalil et al., 1967). Hemopexin levels were found to average 31 mg. per 100 ml. in term infants and 12 mg. per 100 ml. in premature infants (normal adult value 75 to 115 mg. per 100 ml.) by Lundh and co-workers (1970). No relationship between the level of either haptoglobin or hemopexin and the presence or absence of a hemolytic process could be demonstrated by these workers.

THE DEVELOPMENT OF RED CELL ANTIGENS AND ISOAGGLUTININS

Red cell antigens in the ABH, MN, Rh, Kell, Duffy and Vel systems have been found to be well developed in early intrauterine life. (See review by Toivanen and Hirvonen, 1969.) They may be demonstrated in the fifth to seventh gestational weeks and remain constant during the remainder of intrauterine development. The antigens in the Lutheran and Xg^a systems develop more slowly, but are present at birth.

ABH isoagglutinin production occurs in utero (Thomaidis et al., 1969; Fong et al., 1970). Approximately one-half of all term and premature infants of 34 to 36 weeks' gestation can be shown to have anti-A or anti-B antibodies. The fetal production of isoantibodies does not appear to be related to maternal ABO type or isoantibodies (Fong et al., 1970). Intrauterine exposure to gram-negative organisms whose antigens are chemically related to those of blood groups A and B may provide a stimulus for the development of these antibodies.

Isoagglutinin antibodies should be demonstrable in all normal infants by six months of age, reach at least a titer of 1:4 by one year of age, and approach normal adult values by two years of age (Gartner et al., 1967). A persistently low titer is suggestive of a disturbance of immunoglobulin production.

Chapter Two

THE HEMATOLOGIC ASPECTS OF THE MATERNAL-FETAL RELATIONSHIP

The fetus also takes its mother "for better or for worse, in sickness and in health." Although it is nourished and protected during gestation, the fetus may suffer the adverse effects of maternal malnutrition, illness, infection, and drug ingestion. The proximity of the two circulatory systems also permits the passage of formed blood elements between mother and fetus, and on occasion frank hemorrhage may occur. This chapter reviews the abnormalities of the maternal-fetal relationship that may produce disorders with hematologic manifestations in the newborn infant.

NUTRITIONAL FACTORS

Iron

The iron content of the newborn infant is approximately 75 mg./kg. of body weight, as determined by carcass analysis of stillbirths (Iob and Swanson, 1934; Widdowson and Spray, 1951). Studies performed during various stages of pregnancy indicate that the iron content and the weight of the fetus increase proportionately with age; thus, throughout gestation the fetus tends to maintain a constant iron

31

content of about 75 mg./kg. (Osgood, 1955; Friedenthal, 1914) (Fig. 2–1).

In the fetus, iron is present in three forms: hemoglobin iron, tissue iron, and storage iron. The bulk of it is present as hemoglobin iron. One gram of hemoglobin contains 3.4 mg. of elemental iron. An infant, weighing 3 kg. with a blood volume of approximately 270 ml. and a hemoglobin concentration of 17 gm./100 ml., requires 156 mg. of iron for hemoglobin from his total complement of 225 mg.

Tissue iron accounts for about 7 mg./kg. of body weight (Josephs, 1953). Storage iron in the liver and spleen, although subject to great variability, averages 10 mg./kg. (Lintzel et al., 1944; Widdowson and Spray, 1951).

The fetus receives its iron from the maternal circulation. The maternal iron is transported to the placental villi bound to transferrin, a beta-1-globulin. Maternal transferrin does not cross the placenta. The iron is believed to be taken up in the chorionepithelium of the placenta and stored as ferritin or hemosiderin. From these depots the iron, bound to transferrin, is then transported to fetal tissues

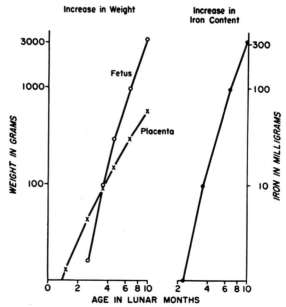

Figure 2–1 Increase in weight and increase in iron content in the human fetus. (From Pribilla, W., Bothwell, T. H., and Finch, C. A.: Iron transport to the fetus in man. In *Iron in Clinical Medicine*, Wallerstein, R. O., and Mettier, S. R., eds. Berkeley, University of California Press, 1958.)

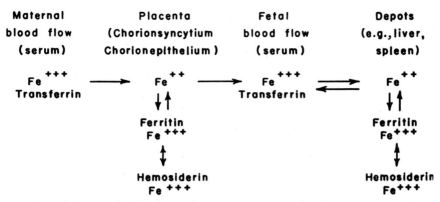

Figure 2–2 A model for placental iron transport. (From Wöhler, F.: *Current Therapeutic Research*, 6:466, 1964.)

(Wöhler, 1964) and initially most of it can be found in the liver (Dyer et al., 1969). Transferrin is synthesized within the fetus for this iron transport (Rausen et al., 1961). This scheme is illustrated in Figure 2–2.

Iron transport appears to be unidirectional and can occur against a steep concentration gradient. When radioactive iron is injected into the fetal circulation, none passes back into the maternal circulation (Pribilla et al., 1958). Within six hours of the injection of radioactive iron into the maternal plasma, 75 per cent or more of the iron extracted by the placenta has been deposited in fetal tissues (Pritchard et al., 1969).

The serum iron levels in the newborn are considerably higher than maternal levels, and the transferrin is more nearly saturated (Table 2–1).

Table 2–1 Serum Iron and Iron-binding Capacity in the Newborn and Mother

SERUM IRON (μG./ 100 ML.)		TOTAL IRON-BINDING CAPACITY (μG./100 ML.)		AUTHOR
Infant	*Mother*	*Infant*	*Mother*	
173	98	259	470	Hagberg (1953)
147	80	226	446	Laurell (1947)
193	–	240	–	Sturgeon (1954)
(145–240)		(147–468)		
159	–	–	–	Vahlquist et al. (1941)
(106–227)				

During the first day of life, a rapid fall in serum iron occurs (Vahlquist, 1941; Sturgeon, 1954; Smith et al., 1952). Serum iron then gradually increases, so that by the end of the second week of life it ranges from 125 to 141 μg./100 ml. (Sturgeon, 1954; Vahlquist, 1941).

Controversy still exists as to the role maternal iron deficiency may play in the iron endowment of the fetus. The hemoglobin concentration in the cord blood of infants born to anemic, iron deficient mothers does not differ from that of infants born to iron sufficient mothers (Fullerton, 1937; Woodruff and Bridgeforth, 1953; Lanzkowsky, 1961; De Leeuw et al., 1966), although Sisson and Lund (1957) found that the red cell volume and total hemoglobin mass were significantly reduced.

Zachau-Christiansen and associates (1962), Lund and Sisson (1957) and Shott (1971) observed that women with low serum iron values tended to have infants with lower than normal serum irons. In 1933, Strauss observed iron deficiency anemia at about one year of age in infants of women who had been severely iron deficient at term. The average hemoglobin of these six women was 5.2 gm./100 ml. In slightly less anemic mothers, a tendency of their offspring to develop iron deficiency anemia in late infancy has not been observed (Fullerton, 1937; Woodruff and Bridgeforth, 1953; Lanzkowsky, 1961). Sturgeon (1959) could find no differences in the state of iron nutrition in infants at 6, 12, and 18 months of age, irrespective of whether their mothers had received iron supplements during pregnancy. Similarly, De Leeuw and associates (1966) could find no effect of iron supplementation during pregnancy on cord blood serum iron values or on the infant's hemoglobin level, red cell count, mean corpuscular hemoglobin concentration, or reticulocyte count during the first year of life.

Guest and Brown (1957) noted that iron deficiency anemia is less common in first born children than in later siblings. It has been postulated that later siblings receive less iron endowment at birth as a consequence of maternal depletion through repeated pregnancies.

Except in the most unusual circumstances, maternal iron deficiency by itself apparently does not result in iron deficiency anemia in later infancy. Factors such as birth weight, rate of growth, subsequent nutrition, and incidence of infections seem to be far more important in determining the later appearance of anemia.

Folic Acid and Vitamin B_{12}

Both serum folic acid (Grossowicz et al., 1960; Zachau-Christiansen et al., 1962; Shojania and Gross, 1964) and serum vitamin B_{12} levels (Killander and Vahlquist, 1954; Boger et al., 1957; Baker et

Table 2-2   Serum Folic Acid and Vitamin B_{12} Levels in the Newborn

FOLIC ACID[°] ($M\mu G./ML.$)		VITAMIN B_{12}[°] ($\mu\mu G./ML.$)		AUTHORS
Infant	Maternal	Infant	Maternal	
40	7	390	190	Baker et al. (1958)
		560	310	Boger et al. (1957)
		1020	500	
		450	380	Killander et al. (1954)
9.8	2.8	373	240	Zachau-Christiansen et al. (1962)

°Mean values.

al., 1960; Zachau-Christiansen et al., 1962) are elevated at birth and in the early neonatal period. Values in the newborn are generally considerably higher than maternal levels (Table 2-2), and there appears to be a certain degree of positive correlation between serum B_{12} levels in mother and infant (Zachau-Christiansen et al., 1962). Grossowicz and co-workers (1966) observed that whole blood folate levels were markedly decreased in the cord blood of infants born to anemic, folate deficient mothers, but that the cord blood levels of the reduced forms of folates, those that are coenzymatically active, were normal. These workers concluded that an efficient mechanism operates to supply the fetus with the required concentrations of meta-bolically active folate regardless of the state of the maternal folate stores.

At the present time, there seems to be no evidence that folic acid (Giles, 1966; Grossowicz et al., 1966; Pritchard et al., 1969) or B_{12} deficiency in the mother results in anemia in the infant in the im-mediate newborn period. Prolonged breast feeding by mothers who have vitamin B_{12} deficiency, owing either to poor diet (Jadhav et al., 1962) or to untreated pernicious anemia (Lampkin et al., 1966), can eventually produce megaloblastic anemia in the infant.

MATERNAL INFECTIONS

Maternal infections acquired during pregnancy may be passed on to the fetus in utero. Congenital syphilis, toxoplasmosis, cyto-megalic inclusion disease, rubella, and generalized Coxsackie B in-fections are examples of transplacentally acquired diseases. The hematologic manifestations of congenital syphilis, toxoplasmosis, and cytomegalic inclusion disease are similar, and each may mimic

Table 2–3   Diagnostic Features of Some Transplacentally Acquired Infections Compared to Erythroblastosis Fetalis

FINDING	CONGENITAL SYPHILIS	TOXOPLASMOSIS (GENERALIZED FORM)	CYTOMEGALIC INCLUSION DISEASE	RUBELLA SYNDROME	ERYTHROBLAS-TOSIS FETALIS
Jaundice	+++	+++	+++	+	+++
Anemia	++++	+++	++	++	+++
Thrombo-cytopenia	++	+	+++	+++	+
Hepatomegaly	++++	+++	++++	++	++
Splenomegaly	++++	++++	++++	++	+++
Purpura	++	+	+++	+++	+
Skin rash	+	+	0	+	0
Chorioretinitis	+	+++	+	+	0
Intracranial calcifications	0	+	+++	?	0
Generalized edema	++	+	+	?	+

SPECIAL FEATURES

	Mucocutaneous lesions Periostitis Snuffles Positive serology	Convulsions Microcephaly Hydrocephaly Positive dye test Lymphadeno-pathy	Pneumonia Cytomegalic inclusion cells in urine	Cataract Glaucoma Heart defects Deafness Microcephaly Hydrocephaly Bone lesions Rubella virus recoverable	Pos. Coombs' test Evidence of blood group incompati-bility between mother and child

0	not described
+	present in approximately 1– 25% of cases
++	present in approximately 26– 50% of cases
+++	present in approximately 51– 75% of cases
++++	present in approximately 76–100% of cases

the findings in erythroblastosis fetalis. Table 2–3 lists the clinical and laboratory features of these diseases.

Cytomegalic Inclusion Disease

In 1904, the first report was made of an unusual disease of infancy associated with the presence of large cells containing intranuclear and, occasionally, intracytoplasmic inclusion bodies (Jesionek and Kiolemenoglou). In 1950, Wyatt and associates suggested that the antemortem diagnosis of this disease might be made by cytologic examination of the urinary sediment. In 1952, Fetterman made the first antemortem diagnosis, and shortly thereafter reports appeared of infants who survived the neonatal period despite infection (Margileth, 1955; Birdsong et al., 1956). In 1956, the etiologic agent was discovered when several related viruses were isolated from infants with the disease (Smith, 1956; Weller et al., 1957). These agents have been variously termed human salivary gland viruses, cytomegalic inclusion disease viruses, or cytomegaloviruses. The disease in the neonate is acquired transplacentally from an asymptomatic mother. Placental infections may occur without fetal involvement (Hayes and Gibas, 1971).

Surveys indicate that between 0.5 and 1.0 per cent of newborns may be harboring this virus (Birnbaum et al., 1969). The vast majority of these infants show no clinically recognizable evidence of disease during this period of life, although many may have elevations in their levels of immunoglobulin M (IgM). Virus excretion may persist for months after birth and virus may also be isolated from the patient's leukocytes (Lang and Noren, 1968). Embil and associates (1970) have observed congenital infections in two siblings from consecutive pregnancies.

Clinical manifestations of the disease in the newborn period may include hepatosplenomegaly, jaundice, purpura and ecchymoses, microcephaly, intracranial calcifications, pneumonia, and chorioretinitis.

Hematologic Manifestations. The hematologic manifestations are variable. Pertinent findings in 29 infants in whom the disease manifested itself in the first week of life and was confirmed by virus isolation, appear in Table 2-4. Enlargement of the liver and spleen is almost always present, and the spleen is frequently larger than the liver. Jaundice was present in approximately 75 per cent of the patients and generally was noted during the first 48 hours of life. Bilirubin values in excess of 30 mg./100 ml. have been recorded, and there is usually a significant elevation in the conjugated as well as the unconjugated bilirubin fraction. In only seven of these patients was the hemoglobin value reported for the first few days of life, and in three of these infants anemia was present. Hemoglobin concentrations of 8 to 12 gm./100 ml. have been observed during the first 48 hours of life in other infants who undoubtedly had cytomegalic inclusion disease, although no attempts at virus isolation were made.

Even in infants in whom no anemia is present, the peripheral blood smear frequently reveals large numbers of nucleated red cells and bizarre red cell morphology.

Table 2-4   Hematologic Findings in Newborns with Cytomegalic Inclusion Disease Confirmed by Virus Isolation[*]

Hepatomegaly	29 of 29
Splenomegaly	28 of 29
Anemia	3 of 7
Jaundice	21 of 29
Thrombocytopenia or purpura	20 of 29

[*]Based on the reports of Guyton et al. (1957), Curtis et al. (1962), Medearis (1957), Kluge et al. (1960), and Weller et al. (1962).

Petechiae, purpura, and ecchymoses are common, and platelet counts of 6 to 20,000/cu. mm. have been observed during the first day of life. Bone marrow aspirations reveal virtual absence of megakaryocytes.

If anemia is not present in the first few days of life, it generally develops rapidly during the next several weeks. In many infants, studied at three to six weeks of age because of persistent jaundice, hemoglobin values of 5 to 10 gm./100 ml. have been noted, in association with reticulocyte counts of 10 to 20 per cent.

Diagnosis. The disease must be distinguished from erythroblastosis fetalis, congenital toxoplasmosis, congenital syphilis, bacterial sepsis, and neonatal leukemia. Major points in the differential diagnosis are summarized in Table 2–3. The finding of an elevated IgM level, in the first two weeks of life, suggests the presence of intrauterine infection, but is not specific for any particular agent.

The diagnosis may be strongly suspected if the typical enlarged cells containing intranuclear and cytoplasmic inclusions can be demonstrated in the spinal fluid or freshly voided urine. At autopsy these cells may be found in almost all tissues of the body.

The oval, or round, homogenous intranuclear portion usually stains reddish-violet with hematoxylin and eosin, is surrounded by a halo, and is approximately 9 μ in diameter. The cytoplasmic portion is granular and more basophilic.

Not all patients with cytomegalic inclusion disease show these cells in their urine at all times, and other viral infections may simulate this disease by the production of similar appearing cells (Medearis, 1964). Because of this, the most reliable diagnostic test is direct isolation of the virus from the urine.

Toxoplasmosis

Congenital toxoplasmosis results from the transplacental passage of the intracellular protozoan parasite *Toxoplasma gondii*. Fetal infection apparently results from a chance primary infection in a nonimmune mother. Generally the mothers are asymptomatic at this time, but occasionally the primary infection may be associated with fever and lymphadenopathy (Feldman, 1958). During the parasitemia, an infected locus may develop in the placenta, enabling parasites to cross into the fetal circulation (Beckett and Flynn, 1953). Feldman believes that maternal infections acquired just before and soon after pregnancy may not result in congenital infections, even though viable parasites can be demonstrated in the lymph nodes. In contrast, infections that spread to lymph nodes after the third month of pregnancy may also invade the fetus.

Congenital toxoplasmosis may manifest itself during the first week of life by fever, jaundice, lymphadenopathy, hepatospleno-megaly, a diffuse maculopapular rash, microphthalmia, chorioretinitis, seizures, hydrocephaly or microcephaly, intracranial calcifications, anemia, and thrombocytopenia. This clinical picture is very similar to that seen in cytomegalic inclusion body disease and like cyto-megalic inclusion disease it has been rarely observed in successive pregnancies (Garica, 1968).

Hematologic Manifestations.   Congenital toxoplasmosis may mimic erythroblastosis fetalis. Pale hydropic infants with marked hepatosplenomegaly have been reported. Infants with this severe form of the disease are either stillborn or live only for several minutes (Callahan et al., 1946; Harwin and Angrist, 1948; Hall et al., 1953; Beckett and Flynn, 1953; Bain et al., 1956).

In the series of Eichenwald (1957), anemia was present in 77 per cent of patients with the generalized form of toxoplasmosis and 50 per cent of the patients with the primarily neurologic form of the dis-ease. Very few precise figures are available in the literature as to the severity of the anemia.

Thrombocytopenia has been observed but does not appear to occur as commonly as it does in cytomegalic inclusion disease. The white cell count may range from 5 to 35,000/cu. mm., and immature forms are frequently observed in the peripheral smear. Beckett and Flynn (1953) noted the presence of 8 per cent blast forms in one patient. Eosinophilia has been observed in 18 per cent of infants with the generalized form of the disease (Eichenwald, 1957).

Diagnosis.   A specific diagnosis can be established by demon-stration of the organism or by serologic methods. Serologic confirma-tion is most easily obtained by the use of the Sabin-Feldman dye test, although a complement fixation test has also been devised. The dye test is performed initially on sera from both the mother and infant. If dye titers are elevated, they must be repeated in the infant at four months of age, or later, to make certain that the original elevation was not merely the result of transplacental passage of previously existent maternal antibody. If the high titer is due to infection with toxoplasma, it will still be elevated in the second test. If the second test is negative or the titer is low, it indicates disappearing passively acquired antibody from the mother, and the diagnosis of toxoplas-mosis cannot be made.

Congenital Syphilis

Congenital syphilis is still prevalent, and the consequences of the transplacental acquisition of the spirochete *Treponema pallidum* must be considered in the differential diagnosis of all jaundiced new-borns. It has been estimated that a minimum of 13.9 per cent of infants of untreated mothers and 5.8 per cent of inadequately treated mothers will show the stigmata of congenital syphilis (Nelson and Struve, 1956). Infants with congenital syphilis may demonstrate snuffles, mucocutaneous lesions, pseudoparalysis with osteochondritis and periostitis, hepatosplenomegaly, jaundice, and lymphadenopathy. The hematologic manifestations are frequently more conspicuous and call attention to its presence before other stigmata of the infection are apparent.

Hematologic Manifestations.   Congenital syphilis is frequently misdiagnosed as erythroblastosis fetalis and can easily be confused with congenital toxoplasmosis, cytomegalic inclusion disease, and congenital leukemia.

Anemia is present in the majority of affected infants (Tudos and Kiss, 1926; Risel, 1908; Whitaker et al., 1965), and hemoglobin values as low as 8.7 gm./100 ml. have been recorded on the first day of life (Whitaker et al., 1965). The associated anemia in most instances is apparently a result of an intense hemolytic process and is associated with reticulocytosis, a marked increase in the number of nucleated red cells, and distortion of red cell morphology. On occasion, the anemia may be a consequence of marrow hypoplasia or aplasia (Baar et al., 1963; Whitaker et al., 1965).

Jaundice may be present on the first day of life, and the bilirubin may exceed 40 mg./100 ml. at its peak. The jaundice is usually associated with elevation of both the conjugated and unconjugated bilirubin fractions.

Hemorrhagic manifestations have been described in infants with congenital syphilis. Freiman and Super (1966) observed platelet counts of less than 100,000/cu. mm. in 13 of 46 infected infants, while Whitaker and associates (1965) found thrombocytopenia in four of nine infants with the disease. Platelet counts as low as 17,000/cu. mm. were recorded, and bone marrow examination revealed adequate numbers of megakaryocytes suggesting the presence of disseminated intravascular coagulation as being responsible for the thrombocytopenia. Whitaker and associates (1965) concluded that the spleen played no important role in platelet depression because thrombocytopenia was observed in patients with minimal or no splenomegaly.

The total white cell count may be subnormal, normal, or elevated. The differential count may reveal an absolute lymphocytosis (Nitschke, 1924) or an increase in the myelocytic series (Ruedda, 1963). It is not uncommon to observe an increase in immature white cell forms in the peripheral blood, and blasts may be present.

Diagnosis.   The diagnosis is established by demonstrating a positive serologic titer and the persistence of this titer after three to six months of age. The diagnosis also can be made by finding the *Treponema* in scrapings from the moist cutaneous lesions.

The diagnosis can be strongly suspected in an infant who exhibits the clinical and radiographic abnormalities and who is born of a mother with a positive serology.

Congenital Rubella

Although it had been previously recognized that purpura was one of the manifestations of intrauterine rubella infection (Prendergast, 1948; Brown and Nathan, 1954; Oxhorn, 1959; Manson et al., 1960; Hugh-Jones et al., 1960; Lundstrom, 1962; and Berge et al., 1963), it was not until the rubella epidemic of 1964–1965 that its frequent occurrence was generally appreciated.

The well recognized consequences of fetal rubella infections occurring during the first 12 weeks of pregnancy are low birth weight, cataract, glaucoma, retinitis, deafness, brain lesions associated with microcephaly, meningoencephalitis, or hydrocephalus, and cardiac defects, especially patent ductus arteriosus and ventricular septal defects. To this list must now be added thrombocytopenic purpura, hepatosplenomegaly, neonatal hepatitis, intrahepatic biliary atresia, jaundice, bone lesions, dermal erythropoiesis (Brough et al., 1967), and a hemolytic anemia.

Hematologic Manifestations.   Thrombocytopenia appears to be the most common hematologic manifestation of congenital rubella. Its incidence has varied from 40 to 80 per cent in the most recently reported series (Rudolph et al., 1965; Cooper et al., 1965; Korones et al., 1965; Plotkin et al., 1965; Banatvala et al., 1965). Platelet counts are frequently below 50,000/cu. mm., and values as low as 3000/cu. mm. have been observed (Banatvala et al., 1965). The platelet count generally returns to normal levels by the end of the second week of life, but thrombocytopenia has persisted in some instances for as long as two months (Rausen et al., 1965) and may progress to a transient hypoplastic anemia (Lafer and Morrison, 1967). Bone marrow aspirates usually reveal a decrease in the number of megakaryocytes. Zinkham and Medearis (1965) observed increased numbers of phagocytic reticulum cells in the marrow aspirates of these infants.

In most instances, petechiae and purpura are present on the first day of life and have largely faded by the end of the second week despite persistent thrombocytopenia. Serious hemorrhage is uncommon.

The white cell count is variable. Either leukopenia or leukocytosis may occur. Examinations of the peripheral blood usually reveals an increase in the number of nucleated red cells and anisocytosis of the erythrocytes.

Anemia may be present, and hemoglobin values in the range of 10 gm./100 ml. have been observed during the first week of life. Red cell survival was reduced to 50 per cent of normal in the one infant so studied (Zinkham and Medearis). This hemolytic anemia may persist for several months and may be associated with alterations in red cell morphology that include fragmented cells, burr cells, tear drop forms, microspherocytes, target cells, basophilic stippling, and the presence of Howell-Jolly bodies (Rausen et al., 1967). It remains to be determined if these red cell alterations are a direct result of virus-induced membrane injury, secondary to the associated liver disease, or are a consequence of mechanical injury to the red cells resulting from an associated process of disseminated intravascular coagulation. In one of 56 infants reported by Cooper et al. (1965) erythroid hypoplasia was present.

Enlargement of the liver and spleen occurs in 33 to 75 per cent of the patients. Jaundice is present in approximately 25 per cent of patients and may have a significant obstructive component with an elevation of the conjugated bilirubin fraction. Jaundice may persist into the second month of life, and biopsies have revealed evidence of giant-cell hepatitis (Plotkin et al., 1965).

Diagnosis.   Congenital rubella should be included in the differential diagnosis of thrombocytopenia in all newborn infants in whom hepatosplenomegaly is present. When these hematologic manifestations are present in an infant with other recognized stigmata of congenital rubella, the diagnosis can be strongly suspected. Confirmation depends on isolation of virus from the newborn or the demonstration of a persistent titer of neutralizing antibody in the infant.

Other Infections

Other transplacentally acquired infections may also be associated with hematologic abnormalities. Coxsackie B virus infections in the newborn infant produce a generalized disease characterized by the presence of encephalomyelitis and myocarditis (Kibrick et al., 1958; 1961). Purpura and hemorrhage occur in about 13 per cent of cases. Hemorrhage appears to be a result of a depletion of coagulation factors and platelets secondary either to the virus-induced process of disseminated intravascular coagulation (Desmond, 1968) or to virus-induced hepatic injury with resultant inability to synthesize certain of the clotting factors. Jaundice, mild anemia, and hepatic and splenic enlargement may also be observed.

Generalized herpes simplex infections in the newborn infant may produce anemia, jaundice, hepatosplenomegaly, thrombocytopenia, (Zuelzer and Stulberg, 1952; Schaffer, 1960) and disseminated intravascular coagulation. There is no conclusive proof that this infection is transplacentally acquired, but it may be contracted from the mother during the birth process by direct contact with herpetic lesions on the mother's genitalia (Eichenwald and Shinefield, 1962). Approximately 40 per cent of severely infected patients demonstrate hemorrhagic phenomena (Miller et al., 1970). In this infection the bleeding also appears to be a result of the associated disseminated intravascular coagulation (Miller et al., 1970; Lascari and Wallace, 1970) and is discussed in detail in Chapter Eight. Cytosine arabinoside may be useful in the treatment of the infection (Hryniuk et al., 1971).

Malaria may be transmitted from mother to fetus and may result in anemia and hepatosplenomegaly in the neonate (Harvey et al., 1969).

Conflicting data exist in the literature concerning the transplacental transmission of serum hepatitis, at least as reflected by the presence of Australia antigen in both mother and infant. Several groups of investigators (London et al., 1969; Smithwick and Go, 1970; Lyons and Guze, 1971) failed to find the antigen in the infants of antigen-positive mothers, while Schweitzer and Spears (1970), Gillespie and associates (1970) and Turner et al. (1971) demonstrated the presence of the antigen, the presumed viral particle, in both mother and infant. In these cases the antigen was first found one to two months after birth and may have been orally acquired during the delivery process.

PLACENTAL TRANSFER OF FORMED BLOOD ELEMENTS

Accumulated evidence indicates that leukocytes, platelets, and erythrocytes traverse the placental barrier. The transfer of platelets and leukocytes and its consequences are discussed in detail in Chapters Nine and Ten, respectively. Fetal red cells can be demonstrated in the maternal circulation in approximately 50 per cent of all pregnancies (Cohen et al., 1964), and on occasion this form of transplacental hemorrhage may be sufficient to produce severe anemia in the newborn infant, as described in Chapter Three.

Maternal-to-Fetal Erythrocyte Transfer

Maternal red cells may also appear in the fetal circulation, and maternal-to-fetal hemorrhage may be responsible for plethora in the newborn infant.

Hedenstedt and Naeslund (1946) were able to demonstrate elliptocytes in the cord blood after infusing these "naturally" marked cells into the mother. Naeslund (1951) was subsequently able to demonstrate the passage of red cells labeled with phosphorus or iron from the maternal circulation to the fetal circulation.

Mengert and associates (1955) tagged erythrocytes with iron-59 and infused them into mothers 13 minutes to 10 days prior to delivery. In 25 of 29 infants, radioactive red cells could be recovered. Macris and co-workers (1958) infused pregnant women with blood from individuals with sickle cell trait 40 minutes to 153 hours prior to delivery. In three of 25 instances sickled cells were found in cord blood specimens. In one mother with naturally occurring sickle cell trait, no sickled cells were observed in her offspring.

Duhring and associates (1960) injected chromium labeled red cells into pregnant women 13 to 15 hours prior to cesarean section. In eight of 12 infants, radioactive red cells could be recovered, and transplacental blood loss was estimated to be between 0.3 and 1.0 ml.

Using immunofluorescent techniques, Lee and Vazquez (1962) were able to demonstrate maternal erythrocytes in two of 27 infants at term.

Cohen and Zuelzer (1965), using immunofluorescent techniques, searched for maternal cells in the offspring in 154 suitable mother-child pairs. The incidence of positive cells in cord and placental vein blood varied from 36.7 to 11.3 per cent in their two studies, the number of positive cells decreasing markedly as precautions against contamination were increased. In only 2.8 per cent of infants were maternal red cells demonstrable when samples of heel blood were taken within hours after birth. In each positive case, only minute numbers of maternal cells were found. Cohen and Zuelzer concluded that generally the presence of maternal cells in the cord blood reflects unavoidable contamination, and that passage of such cells into the fetus is exceptional and of minimal quantitative significance. Donovan and Lund (1966) reached similar conclusions following the injection of chromium-labeled red cells into pregnant women of 12 to 22 weeks' gestation and after examining the abortuses 16 to 24 hours later, at the time of hysterotomy.

Although cord samples may easily become contaminated with maternal blood, the presence of large numbers of maternal cells in infant venous samples obtained days after birth should be regarded as highly significant. The role of maternal to fetal erythrocyte transfer in the etiology of neonatal polycythemia is discussed in Chapter Four.

MATERNAL DISEASES

Systemic Lupus Erythematosus

Bridge and Foley (1954) were the first to describe the presence of lupus erythematosus (L.E.) cells in the blood of infants born to mothers with systemic lupus erythematosus. Both infants were well. Positive L.E. preps could be demonstrated at seven weeks of age, but they were negative at age four months. Several other investigators have reported instances of placental passage of L.E. factor (Jackson, 1964; Cruveiller et al., 1970). L.E. cells could be demonstrated for as long as seven weeks in some of these infants, and antinuclear antibody was shown to persist for 15 weeks (Beck and Rowell, 1963).

In at least two instances hematologic manifestations in the infant have been attributed to the presence of this passively acquired antibody. Nathan and Snapper (1958) observed thrombocytopenia in one infant. This persisted for approximately one month. The infant's platelet count on the second day of life was 30,000/cu. mm., and it gradually rose to 176,000/cu. mm. by four weeks of age. L.E. cells could be demonstrated only on the second day of life. The mother was thrombocytopenic at the time of delivery, and platelet antibodies were present in both the mother and child.

Seip (1960) observed anemia, leukopenia, and mild thrombocytopenia in a two month old infant who was born to a mother with similar hematologic abnormalities in association with her systemic lupus erythematosus. At two months of age, the infant had a hemoglobin of 3.3 gm./100 ml.; a reticulocyte count of 22.8 per cent; leukocytes, 1800/cu. mm.; platelets, 114,000/cu. mm. No. L.E. cells could be found at this time. The patient was treated with prednisone; within two weeks the blood picture became normal and remained so after steroids were discontinued. Hull and associates (1966) observed gross edema in an infant born to a mother with systemic lupus erythematosus. The child died shortly after birth and at autopsy was found to have endocardial fibroelastosis, widespread fibrosis of the liver, spleen, kidneys, and adrenals, and marked extramedullary erythropoiesis. The role of the transplacentally acquired antibody in the production of these abnormalities is not clear.

Discoid lupus erythematosus has been observed in the offspring of mothers with systemic lupus (McCuiston and Schoch, 1954; Epstein and Litt, 1961; Jackson, 1964). L.E. cells were present only in the infant described by Jackson (1964), and no other hematologic abnormalities were noted. East and Lumpkin (1969) described an infant with discoid lupus whose mother was free of disease. By age four months the child had developed signs of systemic lupus.

It is not clear why only some infants with passively acquired L.E. factor, an IgG globulin, demonstrate hematologic abnormalities. It is generally held that these antibodies are a reflection of disease and not etiologic agents. Transfusion of serum containing L.E. factor into human patients does not produce any evidence of systemic L.E., although it may induce a temporary L.E. phenomenon (Bencze et al., 1959).

Leukemia

Over 250 cases of leukemia in association with pregnancy have now been reported (Maloney, 1964); in no instance has leukemia been recognizable in the newborn infant. Fetal loss occurs in approximately 14 per cent of women with chronic granulocytic leukemia and in 34 per cent of women with acute leukemia (Maloney, 1964).

In only two instances has leukemia subsequently developed in an infant of a mother with the disease (Cramblett et al., 1958; Bernard et al., 1964). In the patient described by Cramblett, the diagnosis of acute lymphatic leukemia in the mother was established on the eighth postpartum day, although symptoms and signs attributable to leukemia were present at the seventh month of pregnancy. The infant was hematologically normal at one week of age and remained well until nine months of age, when anorexia, irritability, easy bruising, and hepatosplenomegaly were recognized and led to a diagnosis of acute lymphatic leukemia. Lymphoblastic leukemia was diagnosed at term in the mother described by Bernard and co-workers, and her child manifested the same form of the disease at five months of age. In this infant, an abnormal karyotype was demonstrated in association with the leukemia, but unfortunately no chromosome studies had been performed in the mother. Although the occurrence of leukemia in an infant of a mother with the disease appears to be a distinct rarity, sufficient long-term follow-up of these infants is not available; thus, firm conclusions as to the true incidence of this event cannot be drawn (Diamandopoulos and Hertig, 1963).

Rigby and others (1964) studied the transplacental passage of quinacrine labeled leukemic cells from a mother with acute myelogenous leukemia. Examination of the placenta revealed increased numbers of probable myeloblasts on the maternal side, with none on the fetal side. An occasional labeled cell was observed in the infant's blood. Of interest, but unexplained, was the observation that the infant's white cell alkaline phosphatase level was considerably lower than normal for his age. The mother's white cell alkaline phosphatase level was also in the low normal range, in contrast to the high values usually found during pregnancy.

MALIGNANCIES

Malignancy in the mother does not usually spread to the fetus. Seventeen cases have been recorded in which a malignant process in the mother has involved either the placenta, the fetus, or both (Freedman and McMahon, 1960; Brodsky et al., 1965). Spread of a malignant melanoma has been observed on seven occasions. Carcinomas of the stomach, breast, adrenal gland, bronchus, and ethmoid bone have also been observed to metastasize, as have sarcomas and a lymphosarcoma (Berghinz, 1900).

In four instances, the malignant melanoma was demonstrated in the infant but did not produce death in the patient reported by Holland (1949) until eight months of age. In the infant described by Brodsky and associates (1965), malignant cells were observed in the peripheral blood on the first day of life, lesions became apparent on the eleventh day of life, and they resulted in death from a generalized process on the forty-eighth day. In this patient, an unusual hematologic picture complicated the first week of life. It was characterized by anemia, normoblastemia, agranulocytosis, and thrombocytopenia. The marrow was hypocellular, but no tumor cells could be identified. It was the impression of the authors that some of the peripheral blood

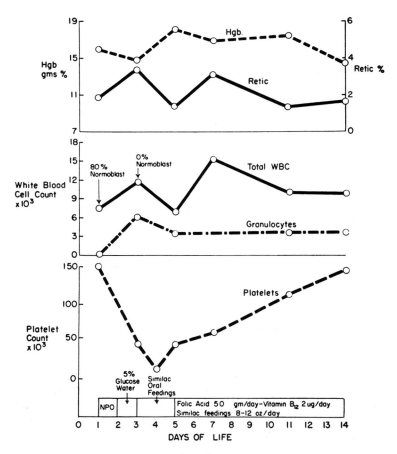

Figure 2–3 Hematologic findings in an infant with transplacental acquisition of malignant melanoma. The first days of life were characterized by normoblastemia, leukopenia, and thrombocytopenia. (From Brodsky, I., et al.: *Cancer,* *18:*1048, 1965.)

findings were related to an associated severe folic acid deficiency. The infant's blood picture during the first 14 days of life is illustrated in Figure 2–3.

Cavell (1963) observed an infant with transplacentally acquired malignant melanoma who recovered despite evidence of metastasis.

Daemen and associates (1961) observed a simultaneous occurrence of a chorionepithelioma in both mother and infant, and they cite two other examples from the literature. Death in these infants occurred at seven weeks, seven months, and eight months.

Hodgkin's disease has developed on two occasions in infants of mothers afflicted with the disease (Kasdon, 1949). One infant died at 4½ months of age and the other at 33 months.

Multiple myeloma in pregnancy has been observed (Kosova and Schwartz, 1966; Radl et al., 1968). In both instances the infants were healthy. In the infant studied by Kosova and Schwartz, no transplacental transmission of the abnormal protein occurred. Radl and associates were able to document a transient paraproteinemia in the offspring, indicating that the nature of the paraprotein determines its placental passage.

Tumors may spread from the fetus to the placenta. Strauss and Driscoll (1964) described two instances in which a congenital neuroblastoma acted in such a fashion. There was no evidence of maternal spread. Clinically, both infants resembled the picture of hydrops fetalis, with pallor, enlargement of the abdomen, hepatosplenomegaly, and peripheral edema. Congenital neuroblastoma must now be added to erythroblastosis fetalis, homozygous alpha thalassemia, severe congenital syphilis, toxoplasmosis, cytomegalic inclusion disease, and protracted fetal-to-maternal hemorrhage as a cause of hydrops fetalis.

HEART DISEASE

Kravkova (1962) noted that fetuses from mothers with severe decompensated heart disease tended to have higher hemoglobin and white cell counts, with marrows showing increased erythropoietic activity.

Bromberg and associates (1956) recorded higher fetal hemoglobin values in infants of mothers with chronic hypoxia. Included in this group were four women with heart failure, two with severe asthma and cyanosis, and six who were profoundly anemic (see Chapter Five).

Anoxemia in the fetus may also reflect itself in the mother. Mothers of infants with fetal distress were noted to have elevated reticulocyte counts (Rolandi and Signorelli, 1962).

HYPERTHYROIDISM

Maternal hyperthyroidism may be associated with neonatal thyrotoxicosis. This is believed to be a consequence of the placental passage of long-acting thyroid stimulator (LATS) from mother to infant. Infants with neonatal thyrotoxicosis may manifest plethora, congestive heart failure, hepatosplenomegaly, hyperbilirubinemia, and thrombocytopenia (Elsas et al., 1967). The mechanism of the thrombocytopenia is unknown, but it is also observed, on occasion, in adults with hyperthyroidism (Woodruff, 1940).

PERNICIOUS ANEMIA

An antibody to intrinsic factor can be demonstrated in approximately 60 per cent of patients with pernicious anemia. It has not been established whether the antibody plays an etiologic role in the disease or is a secondary manifestation of gastric injury. The circulating antibody is an IgG globulin and thus may be transferred from mother to fetus. Two instances of transplacental transmission of intrinsic factor antibody have been documented in women with known pernicious anemia (Bar-Shany and Herbert, 1967; Goldberg et al., 1967). The circulating antibody appeared to suppress intrinsic factor secretion in the stomach of the infants for periods of one to three months. In neither infant did anemia develop, but in one infant (Bar-Shany and Herbert, 1967) the serum B_{12} level had fallen to an abnormally low level by age 3 months.

AUTOIMMUNE HEMOLYTIC ANEMIA

A Coombs positive hemolytic anemia may occur in both mother and infant. Letts and Kredenster (1968, 1969) described a woman with both a severe Coombs positive hemolytic anemia and thrombocytopenia ("Evan's syndrome," 1949) who was observed during the course of three pregnancies. The first pregnancy ended with the birth of a hydropic stillborn infant. The second pregnancy produced a normal infant at a time when the mother's illness appeared to be in remission, and the third pregnancy resulted in the birth of a child with thrombocytopenia. Zuelzer and associates (1970) observed a woman with a history of intermittent thrombocytopenic purpura and a chronic Coombs positive hemolytic anemia who gave birth prematurely to an infant with both a Coombs positive hemolytic anemia and thrombocytopenia. Cytomegalovirus was found in the urine of the infant and his mother.

MATERNAL DRUG ADMINISTRATION

Neonatal hemorrhage, thrombocytopenia, leukopenia, and hemolytic anemia have all been reported as consequences of maternal drug administration. During the last trimester of pregnancy women have been found to take an average of 8.7 different drugs and vitamins. Approximately 80 per cent of these medications are taken without medical supervision or knowledge (Bleyer et al., 1970). A careful history of maternal drug ingestion is always necessary in the evaluation of a neonate with a puzzling condition.

Hemorrhage

Although prenatal heparin administration has not been implicated as a cause of neonatal coagulation disturbances, the use of the coumarin derivatives have.

Flessa and others (1964) compared prothrombin times, recalcification times, thrombin times, and clotting times in infants of mothers who received heparin during the first stage of labor with those of controls; they could demonstrate no differences. One patient in their study had been on long-term heparin therapy; her infant experienced no difficulties. The authors conclude that heparin either does not cross the placenta because of its large molecular size, or if it does, it is rapidly inactivated in the fetus. It does not appear in the breast milk.

Fetal and neonatal deaths have occurred in mothers receiving Dicumarol derivatives (Fillmore and McDevitt, 1970; Sachs and Labati, 1949; von Sydow, 1947; Gordon and Dean, 1955). In one infant, subcutaneous hemorrhages occurred several hours after birth, and a massive intracranial hemorrhage occurred with subsequent hydrocephalus despite vigorous therapy with vitamin K (von Sydow, 1947). While on Dicumarol therapy, a mother gave birth to a macerated fetus with a large hemopericardium (Sachs and Labati, 1949). Two cases have been reported by Gordon and Dean (1955). One mother receiving Dicumarol therapy delivered a stillborn infant with cerebral, pericardial, gastric, and testicular hemorrhages. The second patient hemorrhaged from the cord at two hours of age; this was quickly followed by hemorrhages in the lip and skin. A large organized clot, believed to have been present in utero, was found in the cerebral ventricle. The ingestion of anticoagulants by women who are breast-feeding their infants may result in hemorrhages in these children (Eckstein and Jack, 1970).

Maternal barbiturate medication may prolong the prothrombin time (Dyggve, 1950). Van Creveld (1957) and Mountain and coworkers (1970) have observed that administration of antiepileptics to the pregnant woman produces abnormalities in prothrombin, factor

VII, and factor X levels in the infant up to the fourth day of life. These abnormalities and the associated hemorrhage respond rapidly to vitamin K therapy. Hemorrhage seems to be more common in infants born to epileptic mothers receiving anti-convulsant medications (Köhler, 1966; Douglas, 1966). Large doses of salicylate to the mother may also result in prolongation of the newborn's prothrombin time (Earle, 1961).

Thrombocytopenia and Thrombocytopathy

Rodriguez and associates (1964) observed thrombocytopenia in seven infants of mothers receiving thiazide drugs. Bone marrow examinations performed in four of these patients showed that the megakaryocytes were markedly reduced in number. Maternal quinine administration has also resulted in thrombocytopenia in a neonate (Mauer et al., 1956).

Merenstein and associates (1970) found the platelet count to be normal in 37 infants born to mothers receiving thiazides. These authors speculate that the thrombocytopenia observed by Rodriguez and co-workers may have been a manifestation of disseminated intravascular coagulation in the infants of mothers with either eclampsia or preeclampsia and not a direct result of the drug ingestion.

Pantarotto (1965) observed thrombocytopenia as part of a transient aplastic anemia in an infant born to a mother who was receiving a hydantoin-containing anticonvulsant.

Aspirin, the most commonly used drug in the United States, produces platelet dysfunction by impairing platelet aggregation and thus prolonging the bleeding time (See Chapters Eight and Nine). The ingestion of as little as one tablet (5 grains) of aspirin by the mother in the week prior to delivery can produce abnormalities of platelet function in the newborn infant (Corby et al., 1971; Bleyer and Breckenridge, 1970; Mull and Hathaway, 1970). The incidence of cephalohematoma, melena, and purpura may be higher in these babies (Bleyer and Breckenridge). Other drugs such as glyceryl guaiacolate, phenylbutazone, dipyridamole, and antihistaminics also impair platelet function and thus perhaps will be found to be associated with bleeding problems in newborn infants of mothers who have recently received such drugs.

Leukopenia

Rodriguez and associates (1964) observed leukopenia in three of the seven thrombocytopenic infants whose mothers had received thiazide derivatives near term. The white count was 2600/cu. mm. in one patient.

Hemolytic Agents

It is theoretically possible for all drugs that initiate hemolysis in patients with G-6-PD deficiency (p. 106) to trigger a hemolytic episode in a newborn infant, if these drugs have been administered to the mother in sufficient dosage at or near term. Most commonly employed are the sulfonamides and the nitrofurantoins. The ingestion of

Table 2–5   Maternal Events Associated with Hematologic Abnormalities in the Newborn Infant

	MATERNAL EVENT	HEMATOLOGIC ABNORMALITIES IN THE INFANT
Infection	Cytomegalic inclusion disease Toxoplasmosis Syphilis Rubella Coxsackie B. Herpes simplex Malaria	Jaundice, hemolytic anemia, and thrombocytopenia
Illness	Lupus erythematosus	Thrombocytopenia, leukopenia, and anemia
	Malignant melanoma	Melanoma, hemolytic anemia, and thrombocytopenia
	Hodgkin's disease	Hodgkin's disease in infant
	Leukemia	Leukemia in late infancy (rare)
	Chronic hypoxia	Increased cord blood hemoglobin, and increased concentration of fetal hemoglobin
	Hyperthyroidism	Thrombocytopenia, jaundice, plethora
	Idiopathic thrombocytopenic purpura	Thrombocytopenia
	Eclampsia	Disseminated intravascular coagulation
	Autoimmune hemolytic anemia	Hemolytic anemia, thrombocytopenia
Sensitization in infants	Erythrocytes	Hemolytic anemia
	Leukocytes	Leukopenia
	Platelets	Thrombocytopenia
Drug ingestion	Thiazides	Thrombocytopenia, leukopenia, hemolytic anemia (?)
	Quinine	Thrombocytopenia
	Moth balls, antimalarials, sulfonamides, fava beans, nitrofurantoins (see page 49 for complete list)	Hemolytic anemia if infant has G-6-PD deficiency
	Dicumarol	Hemorrhage
	Barbiturates	Prolongation of the prothrombin time
	Salicylates	Prolongation of the prothrombin time
	Hydantoins	Aplastic anemia
	Penicillin	Coombs positive hemolytic anemia (Clayton et al., 1969)
	Epidural analgesics (prilocaine)	Methemoglobinemia
	Aspirin, glyceryl guiacolate, dipyridamole, antihistamines	Impaired platelet aggregation, prolonged bleeding time

naphthalene-containing moth balls by pregnant mothers of G-6-PD deficient infants also causes a hemolytic episode in the newborn (Zinkham and Childs, 1958).

Lucey and Dolan (1959) observed that the administration of large doses (72 mg.) of the vitamin K analogue, menadione sodium bisulfite, to mothers in labor was associated with early marked hyperbilirubinemia in premature infants. It was not established in this study whether hemolysis or hepatic toxicity was responsible for the profound hyperbilirubinemia, although other workers have observed hemolytic anemia in prematures following administration of large doses of water-soluble vitamin K analogues (Gasser, 1953; see Chapter Five).

Thiazides may produce a hemolytic anemia in newborns who are not deficient in G-6-PD. Two possible cases were observed by Harley and associates (1964).

It is apparent that disease in the newborn infant can only be interpreted after careful questioning and study of the mother. Apparently insoluble diagnostic problems often become clear after a few well spent minutes with the mother (see summary in Table 2–5).

Chapter Three

ANEMIA IN THE
NEONATAL PERIOD

Anemia in the newborn can result from many causes. Many times, anemia is complicated by circulatory collapse due to acute blood loss, or serious hyperbilirubinemia due to hemolysis. Both of these situations may be life-threatening and require prompt rational efforts at diagnosis and treatment. To accomplish this goal, a carefully planned investigation must be completed before transfusion therapy temporarily or permanently obscures the diagnosis.

The purpose of this chapter is to review the many types of anemia in the neonatal period and to offer a procedure for their differential diagnosis. Anemia can result from one of three causes: hemorrhage, hemolysis, or failure of red cell production.

Profound anemia at birth is usually the result of either hemorrhage or hemolysis due to isoimmunization. When anemia becomes apparent after the first 24 hours of life, additional causes must be considered, such as external or internal hemorrhages or a variety of nonimmune hemolytic disorders.

HEMORRHAGE

Hemorrhage leading to anemia at birth or in the early neonatal period may be broadly divided into three major etiologic categories: (1) hemorrhage associated with obstetric accidents or malformations of the placenta and cord; (2) occult hemorrhage from the fetus into the maternal circulation or from twin to twin; and (3) internal hemorrhages. Rapid loss of 30 to 50 ml. of blood in a newborn infant is sufficient to produce pallor and shock. Acute hemorrhage must be promptly recognized and treated in order to save the neonate.

Table 3–1   Types of Hemorrhage in the Newborn

Obstetric Accidents, Malformations of the Placenta and Cord

Rupture of a normal umbilical cord
  Precipitous delivery
  Entanglement

Hematoma of the cord or placenta

Rupture of an abnormal umbilical cord
  Varices
  Aneurysm

Rupture of anomalous vessels
  Aberrant vessel
  Velamentous insertion
  Communicating vessels in multilobed placenta

Incision of placenta during cesarean section

Placenta previa

Abruptio placentae

Occult hemorrhage prior to birth

Fetomaternal
  Traumatic amniocentesis
  Spontaneous
  Following external cephalic version

Twin to twin

Internal hemorrhage

Intracranial

Giant cephalohematoma, caput succedaneum

Retroperitoneal

Ruptured liver

Ruptured spleen

OBSTETRIC ACCIDENTS AND MALFORMATIONS OF THE PLACENTA OR CORD

Rupture of the Normal Cord

The normal umbilical cord may rupture from sudden tension during an unattended precipitous delivery in which the infant falls to the floor (Klein, 1817). In 1913, Nebesky was able to collect from the literature 246 instances of ruptured cords in 754 precipitous deliveries. When the cord ruptures, the tear generally occurs in the fetal third, bleeding is immediate and profuse, and bleeding usually stops spontaneously. Anemia in the infant may result from both external and internal hemorrhages, the latter resulting from trauma due to the fall. Fortunately, this type of hemorrhage is uncommon today, but the physician must consider it when he is confronted with a pale infant who was the product of an unattended delivery.

If excess traction is applied to a normal cord, it may rupture during a normal delivery. This has been observed when the cord is entangled or unusually short.

Kirkman and Riley (1959) described eight instances of hemorrhage due to rupture of a varix or aneurysm of the cord. In this type of abnormality, the site of bleeding may be difficult to find. These same authors collected from the literature 33 cases of cord rupture for which no obvious explanation was available. Obvious external hemorrhage may be absent when the bleeding occurs into the substance of the placenta. Careful inspection in such cases may reveal a large hematoma (Dippel, 1940).

Hematomas of the cord occur uncommonly, but may contain large volumes of blood (Toland et al., 1959; Ratten, 1969). Irani (1964) reported a fetal mortality of 47 per cent with such occurrences.

Rupture of Anomalous Vessels

Rupture of cord vessels in the absence of obvious trauma may occur in certain anomalies, such as aberrant vessels, velamentous insertion of the cord, or a multilobed placenta.

Aberrant Vessels. On occasion, even when the umbilical cord inserts into the central or paracentral area of the placenta the cord may give rise to one or more aberrant vessels before reaching its point of insertion. These aberrant vessels are liable to rupture because of their thinness and lack of protection by Wharton's jelly.

Velamentous Insertion. In a velamentous insertion, the umbilical cord enters the membranes at a point some distance from the placenta. From this point of attachment, the vessels divide into fragile branches that pass unprotected between the amnion and chorion and eventually insert into the edge of the placenta. Approximately 1 per cent of all pregnancies involve such velamentous insertions of the cord (Eastman, 1950; Earn, 1951). This abnormality is ten times more frequent in twins than in single births, and triplet or quadruplet births are almost invariably accompanied by it. Most velamentous insertions of the cord do not rupture. Noldeke (1934) estimated the incidence of hemorrhage to be between 1 and 2 per cent.

Multilobed Placenta. If the placenta is multilobular, each lobe sends out fragile communicating veins to the main placenta and these too are liable to rupture.

If any of these anomalous vessels should overlie the internal os of the cervix, they are termed vasa previa, and they are thus in double jeopardy for they may be also compressed as well as lacerated during the second stage of labor. In vasa previa, the perinatal death rate ranges from 58 to 79.4 per cent (Rucker, 1945; Torrey, 1952). In approximately 88 per cent of such deaths, the infants were stillborn (Kirkman and Riley, 1959). In the remainder death occurred during the first 24 hours of life, often because of severe anemia that was not recognized.

Obstetric Accidents

Severe fetal hemorrhage may accompany placenta previa, abruptio placentae, or accidental incision of the placenta or umbilical cord during a cesarean section. Novak (1953) noted that approximately 10 per cent of all infants born following placenta previa were anemic. Abruptio placentae, in contrast, generally leads to intrauterine death from anoxia rather than to the birth of an anemic infant. Golditch and Boyce (1970) found anemia to be present in 4 per cent of surviving infants born following abruptio placentae.

Novak (1953) reported that the placenta was cut or ruptured with resultant fetal bleeding in 28 out of 879 cesarean sections. Siddall and West (1952) described seven infants who were anemic on the first day of life, and in six of these the anemia appeared to be a consequence of placental incision during section. Neligan and Russell (1954) stressed the frequency with which placental tissue is found beneath lower uterine segment incisions, and they have urged that transverse incisions initially be no longer than one inch when made in this area. Further extension of the incision should be carried out by blunt dissection. Neligan and Russell also suggest that an accurate record be made of the time interval from encountering the placenta to clamping of the cord. They feel that if this interval exceeds 30 seconds the infant will frequently require a transfusion.

Following a cesarean section, the placenta and membranes should always be examined from the fetal side for evidence of damage. If there is any question of injury, the hemoglobin of the infant should be determined at birth and again in 12 to 24 hours because in many cases the initial one is normal. Such determinations should also be performed on all newborns in cases of placenta previa, abruptio placentae, or unusual vaginal bleeding.

In women with late third trimester bleeding, Clayton and associates (1964) were able to anticipate the birth of a possibly anemic infant by examining the vaginal blood for the presence of fetal erythrocytes, detected by employing the acid elution technique of Kleihauer and Betke (1957). No fetal cells were observed in four instances of bleeding that resulted from cervical erosion or a constriction band.

Fetal red cells could be demonstrated in the vaginal blood in association with abruptio placentae, placenta previa, vasa previa, and rupture of a marginal sinus.

Clinical Manifestations

Severe bleeding may result in stillbirth. If the infant is born alive, a picture of acute blood loss is usually evident. Pallor is generally conspicuous and can best be seen in the mucous membranes. The respirations, which usually commence spontaneously or after only a very short delay, are often irregular and gasping. They are not accompanied by marked retractions as in conditions associated with primary pulmonary disease. Cyanosis is minimal, and the infant's color is not improved by oxygen administration. The peripheral pulses are weak and rapid, and the blood pressure is low or unobtainable. There is no edema or hepatosplenomegaly, and on introduction of a catheter into the umbilical vessels the venous pressure is found to be low (Kirkman and Riley, 1959; Mollison, 1961).

These physical findings are in sharp contrast to those of the asphyxiated child, who may appear equally pale. In asphyxia pallida, the pulse is slow, respiration may be absent, and the pallor improves dramatically with oxygen and assisted respiration. In the infant who is severely anemic owing to erythroblastosis fetalis, pallor is generally associated with marked hepatosplenomegaly, edema, and a high venous pressure.

Diagnosis

The hemoglobin concentration is often quite low, even after a recent hemorrhage. Values below 5 gm./100 ml. have been observed, although generally the hemoglobin ranges between 5 and 10 gm./100 ml. It should be emphasized that, if the infant is in shock, capillary hemoglobins may be misleadingly high owing to peripheral stasis. In this situation, hemoglobin determinations should be performed on venous blood samples obtained at the time blood is drawn for cross-matching procedures.

If the hemoglobin is initially high, determinations should be repeated and followed closely during the next 12 to 24 hours of life, despite evidence or history of hemorrhage. One may then observe the expected fall due to the hemodilution that accompanies recent blood loss.

An essential part of the diagnosis is the careful examination of the placenta and cord in an attempt to ascertain the site of blood loss.

FETAL HEMORRHAGE INTO THE MATERNAL CIRCULATION

The passage of fetal erythrocytes into the maternal circulation occurs commonly during pregnancy. It has been estimated that feto-maternal transfusions occur in about 50 per cent of all pregnancies (Cohen et al., 1964; McLarey and Fish, 1966; Jones et al., 1969). Although the majority of such hemorrhages are small, some are of sufficient degree to cause anemia, shock, or even stillbirth. This form of occult blood loss is probably the commonest cause of anemia in the newborn.

Historical Aspects

As early as 1941, when the pathogenesis of erythroblastosis due to Rh immunization was first elucidated, Levine and associates postulated that the cause of the maternal sensitization is the passage of fetal blood into the maternal circulation in sufficient quantities to induce immunization. In 1948, Weiner suggested that massive feto-maternal hemorrhage might be the cause of obscure cases of neonatal anemia. Weiner proposed this hypothesis after observing an infant with a hemoglobin of 7.4 gm./100 ml. and minimal jaundice. The mother was Rh-negative, but she had only developed antibodies in the last two weeks of pregnancy. Weiner felt it unlikely that the antibodies had produced sufficient sensitization in the child to result in such a severe anemia. He speculated instead that the anemia in the infant was a result of hemorrhage into the maternal circulation and was actually the cause of antibody production late in pregnancy.

In 1954, Chown was able to demonstrate the presence of fetal erythrocytes in the maternal circulation by differential agglutination, thus confirming the earlier hypothesis of Weiner. Since the initial report of this entity by Chown, many other cases have been described, and massive fetomaternal hemorrhage is now recognized as a common cause of anemia in the newborn period.

Incidence. In approximately 50 per cent of all pregnancies, some fetal cells can be demonstrated in the maternal circulation (Zipursky et al., 1963; Cohen et al., 1964). Cohen and associates (1964) estimated that, in about 8 per cent of pregnancies, 0.5 to 40.0 ml. of fetal blood may enter the maternal circulation and in almost 1 per cent of pregnancies the blood loss exceeds 40 ml., thus being of sufficient magnitude to produce anemia in the newborn. Previously, O'Connor et al. (1957) had observed that infants who are born of mothers with a significant increase in fetal hemoglobin levels have lower hemoglobin values than infants born of mothers with no increase in fetal hemoglobin.

Transplacental passage of cells may occur as early as the fourth to eighth week of gestation (Zipursky et al., 1963), and therefore such blood loss may be chronic as well as acute.

Effect of Diagnostic Amniocentesis. Transabdominal amniocentesis is now widely employed in the management of fetuses with erythroblastosis fetalis and for the prenatal diagnosis of inherited abnormalities. The probing needle may traumatize the placenta and produce bleeding. Woo Wang and associates (1967) observed a 10.8 per cent incidence of fetomaternal hemorrhage following diagnostic amniocentesis. No hemorrhages occurred when the amniotic fluid was easily obtained, but when no fluid was obtained or the fluid was bloody or was obtained only with difficulty, the incidence was 32 per cent. Fatal hemorrhages following the loss of more than 100 ml. of fetal blood as a result of traumatic amniocentesis have been observed (Misenheimer, 1966). Because of the risks of such procedures all infants born after one or more diagnostic amniocenteses, particularly those that are believed to be traumatic, should be immediately evaluated for the presence of anemia.

External cephalic version prior to delivery may also produce a significant transplacental hemorrhage (Pollock, 1968).

Clinical Manifestations. It is now recognized that fetomaternal hemorrhage may present in two ways. If the hemorrhage has been prolonged or repeated during the course of the pregnancy, anemia slowly develops, giving the fetus an opportunity to adjust hemodynamically. Infants born after chronic hemorrhage may present merely with pallor and unexplained anemia. This type of anemia is not commonly recognized.

Following an acute hemorrhage, the infant may be pale and sluggish with irregular gasping respirations, or shock may be present (Raye et al., 1970). The typical laboratory and physical findings in these two forms of hemorrhage are summarized in Table 3-2.

Exceptions to these usual clinical pictures have been observed. Cohen and associates (1964) reported the case of a stillbirth that they felt was the result of a massive fetomaternal hemorrhage. Weisert and Marstrander (1960) observed generalized edema and ascites in an infant born with a hemoglobin of 3.7 gm./100 ml. In this infant, fetomaternal hemorrhage of a chronic nature apparently had occurred.

Chronic blood loss may lead to iron deficiency and the appearance of a hypochromic microcytic anemia. Many of these infants with chronic blood loss are quite vigorous despite their pallor. Hemoglobin values may range from 4.0 to 6.0 gm./100 ml. (Pearson and Diamond, 1959; Eshaghpour et al., 1966; Schwartz et al., 1966; Miles et al., 1971).

A clinical manifestation that may be noted in the mother rather than the infant is the presence of shaking chills and fever as a consequence of a transfusion reaction. This reaction will occur shortly after the fetomaternal hemorrhage in women who have received

Table 3–2 The Characteristics of Acute and Chronic
Blood Loss in the Newborn

Characteristic	Acute Blood Loss	Chronic Blood Loss
Clinical	Acute distress; pallor; shallow, rapid, and often irregular respiration; tachycardia; weak or absent peripheral pulses; low or absent blood pressure; no hepatosplenomegaly.	Marked pallor disproportionate to evidence of distress. On occasion signs of congestive heart failure may be present, including hepatomegaly.
Venous pressure	Low	Normal or elevated
Laboratory		
Hemoglobin concentration	May be normal initially; then drops quickly during first 24 hours of life.	Low at birth
Red cell morphology	Normochromic and macrocytic	Hypochromic and microcytic. Anisocytosis and poikilocytosis.
Serum iron	Normal at birth	Low at birth
Course	Prompt treatment of anemia and shock necessary to prevent death.	Generally uneventful
Treatment	Intravenous fluids and whole blood. Iron therapy later.	Iron therapy. Packed red cells may be necessary on occasion.

incompatible blood from their infant (Goodall et al., 1958). The hemolytic transfusion reaction in the mother may be of such magnitude as to result in acute renal failure (Pasternak et al., 1966).

Laboratory Findings. The degree of anemia is variable. Generally the hemoglobin is below 12 gm./100 ml. before signs and symptoms of anemia are recognized by the physician. Hemoglobin values as low as 3 to 4 gm./100 ml. have been recorded in viable infants. If the hemorrhage has been acute and shock is present, the hemoglobin value may not accurately reflect the magnitude of the blood loss; several hours may elapse before the profound anemia can be documented. In infants with slower forms of bleeding, anemia is evident at birth.

Examination of a peripheral blood smear provides valuable information in establishing the nature of the anemia. In acute hemorrhage, the red cells appear normocytic and normochromic; in chronic hemorrhage, hypochromia and microcytosis may be observed (Fig. 3–1). Increased numbers of nucleated red blood cells may be seen in both acute and chronic hemorrhage.

The direct Coombs test is negative. Fetomaternal hemorrhage may also occur in infants with erythroblastosis fetalis and thus accentuate the degree of anemia present at birth (Weiner, 1948).

Jaundice is absent and bilirubin levels are very low. In chronic

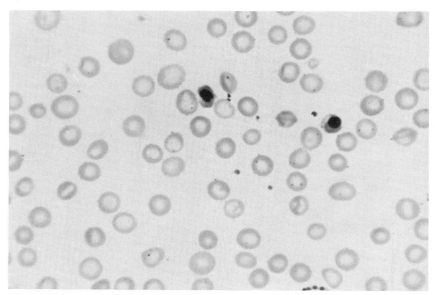

Figure 3–1   Peripheral smear from an infant born with a hemoglobin of 5 gm./100 ml. and found to be iron deficient. Note hypochromic microcytic erythrocytes and normoblasts.

hemorrhage, the serum iron value is decreased and the bone marrow may contain no stainable iron (Eshaghpour et al., 1966).

Diagnosis.   The diagnosis of a fetomaternal hemorrhage of sufficient magnitude to result in anemia at birth can be made with certainty only by demonstrating the presence of fetal red cells in the maternal circulation.

Fetal red cells may be demonstrated in the maternal circulation by one of several techniques. These include direct differential agglutination (Jones and Silver, 1958), mixed agglutination (Jones and Silver, 1958), fluorescent antibody techniques (Cohen et al., 1960), and the acid-elution method of staining for cells containing fetal hemoglobin (Kleihauer et al., 1957).

All these techniques are very sensitive and are capable of detecting as little as 0.1 ml. of fetal blood in the maternal circulation. This degree of sensitivity is unnecessary when attempting to confirm a hemorrhage sufficient to cause anemia in the newborn. This anemia only results from hemorrhages of approximately 50 ml. or more in the average-sized infant.

The Kleihauer technique of acid elution is the simplest method and the one most commonly used for the detection of fetal cells (Table 3–3).

The test is based on the property of fetal hemoglobin to resist elution from the intact red cell in an acid medium (Fig. 3–2). After

Table 3–3 Acid Elution Technique to Demonstrate
Erythrocytes Containing Fetal Hemoglobin on Blood Smear*

Principle:
At low pH, adult hemoglobin is eluted from erythrocytes, whereas fetal hemoglobin
resists elution and may be demonstrated by subsequent staining.

Reagents:
Ethanol, 80%
Citric acid, 0.1 M (stock solution A)
Disodium hydrogen phosphate, 0.2 M (stock solution B)
Working buffer of pH 3.3 is made by mixing 73.4 parts A with 26.6 parts B
Stains:
Acid hematoxylin (Ehrlich's)†
Eosin B, 0.1%

Procedure:
1. Either capillary or oxalated venous blood may be used. Oxalated venous blood
   may be stored in the refrigerator for three to four days before making smears. In
   newborns, it is wise to dilute the blood first with normal saline to enable thin
   smears to be made.
2. Filling staining dish (or Coplin jar) with working citrate-phosphate buffer (pH 3.3)
   and preincubate to 37° C.
3. Using clean glass slides previously marked with a diamond pencil, make a thin
   blood smear. Simultaneous positive and negative control smears should be made
   from newborn (or young infant) and adult blood. Air dry the smears for approximately ten minutes.
4. Fix the slides by covering with 80% ethanol for five minutes. Rinse thoroughly in
   tap water and dry in air (or with bibulous paper).
5. Immerse slides in citrate-phosphate buffer in 37° C. incubator for five minutes,
   agitating at one and three minutes.
6. Rinse slides thoroughly in tap water and blot gently with bibulous paper. Dry
   completely.
7. Slides are stained for three minutes in acid hematoxylin, rinsed in water, and then
   stained for four minutes in eosin.
8. After final rinse, slides are dried and covered with coverglasses.
9. The proportion of erythrocytes containing fetal hemoglobin may be estimated in
   several ways. When studying maternal blood for evidence of fetal cells, we have
   used the following method: Count the total number of erythrocytes in five high-
   power fields and determine the average number per high-power field. Then count
   the number of deeply staining (fetal) erythrocytes in about 30 high-power fields
   and calculate their percentage on the basis of the total number of cells (obtained
   from the above figure for the average multiplied by the number of fields counted).

---

*Kleihauer and Betke technique, from Shepherd et al., 1962.
†May be obtained in solution from Hartman-Leddon Co., Philadelphia, Pa.

staining a maternal blood smear, the number of cells containing
fetal hemoglobin can be counted and a rough calculation made as
to the degree of hemorrhage that has occurred.

The measurement of fetal hemoglobin in the maternal blood by
the alkali denaturation technique of Singer et al. (1951) is a less sensitive estimate of the degree of fetal hemorrhage and is more time-
consuming. A large hemorrhage results in only a modest increase in
the mother's fetal hemoglobin level.

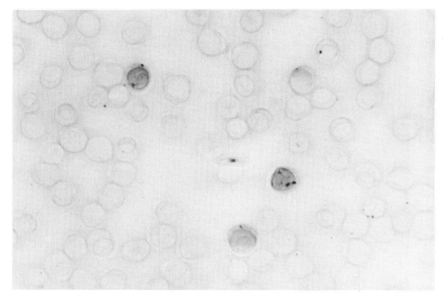

Figure 3–2 Fetal erythrocytes in the maternal circulation as demonstrated by the acid-elution technique. The darkly staining cells contain fetal hemoglobin (HbF).

Only fair correlation exists between estimation of the degree of fetomaternal hemorrhage by these two techniques. By the acid-elution technique, only if each fetal cell contained 100 per cent fetal hemoglobin could strict proportionality be expected. Even then, a fetal cell count of 1 per cent in the maternal circulation, which would be indicative of a hemorrhage in the range of 50 ml. (1 per cent of a maternal blood volume of approximately 4500 ml.), would raise the concentration of alkali-resistant hemoglobin in the mother's blood by only 1 per cent. Small changes of this nature are difficult to interpret by the Singer technique. Because the average concentration of fetal hemoglobin in cord blood ranges from 60 to 80 per cent and very few erythrocytes at term contain 100 per cent fetal hemoglobin, it is understandable why the chemical method does not show proportionality with the cell count and can be used only to detect the most massive transplacental losses.

The acid-elution technique can be relied on with certainty for diagnosis only when other conditions capable of producing elevations in maternal fetal hemoglobin levels are absent. In the presence of maternal thalassemia minor, sickle cell anemia, or hereditary persistence of fetal hemoglobin, other techniques based on differential agglutination should be employed. Because these disorders are relatively uncommon, they generally do not cause confusion.

Diagnosis of a fetomaternal hemorrhage may be missed in situations in which the mother and infant are incompatible in the ABO blood group system. In such instances, the infant's A or B cells are rapidly cleared from the maternal circulation by the maternal anti-A or anti-B, thus becoming unavailable for staining. The staining technique therefore must be carried out within several hours of birth to diagnose such hemorrhages. A presumptive diagnosis may be made by demonstrating either marked erythrophagocytosis in smears of the maternal buffy coat (Goodall et al., 1958) or a rise in maternal immune anti-A or anti-B titers in the weeks following delivery.

A search for fetomaternal hemorrhage should be made in all anemic newborns in whom no obvious blood loss has occurred and in whom isoimmunization has been excluded. The diagnosis can be made by estimating the number of fetal cells in the maternal circulation. ABO and Rh typing of the mother and child as well as performing of a direct Coombs test on the infant's cells provides valuable information for the interpretation of the results.

The placenta should also be examined carefully, because the hemorrhage from the infant may not have entered the maternal circulation but instead may have accumulated in the substance of the placenta (Chown, 1955) or retroplacentally (Kevy, 1962).

HEMORRHAGE FROM ONE TWIN INTO THE OTHER

Herelitz (1942) first described the simultaneous occurrence of anemia in one and polycythemia in the other of a pair of newborn monozygotic twins. Since that time, numerous other cases have been reported and the subject has been recently reviewed (Pochedly and Musiker, 1970). This syndrome has also been recognized in a quadruple birth (Cortes, 1964). It is estimated that a significant twin-to-twin transfusion occurs in at least 15 per cent of all monochorial twins (Rausen et al., 1965). The twin transfusion syndrome results in significant morbidity and mortality for both the donor and the recipient.

There are four types of twin placentas. They may be: (1) separate—diamnionic and dichorionic; (2) fused—diamnionic and dichorionic; (3) fused—diamnionic and monochorionic; or (4) fused—monoamnionic and monochorionic. Monochorionic twins are monozygotic and thus identical twins. Approximately 70 per cent of monozygous twin pregnancies have monochorial placentas (Benirschke, 1961).

In the dichorionic placenta, vascular anastomosis is uncommon, while in the monochorionic placenta twin-to-twin anastomosis occurs in almost every instance (Benirschke, 1961). The anastomosis of the fetal blood vessels in the placenta may be artery to artery, vein to vein, or artery to vein. Bleeding from one twin into the other occurs in the artery-to-vein type of communication. These abnormal communications can be easily visualized by injecting milk into the vessels on one side of the placental "vascular equator" and demonstrating its emergence from the other side (Coen and Sutherland, 1970).

Clinical Manifestations. Stillbirths are common following intrauterine twin-to-twin transfusions; a smaller number die early in the neonatal period. In the series of Rausen and associates (1965), 13 of 26 infants weighing 500 gm. or more at delivery were either stillbirths (11) or early neonatal deaths (2).

The donor twin may be strikingly pale at birth with evidence of listlessness or shock. In many instances, compensatory erythropoiesis may result in only minimal degrees of anemia with no apparent clinical symptoms. The donor twin is usually, although not invariably, smaller then the recipient. The donor twin also has an associated oligohydramnios.

The recipient twin, when born alive, is plethoric owing to polycythemia, and it has an associated polyhydramnios. Polycythemia may result in respiratory difficulty, congestive heart failure, venous thrombosis, hyperbilirubinemia, and kernicterus (Sacks, 1959) and is discussed in detail in Chapter Four. At postmortem examination, the recipient twin frequently demonstrates cardiomegaly, renal glomerular hypertrophy, and an increase of muscle about pulmonary and systemic arteries suggestive of antenatal hypertension in both circulatory beds (Naeye, 1963). The donor twin may show evidence of renal cortical necrosis (Dimmick et al., 1971).

Laboratory Findings. A twin-to-twin transfusion should be suspected when a hemoglobin difference greater than 5 gm./100 ml. exists between identical twins. Rausen et al. (1965) found no hemoglobin difference greater than 3.3 gm./100 ml. in 43 dizygous twin pairs. Hemoglobin determination should be performed on venous blood in order to avoid sampling errors that might lead to misinterpretation of results.

In the donor twin, the hemoglobin may range from 3.7 to 18 gm./100 ml. The peripheral blood reflects the response to hemorrhage with an elevated reticulocyte count and increased numbers of nucleated red blood cells. Thrombocytopenia may accompany the profound anemia (Corney and Aherne, 1965).

Hemoglobin values ranging from 20 to 30 gm./100 ml. have been recorded in the recipient twin, with hematocrits as high as 82 per cent (Hodapp, 1962). In these plethoric infants, the increased red cell mass results in increased bilirubin production from the normally occurring red cell breakdown, and many recipient twins develop hyperbilirubinemia. Bilirubin levels of over 20 mg./100 ml. have been recorded (Betke et al., 1958; Bergstedt, 1957), and kernicterus has occurred (Bosma, 1954; Sacks, 1959).

When a twin-to-twin transfusion is suspected, attempts to confirm it by placental examination should be made. When hematologic evidence has not been obtained and death of the infants has occurred, other findings may suggest the diagnosis. These include hydramnios of one of the amniotic sacs with oligohydramnios of the other, and marked differences in the size and weight of the twins as well as such organs as the heart, kidneys, liver, and thymus. The syndrome of disseminated intravascular coagulation (Chapter Eight) has been observed in the liveborn of three sets of twins, each with a macerated stillborn sibling (Moore et al., 1969).

Polycythemia at birth may be seen in the neonate in the absence of a twin-to-twin transfusion. It has been observed as the result of maternal-to-fetal transfusions, in association with congenital adrenal hyperplasia, and in situations where no suitable explanation can be found.

INTERNAL HEMORRHAGE

Anemia that appears in the first 24 to 72 hours of age and is not associated with jaundice is commonly due to internal hemorrhages. It is well recognized that traumatic deliveries may result in subdural or subarachnoid hemorrhages of sufficient magnitude to result in anemia. Cephalohematomas may also be of giant size and result in anemia (Leonard and Anthony, 1961).

Blood loss into the subaponeurotic area of the scalp tends to be greater than that observed with cephalohematomata. The bleeding is not confined by periosteal attachments and thus is not limited to an area overlying a single skull bone. A subaponeurotic hemorrhage usually extends through the soft tissue of the scalp and covers the whole calvarium. Blood loss in this area can result in exsanguination of the infant (Robinson and Rossiter, 1968). Pachman (1962) observed a hemoglobin of 2.2 gm./100 ml. in an infant 48 hours of age in whom a massive hemorrhage into the scalp had occurred. This form of hemorrhage is more common after difficult deliveries or vacuum extractions. It appears with vitamin K deficiency and may be more frequent in infants of Black parentage. Examination of the infant reveals a boggy edema of the head extending into the frontal region and to the nape of the neck. The edema, which may have a bluish coloration, obscures the fontanelles and swells the eyelids. The infant may be in shock. Robinson and Rossiter (1968) have developed a formula to predict the volume of blood loss in this condition. For each centimeter of increase in head circumference above that expected, a 38 ml. loss of blood has occurred.

When the products of red cell breakdown are absorbed from these entrapped hemorrhages, hyperbilirubinemia may develop (Rausen and Diamond, 1961).

Breech deliveries may be associated with hemorrhage into the adrenals, kidney, spleen, or retroperitoneal area. Blood loss of this type should be suspected in infants found anemic during the first few days of life following a traumatic delivery. Hemorrhage into the adrenals may also be observed in any difficult delivery or following the birth of a large infant. Schaffer (1960) speculates that these adrenal hemorrhages may be more common in infants of diabetic or prediabetic mothers. In adrenal hemorrhage, the clinical picture may include sudden collapse, cyanosis, limpness, jaundice, irregular respirations, elevated or subnormal temperatures, and the presence of a flank mass accompanied by bluish discoloration of the overlying skin.

Rupture of the liver, with resultant anemia, appears to occur more frequently than is clinically appreciated. In stillbirths and neonatal deaths, the incidence of hepatic hemorrhages found at autopsy ranges from 1.2 per cent (Potter, 1940) to 5.6 per cent (Holmberg, 1933). In approximately one-half the cases reviewed by Henderson (1941), the hemorrhage was subcapsular only; in the remainder the capsule had ruptured and free blood was present in the peritoneal cavity.

An infant with a ruptured liver generally appears to be well for 24 to 48 hours, and then he suddenly goes into shock. Shock appears to coincide with the time the gradually increasing hematoma finally ruptures the hepatic capsule and hemoperitoneum occurs. At this time, the upper abdomen may appear distended and a mass contiguous with the liver is often palpable. Shifting dullness can be demonstrated on abdominal percussion. Flat films of the abdomen taken in both the erect and supine position frequently confirm the presence of free fluid in the abdomen. Paracentesis, performed with the infant in the lateral position, reveals free blood in the abdomen. The prognosis is poor, but with multiple blood transfusions and prompt surgical repair of the laceration infants have been saved.

Splenic rupture may also occur after a difficult delivery (O'Neil et al., 1965) or as a result of the extreme distention of the spleen that often accompanies severe erythroblastosis fetalis (Phillipsborn, 1955). The physician should always suspect a rupture of the spleen with associated hemorrhage when at the time of exchange transfusion an anemic and hydropic infant with erythroblastosis fetalis is found to have a decreased, rather than an increased, venous pressure. Rupture of the spleen may also occur during the exchange transfusion.

Splenic rupture occurs, although uncommonly, in healthy infants born after seemingly normal deliveries (Delta et al., 1968; Leape et al., 1971). Many of these infants are of large size. Pallor, abdominal distention, scrotal swelling, and x-ray evidence of peritoneal effusion without free air should alert the physician to the presence of splenic rupture.

Other, less common, sites of neonatal bleeding include hemangiomas of the gastrointestinal tract (Nader and Margolin, 1966) and hemangioendotheliomas of the skin (Svane, 1966).

Treatment

The treatment of the infant depends on the degree of anemia and the acuteness of the hemorrhage. Kirkman and Riley (1959) have proposed one method of management for the severely anemic infant who is in distress at birth. Their program of management embodies all the essentials of good pediatric care:

1. On delivery of a pale infant in distress and without hepato-splenomegaly, ordinary resuscitative measures are provided, such as clearing the airway, administering oxygen, and performing artificial respiration if necessary. During these initial maneuvers, the aid of a second physician should be requested.

2. While attempts at oxygenation are being made, a sample of blood is obtained from the umbilical vein for a hemoglobin determination and for cross-matching. The sample is best obtained by inserting a plastic catheter into the umbilical vein. This catheter is left in place for the measurement of venous pressure and the administration of fluids.

3. Group O, Rh-negative blood, plasma, albumin in saline solution, or dextran is ordered, and the first available solution is administered to the infant when it has become apparent that the pallor is not a result of asphyxia but of profound anemia.

4. Approximately 20 ml./kg. of the available fluid is injected rapidly into the umbilical catheter, and the infant's response is noted. Infants with acute blood loss as a result of an obstetric hemorrhage or a large fetomaternal hemorrhage generally show dramatic evidence of benefit, while infants who have suffered internal hemorrhage secondary to injury may remain limp and unresponsive.

5. A repeat injection of 10 to 20 mg./kg. of whole blood may be given soon after the first injection fluid, particularly if whole blood was not given initially.

6. While the infant is being treated, the second physician should carefully examine the placenta and the umbilical cord for evidence of abnormalities. If a site of bleeding is not obvious, a sample of maternal blood should be obtained for estimation of the percentage of cells containing fetal hemoglobin or of fetal hemoglobin content.

The infant who is mildly anemic at birth as a consequence of chronic blood loss often demonstrates no distress. These infants do not require blood transfusions but instead should be treated with iron. Ferrous sulfate in a dose of 2 mg. of elemental iron per kilogram of body weight administered three times daily for three months is sufficient to replenish body iron stores and return the hemoglobin to normal.

Iron therapy is also needed for the infant who receives a blood transfusion for symptoms of acute distress because the transfusions are generally not sufficient to totally replace the iron lost due to hemorrhage. McGovern and associates (1958) reported iron deficiency anemia in a three month old infant who suffered anemia at birth from hemorrhage into the maternal circulation. Although the baby was transfused on the first day of life, replacement was not adequate to replenish depleted iron stores. Acute or chronic fetomaternal transfusion appears to be an important etiologic factor in many cases of iron deficiency anemia developing in term infants at three to six months of age—a time when dietary factors cannot yet be invoked to explain the presence of iron deficiency.

The treatment of the transfusion syndrome of twins may also present an acute emergency. The donor twin may show evidence of distress at birth; if so, the steps previously outlined should be followed. If transfusion has been chronic, the anemia may be well tolerated. Donor twins with hemoglobin levels as low as 7.5 gm./100 ml. have done well on iron therapy alone (Herelitz, 1942).

The plethoric recipient twin may also require treatment because of respiratory embarrassment, circulatory overload, and hyperbilirubinemia associated with increased blood viscosity when the hematocrit is in the range of 75 per cent. In these situations, a partial exchange transfusion should be performed with plasma to reduce the hematocrit to approximately 60 per cent (see page 81).

Whenever isosexual twin births have occurred, hemoglobin determinations should be performed on both infants during the first several hours of life in order to avoid the complications of prolonged anemia or polycythemia. Attempts should be made to establish zygosity by blood grouping procedures and pathologic examination of the placenta.

CALCULATIONS OF DOSAGE OF BLOOD FOR SIMPLE TRANSFUSIONS

Mollison (1961) has proposed a simple formula for blood transfusion based on the fact that a hemoglobin concentration of 15 gm./100 ml. corresponds to a red cell volume of approximately 30 ml./kg. of body weight. This implies that a transfusion of 3 ml. of packed red cells per kg. of body weight raises the hemoglobin concentration by 1 gm./100 ml. Packed red cells normally have a hematocrit of 66 per cent. If whole blood is used, it should be remembered that the hematocrit is approximately 33 per cent, and thus 6 ml. of whole blood will supply 2 ml. of red cells.

Example: A 3 kg. infant is found to have a hemoglobin of 7 gm./100 ml., and it is desired to raise his hemoglobin to 12 gm./100 ml. Thus, the infant requires 5 (gm./100 ml. hemoglobin increase) × 3 (ml. of red cells supplying 1 gm. of hemoglobin) × 3 (body weight in kg.) = 45 ml. of packed red cells or 90 ml. of whole blood.

HEMOLYTIC ANEMIAS

Anemia as a consequence of a hemolytic process is common in the newborn period and has multiple etiologies. The essential feature of hemolytic anemia is a reduction in erythrocyte life span. Unlike the anemias produced by hemorrhage or by failure of red cell production, a hemolytic anemia in the newborn period is almost always associated with a bilirubin level in excess of 10 to 12 mg./100 ml. In general, a hemolytic process is first detected during the investigation of jaundice occurring during the first week of life.

Jaundice may occur despite minimal changes in the hemoglobin level. Destruction of 1 gm. of hemoglobin results in the production of approximately 35 mg. of bilirubin (Lemberg and Legge, 1949). In an infant with a blood volume of 300 ml., a decrease in hemoglobin of 1 gm./100 ml. would go virtually unrecognized, but it would result in the production of 105 mg. of bilirubin. In many instances, increased red cell destruction is accompanied by increased red cell production; in this situation there may be little or no change in the hemoglobin level despite marked accumulation of bilirubin.

Hemolytic disease in the newborn can be broadly grouped into three large categories: isoimmunization, congenital defects of the red cell, and acquired defects of the red cell. In most parts of the world, isoimmunization as a result of maternal-fetal incompatibilities in either the Rh or ABO blood group systems is the leading cause of hemolytic disease. The entire problem of erythroblastosis fetalis is dealt with in Chapter Seven. Congenital defects of the red cell include those associated with enzymatic defects, those characterized only by alterations in red cell morphology, or those associated with an abnormal hemoglobin. These disorders are discussed in detail in Chapters Five and Six. Acquired defects of the red cell may also result in the production of morphologic abnormalities such as those observed in infantile pyknocytosis or Heinz body anemia.

Acquired hemolytic anemias may result from drugs, toxins, or infections. A hemolytic process frequently accompanies profound acidosis, shock, or asphyxia. The hemolytic anemias observed with infections, acidosis, and asphyxia may be secondary to the process of disseminated intravascular coagulation. This process, described in Chapter Eight, results in the deposition of fibrin in the microcirculation. Red cells undergo mechanical injury and fragmentation as they traverse these partially obliterated capillaries.

Anemia may accompany bacterial septicemia in the newborn period. In 6 of 15 patients reported by Smith and associates (1956), the hemoglobin value was below 15 gm./100 ml. and in three it ranged between 10 and 12 gm./100 ml. Similarly, Silverman and Homan (1949) noted hemoglobin values of less than 15 gm./100 ml. in 12 of 24 infants with sepsis; none had a hemoglobin value of less than 10 gm./100 ml. Although there was no direct correlation between the degree of anemia and the degree of hyperbilirubinemia, both were generally present, and in the jaundiced infants hepatomegaly was a common finding. Smith and co-workers (1951) pointed out that in most infants with sepsis a deviation of the total leukocyte count also may be observed and that, in general, infants with streptococcal or staphylococcal infections tend to have leukocytosis, while those infected with enteric organisms either have a normal count or are leukopenic. Debré and associates (1950) have stated that leukopenia and granulocytopenia occur frequently in generalized *Pseudomonas* infections and that with other enteric infections leukocytosis is extreme. On occasion, histiocytes may be found in the peripheral blood in association with these overwhelming infections.

When sepsis is present, the jaundice is usually associated with elevations of both the conjugated and unconjugated bilirubin fractions. Bernstein and Brown (1962) observed it most commonly in neonates with *Escherichia coli* sepsis, particularly in association with pyelonephritis. The elevation of the direct-reacting bilirubin fraction in the presence of sepsis appears to be a consequence of obstructive disease in the liver produced by hepatocellular damage.

Hemolytic anemia is frequently observed during the course of the respiratory distress syndrome (Inall et al., 1965). Prolonged acidosis may sufficiently alter the metabolism of the red cell, resulting in a decrease in its life span.

The administration of penicillin to the newborn may induce hemolytic anemia. Clayton and associates (1969) observed a positive direct Coombs test in an infant with hemolytic anemia. The positive test was caused by the coating of the erythrocytes with penicillin. The coated cells were sensitized with penicillin antibody which had been transferred across the placenta from the mother. Synthetic penicillin derivatives may be anticipated to cause similar problems.

In marble bone disease, or osteopetrosis, hemolytic anemia may be present during the first week of life. Jaundice has been observed during this period, and a severe anemia with a hemoglobin of 4.6 gm./100 ml. has been recorded as early as the tenth day of life (Gamsu et al., 1962). This disease is characterized by hydrocephalus, hepatosplenomegaly, and a marked increase in the density of the long bones, ribs, and the base of the skull. Examination of a peripheral smear reveals nucleated red cells, early myeloid forms, and bizarre red cell morphology.

IMPAIRED RED CELL PRODUCTION

Congenital hypoplastic anemia, also known as the Blackfan-Diamond syndrome, pure red cell anemia, erythrogenesis imperfecta, or chronic congenital aregenerative anemia, is an uncommon disorder of unknown etiology, in which red cell precursors in the bone marrow are markedly reduced or virtually absent while platelet and leukocyte production remains normal.

Diamond et al. (1961) reported that in 8 of 30 patients with this disorder pallor was noted at birth. In one infant, the hemoglobin was 9.4 gm./100 ml. on the first day of life, and the reticulocyte count was only 0.3 per cent. In 4 of 13 infants reported by Bernard and associates (1962), pallor was also evident at birth. If anemia and pallor are not detected at birth, they are generally noted within the first three months of life. In exceptional cases, however, anemia and pallor may not be evident until after one year of age.

Associated Findings. In infants with congenital hypoplastic anemia, there appears to be an increased incidence of prematurity or abnormalities of pregnancy. In the series of 30 patients referred to in the previous paragraph, seven infants weighed less than 2500 gm. at birth and two others were born prematurely (as calculated by gestational age) and weighed 2693 and 2722 gm. Two mothers had toxemia of pregnancy, one had vaginal bleeding during the early months of gestation, one mother received thyroid, and another received diethylstilbestrol.

In several instances, more than one sibling was affected. Diamond and associates (1970) observed nine patients with this syndrome who exhibited the Turner phenotype. Unlike patients with Turner's syndrome, these patients had a normal chromosomal pattern and three of the patients were males.

Diagnosis. Hypoplastic anemia should be suspected in any anemic newborn with a reticulocyte count less than 2.0 per cent in the absence of some obvious explanation such as overwhelming infection.

This anemia is normocytic and normochromic. The white cell and platelet counts are normal for the age. Diagnosis is confirmed by demonstrating the virtual absence of erythroid precursors in the bone marrow. Erythroid:myeloid ratios ranged from 1:6 to 1:240 in the series of Diamond et al. (1961). Four patients initially had normal numbers of erythroid precursors, but within several months of the first examination these had disappeared.

Treatment. Early diagnosis is important because it apparently increases the prospects of a steroid-induced remission (Allen and Diamond, 1961). All patients treated within three months of onset of the anemia showed a response to steroids, while no patient with a duration of anemia in excess of three years benefited from therapy. Allen and Diamond recommend initial therapy with prednisone in a dosage of 30 mg./day for two weeks. Response as reflected by reticulocytosis generally occurs during this interval. Once a response is obtained, the dosage of steroid is gradually lowered to the minimum necessary to maintain a normal or near normal hemoglobin and reticulocyte levels.

Red cell aplasia has also been observed in association with the congenital deformity of triphalangeal thumb. Aase and Smith (1969) observed two brothers with this syndrome, both of whom were anemic at birth.

DIFFERENTIAL DIAGNOSIS OF ANEMIA IN THE NEONATE

Although seemingly paradoxical, at no other time than the first week of life does such a myriad of disorders result in anemia. The need for rapid treatment often adds to the diagnostic confusion. It is because of these reasons — multiple causes and the need for prompt therapy — that the fundamentals of diagnosis should be appreciated and practiced with precision and without delay. One approach to the differential diagnosis of anemia in the newborn is offered in Figure 3–3.

Attempts at diagnosis properly begin with a history, when the cause is not immediately apparent. In the family history, attention should be paid to the presence of anemia in other members of the

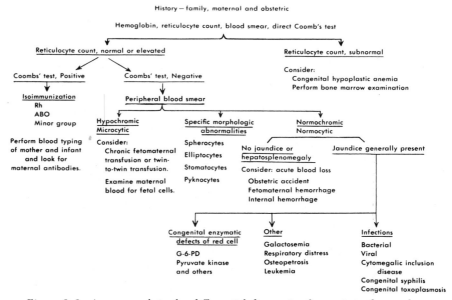

Figure 3–3   An approach to the differential diagnosis of anemia in the newborn.

family, or to unexplained episodes of jaundice or cholelithiasis. A positive family history is frequently obtained in cases of infants with hereditary spherocytosis, while a history indicating affected siblings may be encountered in cases of patients with enzymatic defects of the red cell.

In the maternal history, information should be obtained concerning drug ingestion near term. Information concerning drugs known to initiate hemolysis in G-6-PD deficiency should especially be sought, as well as any history of recent exposure to naphthalene-containing moth balls.

The obstetric history should provide information on vaginal bleeding during pregnancy, the presence or absence of placenta previa, abruptio placentae, vasa previa, or cesarean section. Additional questions to be answered include: was the birth traumatic, was the birth attended by a physician, did the cord rupture, and was it a multiple birth.

The age at which anemia is first noted is also of diagnostic value. Marked anemia at birth is generally the result of either hemorrhage or severe isoimmunization. Anemia manifesting itself during the first two days of life is frequently caused by internal or external hemorrhages, while anemia appearing after the first 48 hours of life is most commonly hemolytic and is generally associated with jaundice.

The basic laboratory studies in the initial investigation of anemia should include hemoglobin determination, reticulocyte count, examination of a peripheral blood smear, a direct Coombs test of the infant's blood, and examination of the maternal blood smear for fetal erythrocytes. From these few studies and the history, a diagnosis often can be made. If the diagnosis has not been made, at least the list of diagnostic possibilities has been greatly shortened.

The reticulocyte count provides the first valuable laboratory clue. If the anemia is a result of either hemorrhage or hemolysis, the reticulocyte count usually is elevated. If the anemia is associated with reticulocytopenia, the diagnosis of congenital hypoplastic anemia must be considered as well as processes that might result in bone marrow infiltration, such as congenital leukemia. In reticulocytopenia, a bone marrow examination is necessary to establish the diagnosis.

When the reticulocyte count is elevated, a variety of diagnostic possibilities remains, if obstetric hemorrhage has already been excluded. A positive direct Coombs test will identify the infants with isoimmunization in the Rh, ABO, or minor blood group systems (see Chapter Seven), after which both infant and mother must be blood typed and a search made for maternal antibodies.

If the Coombs test is negative, other forms of hemolytic disease as well as occult hemorrhage remain to be excluded. At this point, careful attention must be paid to red cell morphology. While examining the smear, attention should be paid to the numbers of platelets present and to any peculiarities of the leukocytes.

If the peripheral smear reveals the presence of hypochromic microcytic red cells, iron deficiency should be considered as a likely cause of the anemia. Iron deficiency anemia can result from chronic fetomaternal hemorrhage or twin-to-twin transfusion. If fetomaternal hemorrhage is suspected, the mother's blood should be examined for cells containing fetal hemoglobin.

The presence of morphologic abnormalities such as spherocytes or elliptocytes aids in establishment of a diagnosis of hereditary disorder of red cell morphology (described in Chapter Five). If pyknocytes are present in large numbers, then this poorly understood acquired defect of red cells must be considered as a distinct diagnostic possibility. Pyknocytes have also been observed in newborns with hemolysis as a consequence of G-6-PD deficiency.

If the red cells are normocytic and normochromic, the anemia may be the result of acute blood loss or a congenital enzymatic defect of the red cell, or secondary to a systemic disease in the infant. In this event, the birth history, the history of the first few days of life, and the physical examination aid in the differential diagnosis.

Anemia as a result of acute hemorrhage is generally not associated with jaundice or hepatosplenomegaly. Pallor is prominent and the infant may be in shock. A search for fetal cells in the maternal circulation helps to establish the commonest cause of occult hemorrhage. Internal hemorrhage must be suspected in infants born after a traumatic delivery.

Pyruvate kinase deficiency, hexokinase deficiency, glucose-6-phosphate dehydrogenase deficiency, and the other enzymatic defects of the red cell may result in a hemolytic anemia during the first week of life. G-6PD deficiency should be strongly suspected in Mediterranean and Oriental male infants. The other anemias show no racial predisposition.

A variety of infections may produce a hemolytic anemia characterized by normochromic cells. Red cell fragmentation and spherocytes also may be observed. Cytomegalic inclusion disease, toxoplasmosis, and congenital syphilis are usually accompanied by prominent hepatosplenomegaly, jaundice, and thrombocytopenic purpura. Diagnosis of cytomegalic inclusion disease is supported by finding the characteristic cells in the urinary sediment, and it is confirmed by isolation of the salivary gland virus from the urine. Serologic studies are necessary to establish a diagnosis of congenital syphilis or toxoplasmosis. Other infections may also be accompanied by anemia and jaundice, and appropriate blood and urine cultures should be performed in all infants with obscure hemolytic anemias during the first weeks of life. Measurement of the serum IgM level may provide useful information. The presence of an elevated IgM level in a newborn infant strongly suggests that an antecedent intrauterine infection has occurred.

When a burr cell anemia is present in an infant who is ill with sepsis, acidosis, or hypoxia, laboratory evidence of disseminated intravascular coagulation should be collected and evaluated. Performance of a platelet count, prothrombin time, partial thromboplastin time, thrombin time, Factor V assay, and measurement of fibrin split products are most useful in establishing this diagnosis (see Chapter Eight).

In most newborn infants with anemia, a diligent search is required to reveal the diagnosis. In certain instances, the diagnosis must be deferred until the infant is older; in others the anemia disappears, the cause remains undetermined, and the curiosity unsatisfied.

Chapter Four

POLYCYTHEMIA IN THE NEONATAL PERIOD

Polycythemia may be less common than anemia in the newborn period, but it too can produce or be associated with undesirable symptoms. A venous hematocrit of greater than 65 per cent or a venous hemoglobin concentration in excess of 22.0 gm./100 ml. anytime during the first week of life should be considered as evidence of polycythemia. For reasons discussed in Chapter One, capillary blood samples should not be relied on for the diagnosis of polycythemia because of their tendency to result in misleadingly high values for both hemoglobin and hematocrit.

Etiology.   Polycythemia, like anemia, has a variety of recognized causes, although in many instances its etiology is obscure (Table 4–1). Placental insufficiency with intrauterine hypoxia appears to play a central role in many of the conditions associated with plethora. The transfer of red cells from mother to fetus, or from twin to twin, may also result in polycythemia.

Michael and Mauer (1961) were the first to demonstrate that this maternal transfer of erythrocytes could produce plethora in the newborn infant. In three infants in whom this syndrome could be demonstrated, the hemoglobins ranged from 21.2 to 24.6 gm./100 ml. and hematocrits ranged from 73 to 80 per cent. Maternal–fetal transfusion was proved by the finding of maternal erythrocytes in the fetal blood using differential agglutination techniques; lower than normal fetal hemoglobin concentration; and the presence of IgM globulin in the fetal blood. Although plethoric, the infants were well and required no phlebotomies other than those employed for the diagnosis.

Andrews and Thompson (1962) examined 207 consecutive infants for evidences of a maternal–fetal transfusion and found two cases.

Table 4–1 Neonatal Polycythemia

May be caused by placental hypertransfusion:
   Twin to twin transfusion
   Maternal–fetal transfusion
   Delayed cord clamping
      Intentional
      Unassisted home delivery

May be associated with:
   Placental insufficiency
      Small for gestational age infants
      Postmaturity
      Toxemia of pregnancy
      Placenta previa

   Endocrine and metabolic disorders:
      Congenital adrenal hyperplasia
      Neonatal thyrotoxicosis
      Maternal diabetes

   Miscellaneous:
      Down's syndrome
      Hyperplastic visceromegaly (Beckwith's syndrome)

Walsh and co-workers (1962) demonstrated by differential agglutination techniques that a maternal–fetal transfusion was responsible for a hemoglobin value of 27 gm./100 ml. in an 11-day-old infant. The infant died on the fourteenth day and was found to have hepatitis at postmortem examination. The authors speculated that the liver damage was the result of the transfer of sensitized leukocytes from the mother to the infant.

Two infants with plethora and convulsions were observed by Wood (1959). In one infant, the fetal hemoglobin concentration was only 26.6 per cent and could have been the result of a large maternal-fetal transfusion, although this was not demonstrated in either baby.

Hematocrits in excess of 75 per cent have been observed in the recipient of twin to twin transfusions (Shorland, 1971). The plethoric recipient may manifest hyperbilirubinemia, kernicterus (Sacks, 1959), and heart failure (Minkowski, 1962).

Infants with Down's syndrome and polycythemia have been found to have increased erythropoietin levels (Naveh, 1971).

Symptoms. The symptoms observed in the polycythemic infant appear to be primarily a consequence of the associated increase in blood viscosity. After the central venous hematocrit reaches 60 to 65 per cent any further increase will result in an exponential increase in blood viscosity (Stone et al., 1968). The resultant hyperviscosity will decrease blood flow and may be responsible for the respiratory difficulties and central nervous system abnormalities observed in these infants. The increased red cell mass results in a greater number of erythrocytes being broken down each day and is reflected in the hyperbilirubinemia so common in this condition. Most infants with polycythemia manifest no symptoms of any type (Gatti et al., 1966). However, certain symptoms occur with sufficient regularity to enable the physician to suspect this entity; they are listed in Table 4–2. For reasons, as yet unexplained, the syndrome is more common in males.

Laboratory Findings.   In addition to the elevation in hemoglobin and hematocrit, other laboratory abnormalities may be present. These include transient thrombocytopenia (Naiman and Schlackman, 1971), an increase in the number of circulating nucleated red blood cells (Gatti et al., 1966), hyperbilirubinemia (Bergstedt, 1957; Kresky, 1964), hypocalcemia and hypoglycemia (Humbert et al., 1969), and an increase in blood viscosity (Baum, 1967; Kontras, 1970). Fetal hemoglobin levels are higher than anticipated for gestational age in small for gestational age infants with polycythemia (Humbert et al., 1969), while fetal hemoglobin values are decreased in infants who have been recipients of maternal–fetal transfusions (Michael and Mauer, 1961). Gross and Hathaway (1971) have observed that the red cells of some infants with polycythemia are not as deformable as those of normal infants. This decrease in deformability may result in impaired blood flow in the microcirculation, which, in turn, could result in a hypoxic stimulus leading to secondary polycythemia.

Although maternal–fetal transfusion is not a common cause of neonatal polycythemia, the search for an etiology should begin with efforts to exclude this possibility. The detection of red cells of maternal blood type in the infant's blood by the mixed agglutination technique is useful in this respect. Similarly, the demonstration of increased quantities of IgA and IgM in the infant's serum, although not diagnostic, is suggestive of an admixture of maternal and infant blood. Although the range of fetal hemoglobin concentration is rather wide at any given gestational age (Chapter Six) the presence of levels of less than 60 per cent in a plethoric infant also suggests the presence of a maternal–fetal transfusion. In a male infant, chromoso-

Table 4–2   Symptoms and Signs of Neonatal Polycythemia

Respiratory distress
Cyanosis
Congestive heart failure
Convulsions (myoclonic, generalized)
Priapism
Jaundice
Renal vein thrombosis
Tetany

mal analysis can be performed to detect the presence of XX cells of maternal origin.

Treatment

Treatment of infants with polycythemia should be reserved for those with respiratory, cardiac, or central nervous system symptomatology, although all plethoric infants should be carefully monitored for evidence of hypoglycemia, hypocalcemia, and hyperbilirubinemia.

Treatment should be designed to reduce the venous hematocrit to approximately 60 per cent. This can be most readily accomplished by the performance of a partial exchange transfusion, using fresh frozen plasma rather than blood for the exchange. This procedure reduces the hematocrit while maintaining the blood volume.

The following formula may be employed to approximate the volume of exchange required to reduce the hematocrit to the desired level:

$$\text{Volume of exchange (ml.)} = \frac{\text{Blood volume} \times (\text{Observed Hct} - \text{Desired Hct})}{\text{Observed Hct}}$$

Example: A two-kilogram infant with a venous hematocrit of 75 per cent requires an exchange transfusion to reduce the hematocrit to 60 per cent.

Assume a blood volume of approximately 100 ml. per kilogram for a newborn infant. Then

$$\text{Volume of exchange (ml.)} = \frac{(100 \times 2) \times (0.75 - 0.60)}{0.75}$$

$$= \frac{200 \times 0.15}{0.75}$$

$$= 40 \text{ ml.}$$

The transfusion may be performed in 10 ml. increments. At the conclusion of the desired exchange, and prior to the removal of the catheter, a blood sample is removed for a repeat hematocrit determination.

Whether asymptomatic children with polycythemia should also undergo exchange transfusions remains open to question. In a review of 44,683 births, Weinberger and Oleinick (1971) found that 418 infants (0.09 per cent) had capillary hematocrit values in excess of 77 per cent between the thirty-sixth and sixtieth hour of life. Morbidity in this group was no different than that of the entire group.

Intelligence quotients at four years were similarly distributed, except for an excess of scores under 70 in the infants with polycythemia. The polycythemia group was found to have an excess of maternal toxemia, increased maternal age, an excess of primiparous and grand-multiparous women, longer gestations, lower birthweights for gestational age, smaller placentas, and increased frequency of placental infarcts. From this study, it would appear that the obstetric conditions leading to the birth of a polycythemic infant are more important determinants of the subsequent development of the infant than is the associated polycythemia.

Chapter Five

DISORDERS OF
RED CELL METABOLISM

Although isoimmunization as a result of blood group incompatibility still remains the leading cause of neonatal hemolytic disease in most parts of the world, other inherited, transient, or acquired defects of the red cell are now being recognized with increasing frequency as causes of anemia, jaundice, and even hydrops fetalis.

A hemolytic disease may be defined as a disorder in which the red cell life span is shortened. A shortening of red cell survival does not necessarily result in an obvious anemia if the increased red cell breakdown is compensated for by increased red cell production. This type of compensated hemolytic disease is unusual during the first few weeks of life.

A variety of disorders may produce hemolytic disease during the newborn period (Table 5–1). In general, those anemias caused by the production of an abnormal type of hemoglobin or those that are a result of defective hemoglobin synthesis rarely manifest themselves in the first weeks of life. The reasons for this and the exceptions to it are discussed in Chapter Six.

Disturbances of red cell metabolism in the newborn period are generally accompanied by jaundice and varying degrees of anemia. The destruction of 1 gm. of hemoglobin results in the production of 35 mg. of bilirubin (Lemberg and Legge, 1949). Therefore, in the newborn possessing an immature liver with limited bilirubin conjugating ability, slight degrees of hemolysis, insufficient to produce marked anemia, can result in considerable pigment accumulation.

Because all hemolytic anemias may result in hyperbilirubinemia, all are capable of producing kernicterus. Profound anemia with its

83

Table 5–1   Causes of Hemolytic Disease in the Newborn

Isoimmunization (erythroblastosis fetalis)

Enzymatic deficiencies of the red cell

      Glycolytic enzymes
        Hexokinase
        Phosphoglucose isomerase
        Phosphofructokinase
        Triose phosphate isomerase
        2, 3-DPG mutase
        Phosphoglycerate kinase
        Pyruvate kinase
        Glucose-6-phosphate dehydrogenase
        6-phosphogluconate dehydrogenase
        Galactose-1-phosphate uridyl transferase deficiency—galactosemia

      Non-glycolytic enzymes
        Glutathione reductase
        Glutathione peroxidase
        Glutathione synthetase
        ATPase
        Adenylate kinase

Drugs and Toxins

      Heinz body anemia

Defects characterized by abnormalities of red cell morphology

      Hereditary spherocytosis
      Hereditary elliptocytosis
      Hereditary stomatocytosis
      Infantile pyknocytosis

Infections

      Bacterial
      Viral (cytomegalic inclusion disease, hepatitis)
      Toxoplasmosis
      Syphilis

Defects in hemoglobin synthesis

      Hemoglobin Barts (alpha thalassemia)
      Unstable hemoglobins (congenital Heinz body anemias)

Miscellaneous

      Erythropoietic porphyria
      Disseminated intravascular coagulation (see Chapter Eight)

associated circulatory manifestations, although less common, is still another complication of hemolytic disease during this period of life. In the hemolytic anemias, there is generally evidence of compensatory red cell regeneration, as reflected in elevations in the reticulocyte count, the presence of increased numbers of nucleated red blood cells in the peripheral blood, and erythroid hyperplasia of the bone marrow. Hepatosplenomegaly is an inconstant feature of hemolytic disease during the neonatal period.

The erythrocytes of the newborn infant differ in many respects from those of the normal adult, and they are particularly susceptible to certain forms of damage. These differences may alter the clinical and laboratory manifestations of the disease from that commonly observed in the adult. For these reasons, a brief discussion of red cell metabolism and its alterations in the newborn period are presented before discussing the individual hemolytic disorders in greater detail.

RED CELL METABOLISM

The mature red cell is strikingly different from all other cells in the body. It has no nucleus and therefore lacks the ability to divide. It has no mitochondria or ribosomes, no ribonucleic or deoxyribonucleic acid synthesis, no Krebs cycle of intermediary metabolism, and no electron transport system for oxidative phosphorylation (Table 5–2). Despite these deficiencies, the red cell is a complex, meta-

Table 5–2 Metabolic Differences Between Red Cells at Various Stages of Maturation*

	NUCLEATED CELL	RETICULOCYTE	ADULT CELL
Replication	+	0	0
DNA synthesis	+	0	0
RNA synthesis	+	0	0
RNA present	+	+	0
Lipid synthesis	+	+	0
Heme synthesis	+	+	0
Protein synthesis	+	+	0
Cytochrome and electron transfer system	+	+	0
Carbohydrate metabolism			
Krebs cycle	+	+	0
Embden-Meyerhof pathway	+	+	+
Pentose phosphate pathway	+	+	+

+ = Present
0 = Absent
*From Harris, J. W. and Kellermeyer, R. W.: *The Red Cell.* Cambridge, Mass., Harvard University Press, 1970, p. 464.

bolically active cell with a measurable, finite life span of approximately 120 days in the normal adult.

Three interacting cellular units serve to maintain the integrity of the cell and enable it to perform its primary functions of oxygen and carbon dioxide transport. These three cellular units consist of hemoglobin, the cell membrane, and the intracellular soluble elements — notably the enzymes, coenzymes, and substrates of glucose metabolism. A disturbance in one cellular unit generally reflects itself in alterations in the other two units.

GLYCOLYSIS

Because glycogen is virtually absent from the normal mature red cell (Wagner, 1946), the red cell must rely on a constant supply of carbohydrate in order to maintain its energy potential. Although glucose is the preferred carbohydrate for red cell energy production, the cell can metabolize fructose and mannose almost as readily and galactose much more slowly. Pentoses and disaccharides cannot serve as energy-yielding substrates (Maizels, 1951). Glucose enters the human erythrocyte by a process of facilitated transfer, and at glucose levels in the physiological range of the blood concentration, equilibration occurs in a matter of seconds. Normally, its concentration within the red cell approximates, on a water basis, its concentration in the surrounding medium and is far in excess of the requirements of the hexokinase reaction, the first step in red cell glycolysis.

Within the red cell glucose is then either phosphorylated to glucose-6-phosphate or reduced to its polyol derivative sorbitol (Figure 5–1), which is then converted to fructose (Travis et al., 1971).

The glucose-6-phosphate formed is metabolized via one of three well-documented pathways (Figure 5–1):

1. Metabolism by way of the Embden–Meyerhof pathway in which it is catabolized to lactate or pyruvate.

2. Metabolism by way of the pentose phosphate pathway with the evolution of carbon dioxide and the production of a phosphorylated pentose sugar. This pentose, after a series of molecular rearrangements, is returned to the Embden–Meyerhof pathway at either the fructose-6-phosphate or glyceraldehyde-3-phosphate step.

3. The conversion of glucose-6-phosphate to glucose-1-phosphate and then eventually to glycogen. Only approximately 0.5 to 1.0 per cent of the glucose metabolized by the cell under normal circumstances is converted to glycogen (Moses et al., 1968) and, thus, will not be considered in the subsequent discussion.

The Embden–Meyerhof Pathway

Under normal conditions, approximately 89 to 97 per cent of all glucose is metabolized by the red cell via the Embden–Meyerhof

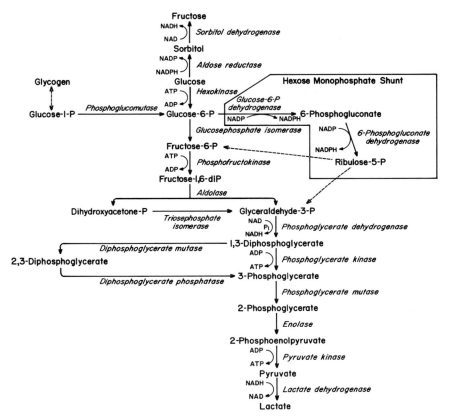

Figure 5-1 Pathways of red cell glucose metabolism.

pathway (Murphy, 1960; Oski, 1966). In this process, one mole of glucose is catabolized to two moles of lactic acid; two moles of adenosine triphosphate (ATP) are degraded to adenosine diphosphate (ADP); while four moles of ADP may potentially be phosphorylated to ATP, resulting in the possible net gain of two high-energy phosphate bonds. This potential is usually not achieved because approximately 20 per cent of the glucose metabolized traverses the 2,3-diphosphoglycerate cycle (Gerlach, 1970), thus by-passing the phosphoglycerate kinase step, one of the sites of ATP regeneration.

The 2,3-diphosphoglycerate (2,3-DPG) cycle, first described by Rapoport and Luebering (1952), provides the red cell with a mechanism for the generation of 2,3-DPG, the organic phosphate of the erythrocyte that is most responsible for determining the affinity of hemoglobin for oxygen (Benesch et al., 1967; Chanutin et al., 1967). The binding of 2,3-DPG to hemoglobin reduces its affinity for oxygen. Its regulatory role in the newborn period is discussed in Chapter Six.

The individual reactions in glycolysis have all been studied and the activity of the individual enzymes measured. In general, younger red cells have higher levels of glycolytic enzyme activity, consume greater amounts of glucose, and have higher ATP stores than do the older cells. Some of the major differences between young and old erythrocytes are described in Table 5–3.

The red cells of newborn infants consume greater quantities of glucose than do the cells of adults (Lachein et al., 1961; Oski and Naiman, 1965). In the newborn infant, the mean age of the erythrocyte population is younger than that found in the adult, and is responsible for the comparatively greater glucose consumption. The erythrocytes of the premature infant appear to consume less glucose than would be expected from their mean cell age (Oski et al., 1968). This apparent decrease in glucose consumption can be overcome by increasing the phosphate concentration (Bentley et al., 1970) or the pH of the incubation medium (Oski, 1971). Betke and co-workers (1960) have demonstrated that the red cells from adults utilize glucose more effectively for the reduction of methemoglobin than do red cells from newborn infants.

Galactose metabolism in the red cells of the newborn seems to differ from that of the adult. Galactokinase activity is three times greater in the erythrocytes of the newborns (Ng et al., 1965), and these cells consume galactose more rapidly than do those of the adult (Lachein et al., 1961). Betke (1960) has observed that methemoglobin reduction in the presence of galactose also proceeds more rapidly in the newborn than in the adult.

The activity of many of the enzymes of the Embden-Meyerhof pathway — hexokinase, aldolase, phosphoglyceraldehyde dehydrogenase, phosphoglycerate kinase, enolase, pyruvate kinase, and lactic dehydrogenase — is increased or equal to that found in the erythrocytes of the normal adult (Gross et al., 1963; Stave et al., 1961; Stewart et al., 1962; Caruso et al., 1963). The activity of phosphoglycerate kinase and enolase appears to be disproportionately elevated (Gross et al., 1963; Cotte et al., 1967; Witt et al., 1968; Oski, 1969). The activity of these enzymes reaches adult levels at varying ages — phosphoglyceraldehyde dehydrogenase reaches adult values within several days after birth, while aldolase activity remains elevated for more than one year.

Of particular interest and possible profound importance are the observations of Gross et al. (1963) and Caruso et al. (1963) concerning the decreased activity of phosphofructokinase. This is the only enzyme of either the Embden-Meyerhof or pentose phosphate pathways

Table 5–3   Some Characteristics of Young Erythrocytes

Enzymes Increased in Young Erythrocytes

Glycolytic
   Hexokinase
   Phosphohexose isomerase
   Phosphofructokinase
   Aldolase
   Glyceraldehyde-3-phosphate dehydrogenase
   Pyruvate kinase
   Glucose-6-phosphate dehydrogenase
   6-phosphogluconic dehydrogenase

Nonglycolytic
   Glutathione reductase
   Glutathione peroxidase
   ATPase
   Methemoglobin reductase
   Cholinesterase
   Glyoxalase
   Acid phosphatase
   Glutamic-oxaloacetic transaminase
   Pyrophosphatase

Enzymes Showing No Apparent Decrease with Age

Glycolytic
   Lactic dehydrogenase
   Enolase
   Phosphoglycerate kinase

Nonglycolytic
   Catalase
   Purine nucleoside phosphorylase
   DPNase
   Isocitric dehydrogenase
   Malic dehydrogenase

Other Characteristics of Young Erythrocytes

Increased glucose consumption
Increased adenosine triphosphate content, increased ATP stability during
   incubation
Slight increase in glutathione levels
Increased total SH group content
Increased total lipid content
Increased potassium content, decreased sodium content
Increased cell water
Decreased osmotic fragility
Increased 2,3-DPG content, decreased oxygen affinity

whose activity has been found to be decreased in the newborn. Its properties appear to be the same as those of the enzyme isolated from the red cells of adults (Whaun et al., 1969).

The Pentose Phosphate Pathway

The pentose phosphate pathway is the main alternate pathway of glycolysis in the erythrocyte (Fig. 5–2). By this pathway, glucose-6-phosphate undergoes oxidative decarboxylation, with the consumption of oxygen and the production of carbon dioxide.

In the first step of this pathway, oxidation of glucose-6-phosphate to 6-phosphogluconolactone is catalyzed by glucose-6-phosphate dehydrogenase. This enzyme in particular, and this pathway in general, has been the focus of extensive study in recent years, since the demonstration by Carson et al. (1956) that the erythrocytes of individuals susceptible to acute hemolysis after ingestion of the antimalarial primaquine were deficient in glucose-6-phosphate dehydrogenase.

The second step in the pentose pathway involves the enzymatic

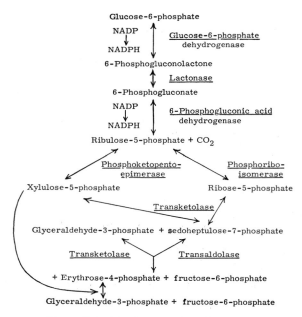

Figure 5–2   The pentose phosphate pathway.

hydrolysis of 6-phosphogluconolactone to 6-phosphogluconate, which is then oxidized in the presence of 6-phosphogluconic dehydrogenase to ribulose-5-phosphate with the production of carbon dioxide. Carbon dioxide is formed from the first carbon atom of glucose in this series of reactions, and in all probability is the only site in the mature erythrocyte for the oxidation of glucose to CO_2 (Brin and Yonemoto, 1958; Johnson and Marks, 1958; Murphy, 1960).

Unlike the Embden-Meyerhof pathway, in which NAD (DPN)[*] serves as an essential cofactor, the pentose pathway requires NADP (TPN) as a cofactor. The reactions catalyzed by glucose-6-phosphate dehydrogenase and 6-phosphogluconic dehydrogenase require NADP (TPN)[*] and result in the generation of the reduced cofactor $NADPH_2$ (TPNH).

Following the production of ribulose-5-phosphate, the remainder of the reactions of the pentose phosphate pathway are nonoxidative. The ribulose-5-phosphate formed is subsequently returned to the Embden-Meyerhof pathway as either fructose-6-phosphate or as glyceraldehyde-3-phosphate by reactions requiring transketolase or transaldolase (Fig. 5–2). The fructose-6-phosphate and glyceraldehyde-3-phosphate formed can then either be metabolized anaerobically to lactic acid or recycled through the pentose phosphate pathway. The factors determining the degree of recycling through the pentose pathway have not been completely determined.

Under normal conditions, approximately 3 to 11 per cent of all glucose metabolized by the cell is cycled through the pentose pathway. Increasing the partial pressure of oxygen or lowering the pH leads to more glucose metabolism via this pathway (Murphy, 1960). Physiological substances such as cysteine, ascorbic acid, and pyruvic acid increase the amount of glucose oxidized to CO_2 (Szeinberg and Marks, 1961), and chemical agents such as methylene blue, primaquine, acetylphenhydrazine, and nitrofurantoin also increase the metabolism of glucose via the pentose pathway (DeLoecker and Prankerd, 1961; Szeinberg and Marks, 1961). It is probable that this increase in pentose phosphate pathway activity is a result of the more rapid reoxidation of $NADPH_2$ to NADP in the presence of these various substances, thus providing more NADP for the glucose-6-phosphate dehydrogenase and 6-phosphogluconic acid dehydrogenase reactions.

Functions of the Pentose Phosphate Pathway. The pentose pathway provides the cell with ribose-5-phosphate, which is a constituent of the vital pyridine nucleotides, NAD and NADP, and the

---

[*]NAD = Nicotinamide adenine dinucleotide
NADP = Nicotinamide adenine dinucleotide phosphate
DPN = Diphosphopyridine nucleotide
TPN   = Triphosphopyridine nucleotide

purine nucleotides, ADP and ATP. Although the mature red cell can utilize preformed purines for nucleotide synthesis, there is no pathway for de novo purine formation. The mature red cell does retain the ability for pyridine nucleotide formation. The precise quantitative contribution to NAD and NADP synthesis by the ribose-5-phosphate formed by the pentose pathway in the mature red cell has not been elucidated.

Perhaps the most vital role of the pentose pathway in the mature erythrocyte is in the generation of NADPH$_2$. Although there is no evidence that NADPH$_2$ oxidation serves as an energy source (Kaplan et al., 1956), NADPH$_2$ is a necessary cofactor in several reactions that are apparently vital to the preservation of red cell integrity (Fig. 5-3), such as glutathione reduction, methemoglobin reduction, and the stabilization of certain enzymes.

NADPH$_2$ serves as a hydrogen donor in the reduction of glutathione mediated by the enzyme glutathione reductase. Reduced glutathione stabilizes certain sulfhydryl-containing enzymes of the erythrocyte as well as stabilizing hemoglobin (Benesch and Benesch, 1954; Allen and Jandl, 1960). Reduced glutathione also serves as a substrate for the enzyme glutathione peroxidase. This enzyme appears to be principally responsible for the detoxification of hydrogen peroxide by the human erythrocyte (see page 95).

NADPH$_2$ plays a role in methemoglobin reduction that is medi-

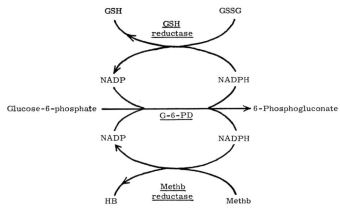

Figure 5-3 The relationship of NADPH$_2$ generation in the presence of glucose-6-phosphate dehydrogenase (G-6-PD) to glutathione and methemoglobin reduction. (GSH = glutathione, reduced; GSSG = glutathione, oxidized; Methb = methemoglobin; HB = hemoglobin.)

ated by the $NADPH_2$-dependent enzyme, methemoglobin reductase (Huennekens et al., 1958). As further detailed in Chapter Five, methemoglobin is also reduced by an NADH-dependent enzyme (Scott, 1960) that seems to play a more important role in methemoglobin reduction under normal conditions.

Szeinberg and Marks (1961) demonstrated that $NADPH_2$ can directly protect hemoglobin from oxidative denaturation and that this protection need not be mediated via reduced glutathione. Marks et al. (1961) also have demonstrated that both $NADPH_2$ and NADP are necessary for the stabilization of glucose-6-phosphate dehydrogenase activity.

In summary, the pentose phosphate pathway, because it is the only source of $NADPH_2$ generation in the mature red cell, is important in the protection of both hemoglobin and vital enzymes from oxidative denaturation. This protection may be mediated by $NADPH_2$ or indirectly by reduced glutathione.

The Pentose Phosphate Pathway in the Newborn. Two enzymes of the pentose pathway — glucose-6-phosphate dehydrogenase, and 6-phosphogluconic dehydrogenase — have been measured repeatedly in the red cells of newborn infants, and their activity has been found to be above adult values (Gross and Hurwitz, 1958; Zinkham, 1959; Fois et al., 1961; Stave et al., 1961; Witt et al., 1967). Only Tada and Watanabe (1962) have reported that premature infants have lower than normal glucose-6-phosphate dehydrogenase activity at birth. The pentose pathway also appears capable of responding to stimulation by menadione (Zinkham, 1959) or methylene blue (Betke et al., 1960). Carbon dioxide production by erythrocytes of the term and premature infants is equal to or greater than that seen in the red cells from adults. This again indicates normal pentose phosphate pathway activity in the newborn (Oski, 1966).

ADENOSINE TRIPHOSPHATE AND RED CELL METABOLISM

The metabolism of one mole of glucose via the Embden-Meyerhof pathway can result in a net gain of two moles of adenosine triphosphate (ATP). This ATP plays a central role in the economy of the red cell. Erythrocytes with low levels of ATP or erythrocytes unable to maintain their ATP levels have a shortened life span (Harris et al., 1957; Oski et al., 1964).

ATP is necessary for the maintenance of the normal biconcave shape of the erythrocyte (Nakao et al., 1960), for pyrimidine nucleotide synthesis, completion of purine nucleotide synthesis, glutathione synthesis (Koj, 1962), incorporation of fatty acids into membrane phospholipids (Oliveira and Vaughn, 1962), active cation transport (Whittam, 1964), and the initial step in the phosphorylation of glucose. Loss of red cell ATP also produces a decrease in red cell deformability (Weed et al., 1969).

Older red cells have lowered ATP levels (Bernstein, 1959). These old cells have lower glucose utilization, greater osmotic fragility on incubation, lower stromal lipid content, lower potassium concentration, greater sodium concentration, less deformability, and a shorter life span. Many of these factors appear to be consequences of lower ATP levels.

Although several workers have been unable to demonstrate elevations of red cell ATP in cord blood samples (Zipursky et al., 1960; Greenwalt et al., 1956; Caruso et al., 1963), others have shown that the red cells of term and premature infants, when studied during the first several days of life, contain higher levels of ATP than do red cells from adults (Stave and Cara, 1961; DeLuca et al., 1962; Gross et al., 1963; Oski and Naiman, 1965). The small premature infants had higher levels of ATP than did the term infants. Unlike those of normal adults, these red cell ATP levels could not be maintained during short periods of in vitro incubation (Oski and Naiman, 1965).

Zipursky et al. (1960) and Greenwalt et al. (1962) have reported that the uptake of labeled orthophosphate by cord blood erythrocytes is much slower than that observed in adults.

In the red cells of both adults and newborns, 2,3-diphosphoglycerate constitutes the major portion of the phosphate-containing glycolytic intermediates. During in vitro incubation, the erythrocytes of the newborn do not synthesize this compound as rapidly as do those of normal adults, so that a more rapid fall in concentration results (Zipursky et al., 1960; Greenwalt and Ayers, 1956; Schroter and Heyden, 1965). The activity of the enzyme responsible for its synthesis, 2,3-diphosphoglycerate mutase, is normal (Schroter et al., 1967) and, thus, the reason for the 2,3-DPG instability is still unknown.

In summary, it appears that the erythrocytes of the newborn infant demonstrate a transient immaturity in their metabolic profile. This results in a disturbance in energy metabolism that is evidenced by a slow uptake of phosphorus, a delayed incorporation into 2,3-diphosphoglycerate, and a marked decline in this compound as well as adenosine triphosphate during short periods of incubation. The precise defect, or defects, responsible for these alterations has not been defined.

Possibly as a consequence of this alteration in energy metabolism, the red cell of the newborn loses potassium at an increased rate, both during incubation at 37°C. or storage at 4°C. (Sjolin, 1954; Zipursky et al., 1960). These erythrocytes also tend to undergo marked morphologic alterations during these short periods of incubation (Sjolin, 1954; Oski and Naiman, 1965) although their rate of autohemolysis does not appear to be increased (Rudolph and Gross, 1966).

Glutathione and Red Cell Metabolism

Glutathione — a tripeptide of glycine, cysteine, and glutamic acid — is believed by many investigators to play a central role in maintaining the integrity of the erythrocyte (Carson and Tarlov, 1963; Allen and Jandl, 1961).

Glutathione is in a dynamic state in the red cell. The human red cell incorporates glycine into its glutathione with a half-life of approximately four days (Elder and Mortensen, 1956). The recent work of Koj (1962) and Sass and Caruso (1964) indicates that in addition to this constant interchange of a constituent amino acid, actual synthesis of glutathione occurs in the human erythrocyte.

In the reduced form of glutathione (GHS), a free sulfhydryl group is provided by the cysteine; GSH appears to be the only nonprotein molecule with free sulfhydryl groups found within the red cell. When glutathione is oxidized (GSSG), two molecules of this tripeptide are joined by a disulfide bond.

Glutathione is kept in the reduced state by the enzyme glutathione reductase, which catalyzes the conversion of oxidized glutathione reductase to reduced glutathione. Glutathione reductase requires $NADPH_2$ (TPNH) as a cofactor in this reaction. The pentose phosphate pathway is the only site in the red cell for the reduction of NADP (TPN) to $NADPH_2$ (TPNH), and this pathway thus provides a link between the metabolism of glucose and glutathione (Fig. 5–3).

It has been proposed that glutathione plays a central role in red cell metabolism by its possession of a free sulfhydryl group. This structure maintains the stability of SH-containing enzymes, such as glyceraldehyde-3-phosphate dehydrogenase and pyrophosphatase (Scheuch et al., 1961); protects free sulfhydryl groups in the red cell membrane (Benesch and Benesch, 1954); protects hemoglobin from oxidative degradation (Allen and Jandl, 1961); and prevents the formation of disulfides which may inhibit glycolysis at the hexokinase step (Eldjarn and Bremer, 1962).

Glutathione apparently also serves as a buffer against the injurious effects of hydrogen peroxide, which is slowly generated within the red cell. Hemoglobin is spared from oxidative denaturation by hydrogen peroxide in the red cell by reduced glutathione and the enzyme glutathione peroxidase. In detoxification of hydrogen peroxide, reduced glutathione rather than hemoglobin is oxidized (Fig. 5–4). The erythrocytes of newborn infants have lower levels of glutathione peroxidase activity than those of adults (Bracci et al., 1965; Whaun et al., 1970). This relative deficiency of glutathione peroxidase appears to render the cell more susceptible to the damaging effects of hydrogen peroxide (Bracci et al., 1965; Bracci et al., 1969).

Although small amounts of hydrogen peroxide are normally

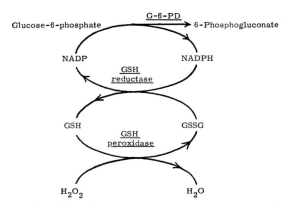

Figure 5-4   Reduced glutathione (GSH) in the presence of glutathione peroxidase converts hydrogen peroxide to water. The oxidized glutathione (GSSG) is reduced again by NADPH$_2$ generated by the pentose pathway.

generated by the red cell, this generation is accelerated when the erythrocyte is exposed to a variety of oxidant drugs (Cohen and Hochstein, 1962).

The erythrocytes of the newborn contain levels of reduced glutathione equal to or greater than those found in adults (Zinkham, 1959; Swierczewski et al., 1961). Levels of reduced glutathione fall more rapidly in the newborn during the first 48 hours of life when these cells are exposed to oxidant compounds, but this glutathione instability can be prevented by the addition of supplementary glucose to the incubation mixture (Zinkham, 1959; Szeinberg et al., 1958).

The exposure of red cells from newborn infants to oxidant compounds, such as acetylphenhydrazine or menadione, in the absence of glucose, produces irreversible metabolic alterations. These include a decrease in the activity of hexokinase, phosphofructokinase, and glyceraldehyde-3-phosphate dehydrogenase, and a reduction in the cell's ability to consume glucose (Lubin et al., 1971). Spennati and associates (1971) observed that oxidant agents produce alterations in the activity and structure of red cell acid phosphatase in newborns, but not in adults.

Glutathione stability requires NADPH$_2$ (TPNH) generation and adequate levels of glutathione reductase (Fig. 5-4). NADPH$_2$ (TPNH) generation appears adequate in the newborn in that the first two enzymes of the pentose pathway—glucose-6-phosphate dehydrogenase and 6-phosphogluconic dehydrogenase—are present in increased quantities. Glutathione reductase levels are also increased in the neonatal period (McDonald and Huisman, 1962). Gross and Schroeder (1963) have suggested that decreased stability of the triphosphopyridine nucleotides may be responsible for the glutathione instability and the tendency to form Heinz bodies in the newborn period. NADP and NADPH$_2$ levels were not increased in the cells of the premature infant despite the fact that the enzymes of the pentose pathway were increased, and on incubation with acetyl-phenylhydrazine, ascorbic acid, and menadione bisulfite, a decrease in NADP (TPN) was observed in the prematures that did not occur in the adults.

Nonglycolytic Enzymes and Red Cell Metabolism

The activity of several nonglycolytic enzymes has been well characterized. Carbonic anhydrase (Stevenson, 1943), catalase (Jones and McCance, 1949; Poblete et al., 1968), cholinesterase (Jones and McCance, 1949; Burman, 1961), and adenylate kinase (Rudolph, 1969) all have less activity in the red cells of the newborn. As yet, no functional significance has been attached to these relative deficiencies.

A nonglycolytic enzyme whose essential cofactor is closely linked to glycolysis is the NADH(DPNH)-dependent methemoglobin reductase, or diaphorase. Diaphorase levels are below adult levels in the newborn period (Ross, 1963; Bartos and Desforges, 1966) and may not reach adult values until the infant is three months of age (Kunzer, 1953). This relative deficiency of diaphorase is probably an important factor in the unusual susceptibility of young infants to methemoglobinemia on their exposure to certain medications and toxic agents such as nitrates, benzocaine, resorcin, or aniline dyes. Levels of methemoglobin are normally slightly elevated in the blood of both term and premature infants (Kravitz et al., 1956) (see also Chapter Six).

The Red Cell Membrane

The membrane of the infant's erythrocytes also differs in many respects from that of the adult.

The red cells of the cord blood of full-term infants contain increased quantities of total lipid, lipid phosphorus, and cholesterol per cell, although the percentages of total lipid comprised by lipid phosphorus and cholesterol are similar to those found in the adult (Neerhout, 1968). These erythrocytes have a greater percentage of their phospholipid as sphingomyelin and less as lecithin (Crowley et al., 1965). Phospholipid fatty acid patterns in cord blood erythrocytes show an increased percentage of palmitic, stearic, arachidonic, and combined 22- and 24-carbon fatty acids and less oleic and linoleic acid (Neerhout, 1968). These cells also contain a much greater quantity of easily peroxidizable lipid (Younkin et al., 1971). Not only is the composition of the membrane different from that of the adult, but electron microscopy reveals that the structure is different as well

(Dervichian et al., 1952; Haberman et al., 1967). Adult red cells appear as regular shapes with uniform cell walls and cytoplasm free of vacuoles. In contrast, neonatal red cells frequently show vacuoles immediately beneath the cell wall, and these occasionally contain internal structures thought to be remnants of cristae of mitochondria. These vacuoles may give the newborn's red cells a "pocked" appearance under the interference-phase microscopy (Holroyde et al., 1969) as shown in Figure 1–3.

From an immunologic standpoint the erythrocyte membrane of the newborn's cell is also different. At birth the Lewis system of absorbed serum antigens is incompletely expressed, partly because the receptor sites of the membrane are weak or absent. In the ABO system, the A and B antigen sites are thought to be incompletely expressed, and in the Ii system the I antigen is weakly developed (Mollison, 1967).

These membranes contain less ouabain-sensitive stromal adenosine triphosphatase (Whaun et al., 1969) and this may explain the decreased rate of active potassium influx observed in the cells of the newborn infant (Blum et al., 1969). These cells are also less permeable to the non-electrolytes glycerol and thiourea (Hollan et al., 1967) and in their kinetics of glucose transfer (Moore and Hall, 1971).

The red cells of the neonate are more prone to acid lysis (Schettini et al., 1971) and do not resemble those of the adult, in this respect, until about the ninetieth day of life.

Gross and Hathaway (1971) have demonstrated that the newborn's erythrocytes are much less deformable than those of the adult. It has not as yet been established whether this reflects a primary membrane abnormality or is a consequence of intra-erythrocytic alterations in metabolism.

SUMMARY OF METABOLIC CHARACTERISTICS OF RED CELLS IN THE NEWBORN

In Table 5-4 are listed many of the characteristics of the newborns' erythrocytes. The red cells produced in utero, and perhaps during the first several months of life, are truly unique. They differ from those of the adult in each of the three interacting cellular units that maintain the integrity of the cell. These cells contain more fetal hemoglobin and methemoglobin, possess striking differences in the activity of many of the glycolytic and nonglycolytic enzymes, and show characteristic variations of their membranes.

The erythrocytes of the newborn differ in their osmotic properties, mechanical fragility, and storage characteristics. Cellular energy metabolism seems to be impaired, and the detoxification of hydrogen peroxide is limited. Which of the observed differences is responsible for the shortened lifespan of these fetal cells remains to be deter-

Table 5–4 Metabolic Characteristics of the Erythrocytes of the Newborn

Carbohydrate Metabolism

Glucose consumption increased.
Galactose more completely utilized as substrate both under normal circumstances and for methemoglobin reduction.°
Decreased activity of sorbitol pathway.°

Glycolytic Enzymes

Increased activity of hexokinase, phosphoglucose isomerase, aldolase, phosphoglycerate kinase,° phosphoglycerate mutase, enolase,° pyruvate kinase, lactic dehydrogenase, glucose-6-phosphate dehydrogenase, 6-phosphogluconic dehydrogenase, galactokinase, and galactose-1-phosphate uridyl transferase.
Decreased activity of phosphofructokinase.°
Distribution of hexokinase isoenzymes differs from that of adults.°

Nonglycolytic Enzymes

Increased activity of glutamic-oxaloacetic transaminase and glutathione reductase.
Decreased activity of NADP-dependent methemoglobin reductase,° catalase,° glutathione peroxidase,° carbonic anhydrase,° and adenylate kinase.°

ATP and Phosphate Metabolism

Decreased phosphate uptake,° slower incorporation into ATP and 2,3-diphosphoglycerate.°
Accelerated decline of 2,3-diphosphoglycerate upon red cell incubation.°
Increased ATP levels.
Accelerated decline of ATP during brief incubation.

Storage Characteristics

Increased potassium efflux and greater degrees of hemolysis during short periods of storage.°
More rapid assumption of altered morphologic forms upon storage or incubation.°

Membrane

Decreased ouabain-sensitive ATPase.°
Decreased potassium influx.°
Decreased permeability to glycerol and thiourea.°
Decreased membrane deformability.°
Increased sphingomyelin, decreased lecithin content of stromal phospholipids.
Decreased content of linoleic acid.°
Increase in lipid phosphorus and cholesterol per cell.
Greater affinity for glucose°

Other

Increased methemoglobin content.°
Increased affinity of hemoglobin for oxygen.°

°Appears to be a unique characteristic of the newborn's erythrocytes and not merely a function of the presence of young red cells.

mined. These differences make the cell more vulnerable to a variety of stresses such as drug exposure and acidosis, and they result in the more rapid appearance of a hemolytic anemia in certain clinical situations. These transient physiologic alterations in red cell metabolism, characteristic of the newborn period, may also contribute to the severity of the anemia due to an associated congenital defect of red cell metabolism.

HEMOLYTIC DISEASES IN THE NEWBORN

In Table 5–1 a classification of hemolytic diseases is presented. All these disturbances are capable of producing symptoms in the newborn period, although not all have as yet been reported as etiologic agents in hemolytic diseases of the newborn. Hemolytic diseases of the newborn must be regarded as a large heterogeneous category of red cell abnormalities. It must be stressed that finding a negative Coombs test in a jaundiced infant is no longer sufficient to exclude hemolytic disease.

The congenital defects responsible for hemolytic disease have been classified into three large categories: enzymatic defects of the red cell, defects characterized by abnormalities of red cell morphology, and defects in hemoglobin synthesis. The other abnormalities responsible for the appearance of a hemolytic anemia in the newborn period are the result of transient, acquired disturbances.

Enzymatic Deficiencies of the Red Cell

For many years, these defects were grouped together as "congenital nonspherocytic hemolytic anemias." With increased understanding of red cell metabolism, many of these disorders have been identified as resulting from specific, distinct enzyme deficiencies. As yet not all the defects capable of producing a congenital nonspherocytic hemolytic anemia have been identified, but some order has been imparted to this once large heterogeneous group of disturbances.

The congenital nonspherocytic hemolytic anemias can be most easily classified into three large groups based on the site of the primary metabolic abnormality. These three groups are: 1. Defects of the Embden–Meyerhof pathway; 2. defects of the pentose phosphate pathway and disorders of glutathione metabolism; and 3. a miscellaneous group which includes disorders of adenosine triphosphate metabolism.

These disorders are characterized by: normal osmotic fragility of unincubated blood, few or no spherocytes, normal hemoglobin type, and the failure of splenectomy to correct the hemolytic process.

Although all these disorders are potentially capable of manifesting themselves in the neonatal period with jaundice and anemia, the hemolytic process may be so mild as to escape detection until later life. With the exception of red cell glucose-6-phosphate dehydrogenase deficiency, a defect of the pentose phosphate pathway which is estimated to affect nearly 100 million individuals throughout the world, these red cell disorders are very uncommon and generally unsuspected, and they are rarely diagnosed during the first weeks of life.

DEFECTS OF THE EMBDEN-MEYERHOF PATHWAY

At the present time deficiencies at eight of the 13 enzymatic steps in this pathway have been reported in association with a congenital hemolytic process. The salient features of these disorders are summarized in Table 5–5. The most common of these disorders is pyruvate kinase deficiency and its manifestations, variability, and genetic heterogeneity are representative of the clinical picture produced by red cell enzymatic deficiencies involving the Embden-Meyerhof pathway of metabolism.

Pyruvate Kinase Deficiency

In 1961, Valentine and co-workers first demonstrated that a deficiency of the erythrocyte glycolytic enzyme, pyruvate kinase, was associated with one form of congenital nonspherocytic hemolytic anemia.

Mode of Inheritance and Racial Incidence. This disease is inherited as an autosomal recessive with great variation in clinical severity. The heterozygote, although generally detectable by enzyme assay, is usually asymptomatic, although Bossu and co-workers (1968) observed a transient hemolytic anemia during the newborn period in an infant who was heterozygous for the defect. The disease has been reported chiefly in individuals of northern European stock, particularly the Amish (Bowman et al., 1964), but it has also been observed in Blacks, Chinese, Japanese, Mexicans, Syrians, and Italians.

Pathogenesis. Pyruvate kinase deficiency is an inborn error of metabolism that illustrates clearly the consequences of a block in red cell glucose metabolism. Pyruvate kinase catalyzes the conversion of phosphoenolpyruvate to pyruvate. During this reaction, adenosine diphosphate is converted to adenosine triphosphate, and for every mole of glucose that enters the Embden-Meyerhof pathway, two moles of ATP are formed from two moles of ADP at this point.

As a consequence of this block, erythrocytes deficient in pyruvate

Table 5-5 Enzyme Deficiencies of the Embden-Meyerhof Pathway

ENZYME	MODE OF INHERITANCE	OTHER TISSUES INVOLVED	ENZYME KINETICS	UNUSUAL FEATURES	REFERENCES
Hexokinase	Autosomal recessive	None	Normal and abnormal	Enzyme activity must be compared to red cells of similar young age	Valentine et al. (1967) Keitt (1969) Necheles (1970)
Glucose-phosphate isomerase	Autosomal recessive	Leukocytes	Normal	Spiculated microspherocytes and increased osmotic fragility may be observed	Baughan et al. (1968) Paglia et al. (1969) Oski et al. (1971)
Phosphofructokinase	Autosomal recessive, sex-linked?	Muscle	Normal and abnormal	Hemolysis may be mild. Glycogen accumulation in muscle may occur	Tarui et al. (1969) Waterbury et al. (1969)
Glyceraldehyde 3-phosphate dehydrogenase	Autosomal recessive?	None	Normal	Hemolysis aggravated by ingestion of oxidant compounds	Oski and Whaun (1969)
Triose-phosphate isomerase	Autosomal recessive	Leukocytes, muscle, serum, spinal fluid	Normal	Progressive neuromuscular disorder, sudden death in early life	Schneider et al. (1968) (a review)
2,3-diphosphoglycerate mutase	Autosomal recessive Autosomal dominant?	None	Unknown	Severe hemolytic anemia in infancy in one patient	Bowdler et al. (1964) Lohr et al. (1963) Schröter (1965)
Phosphoglycerate kinase	Sex-linked, uncertain	Leukocytes	Unknown	May be associated with mental retardation	Kraus et al. (1968) Valentine et al. (1969)
Pyruvate kinase	Autosomal recessive	Liver	Normal and abnormal	Marked clinical variability, splenectomy beneficial	Tanaka and Valentine (1968) (a review)

kinase consume less glucose than other normal erythrocytes of a similar age and generally have low levels of ATP. Concentrations of 2,3-diphosphoglycerate, phosphoenolpyruvate and 3-phosphoglycerate are increased. As a secondary consequence of this enzymatic block, the red cells have low levels of NAD. The levels of NAD are low apparently because decreased amounts of pyruvate are present to be converted to lactate, the step in which NADP is reduced to NAD in the presence of lactic dehydrogenase (Fig. 5–5).

The erythrocytic deficiency of pyruvate kinase also illustrates clearly the relationship between the cation pump and red cell ATP levels. Because of reduced and unstable levels of ATP, there is insufficient energy available for cation transport, and these red cells lose potassium at an accelerated rate. Their survival is shortened, and they are sequestered in both the liver and the spleen (Nathan et al., 1965). The pyruvate kinase deficient reticulocyte is particularly prone to splenic sequestration (Bowman et al., 1963; Nathan et al., 1968). Mentzer and associates (1971) have demonstrated that these reticulocytes, which are primarily dependent upon mitochondrial oxidative phosphorylation as a source of energy, are unable to sustain metabolism at the low oxygen tensions normally present in the spleen.

The unstable ATP levels and the marked cation leak may be responsible for the morphologic abnormalities noted in these cells. Many irregularly contracted cells are present, not only in the circulating blood of these patients, but also after short periods of incubation.

Clinical Manifestations. Jaundice and anemia occur frequently during the newborn period (Bowman and Procopio, 1963; Oski and Diamond, 1963; Valaes, 1969). Splenomegaly may be present during the first weeks of life and appears to be a constant finding in the slightly older patient. Kernicterus may result from the hyperbilirubinemia (Oski et al., 1964).

Laboratory Findings. The laboratory findings include hyperbilirubinemia, anemia, and reticulocytosis. Serum bilirubin levels exceeding 20 mg./100 ml. are not uncommon. The hemoglobin may fall below 10 gm./100 ml. during the first week of life, and values as low as 4 gm./100 ml. have been observed during the first three months of

Figure 5–5 Site of glycolytic block in pyruvate kinase deficiency. Note how the block in glycolysis at this point results in failure of ATP regeneration and decreased pyruvate production with resultant failure of NADH oxidation.

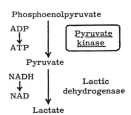

life. The reticulocyte count generally is above 5 per cent and on occasion may exceed 50 per cent.

Examination of a peripheral blood smear often reveals a small number of spherocytes, elongated oval forms, an occasional "tailed poikilocyte," and irregularly contracted cells, in addition to the macrocytosis, polychromasia, and normoblastosis seen in any severe hemolytic process. These morphologic abnormalities may be evident in cord blood samples (Fig. 5–6).

The diagnosis is made by demonstrating the enzyme deficiency by spectrophotometric assay (Tanaka et al., 1962). If the infant has been transfused, the assay should be performed three to four months later, when relatively few transfused cells remain in the circulation. A presumptive diagnosis can be made by demonstrating the carrier state in parents who are otherwise hematologically normal. The heterozygous state can be demonstrated by enzyme assay in approximately 90 per cent of carriers. A colorometric screening test has also been devised for the detection of the homozygous individuals; it will also detect the heterozygous state in many instances (Brunetti and Nenci, 1964; Beutler, 1966). Care must be taken in the interpretation of enzyme values obtained by assays employing high concentrations of the enzyme's substrate, phosphoenolpyruvate. It is now recognized that, in addition to patients who have a simple deficiency

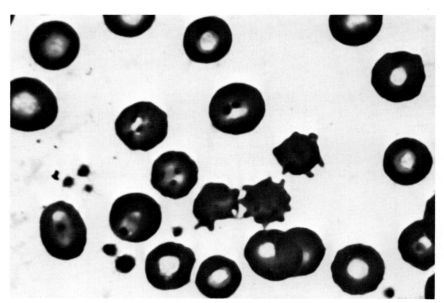

Figure 5–6   Morphologic abnormalities of the erythrocyte observed in an infant with pyruvate kinase deficiency (× 5000). Note cells with irregular surface projections.

of the enzyme, there exist individuals who have a hemolytic anemia as a consequence of the inheritance of an enzyme with mutant properties. These mutants may have either increased requirements for the substrate phosphoenolpyruvate (Paglia et al., 1968; Sachs et al., 1968; Boivin and Galand, 1968) or decreased requirements (Rose and Warms, 1966; Hanel and Brandt, 1968; Oski and Bowman, 1969).

A history of previously affected siblings may be available.

Treatment. Treatment in the newborn period is primarily directed toward avoiding the neurologic complications of hyperbilirubinemia. This has been accomplished successfully by exchange transfusions. Hemoglobin values below 8 gm./100 ml. in the neonatal period may require packed cell transfusions if they are associated with failure to thrive or signs of circulatory failure.

Splenectomy does not "cure" these individuals, as it does patients with hereditary spherocytosis. Although the anemia and reticulocytosis persist following operation, many children have benefited from this procedure owing to a decrease in their transfusion requirements. These infants should be transfused as often as it is clinically necessary in order to maintain relatively normal growth and activity until the age of two, when splenectomy may be considered. The disease varies in severity. Some patients may have no hematologic difficulties and never require transfusions; therefore it is necessary to follow these infants for some time after the neonatal period in order to determine the pattern of the disease before consideration is given to splenectomy.

Deficiencies of Other Embden-Meyerhof Pathway Enzymes

Considerable variability exists in the severity of the hemolysis associated with this group of defects. Pertinent features of these disorders are listed in Table 5–5. Detailed information concerning the clinical and laboratory aspects of these congenital non-spherocytic hemolytic anemias have been recently summarized (Beutler, 1968; Jaffe, 1970; Harris and Kellermeyer, 1970).

Most patients with these forms of anemia are jaundiced at some time in their lives. Anemia and jaundice seem to be aggravated by infections. Splenomegaly is a common finding. In addition to the anemia and reticulocytosis, laboratory findings frequently include the presence of mild to moderate anisocytosis and poikilocytosis, macrocytosis, polychromatophilia, burr cells, and fragmented erythrocytes in peripheral blood smears. Spiculated microspherocytes have been observed in glucose-phosphate isomerase deficiency.

The history, physical findings, routine laboratory tests, and red cell morphologic findings are non-specific, especially in the neonatal period, and diagnosis depends on biochemical analysis of the red cells. Jaffe (1970) has proposed criteria for the diagnosis of an enzyme deficiency as responsible for a hemolytic anemia. These criteria are: "(1) significantly decreased enzyme activity in the hemolysate relative to the activity in a hemolysate of erythrocytes of comparable age, (2) increased concentrations of substrates preceding the metabolic block, (3) decreased concentrations of compounds dependent upon the deficient enzyme activity, and, ideally, (4) similar but less pronounced abnormalities in erythrocytes of blood relatives with minimal or no evidence of hemolysis."

In general, attempts to diagnose these defects should be deferred until it can be established that the hemolytic process observed in the newborn period is of a chronic nature and cannot be attributed to more common causes such as isoimmunization, occult intrauterine infections, or the more frequent forms of congenital hemolytic anemias such as hereditary spherocytosis or those associated with abnormal hemoglobins. Similarly, diagnostic studies should not be attempted until a significant proportion of the patient's circulating erythrocytes are his own and not those acquired as a consequence of either an exchange transfusion or a simple transfusion.

Treatment in the neonatal period is similar to that described for pyruvate kinase deficiency and includes exchange transfusions when necessary for the management of hyperbilirubinemia and packed red cell transfusions for anemia, if the anemia appears severe enough to be responsible for failure to thrive or circulatory failure.

Defects of the Pentose Phosphate Pathway and Disorders of Glutathione Metabolism

Metabolic abnormalities in these pathways appear to produce hemolysis as a consequence of oxidative injury to the erythrocyte. In the absence of "trigger" events, such as drug administration, infections, or acidosis, these defects are associated with less severe hemolysis than that observed with deficiencies in the Embden-Meyerhof pathway. During the newborn period, many of these defects may be associated with a hemolytic anemia and hyperbilirubinemia in the absence of a recognized "trigger" agent or event. The outstanding features of this group of disorders are listed in Table 5–6.

Glucose-6-Phosphate Dehydrogenase Deficiency

While studying the mechanism of primaquine-induced hemolytic anemia, Dern and associates (1954) first provided evidence that this type of drug-induced hemolysis occurred in subjects with an intrinsic abnormality of the erythrocyte. In 1956, Carson and co-workers demonstrated that the major defect in the erythrocytes of these individuals

Table 5-6 Abnormalities of the Pentose Phosphate Pathway and Disorders of Glutathione Metabolism

Enzyme	Mode of Inheritance	Other Tissues Involved	Enzyme Kinetics	Unusual Features	References
Glucose-6-phosphate dehydrogenase	Sex linked	WBC's, lens, platelet, liver, adrenal	Multiple variants	Defects responsible for both drug induced and con-genital hemolytic anemias	Beutler (1969)
6-phosphogluconate dehydrogenase	Autosomal recessive, and also unknown	Unknown	Normal and abnormal	Some patients have no hematologic abnormality	Lausecker et al. (1965)
Glutathione reductase	Uncertain	White cells in some patients	Normal and abnormal	Not always associated with a hemolytic anemia	Carson et al. (1966)
Glutathione peroxidase	Autosomal recessive	Uncertain	Unknown	May be responsible for some drug induced hemolytic anemias	Necheles et al. (1968)
Glutathione synthetase	Autosomal recessive	Unknown	Normal	Not always associated with a hemolytic anemia	Boivin et al. (1966)
γ Glutamyl-cysteine synthetase	Autosomal recessive	Unknown	Unknown	Glutathione levels 5% of normal	Konrad et al. (1971)

was a deficiency of glucose-6-phosphate dehydrogenase (G-6-PD). This enzyme governs the first step in the pentose phosphate pathway.

It is now recognized that many drugs, as well as other metabolic disturbances, may precipitate a hemolytic episode in individuals deficient in G-6-PD (Table 5–7). The incidence and severity of the disease, and the agents capable of initiating hemolysis in this condition differ in the racial and ethnic groups in which this disease occurs. Because of this genetic heterogeneity, it is necessary for any individual caring for newborns in a cosmopolitan nursery to be familiar with the variable characteristics of this deficiency state. Neonatal jaundice and kernicterus secondary to hemolytic disease have frequently been observed in newborns deficient in G-6-PD.

Mode of Inheritance and Racial Incidence. G-6-PD deficiency is genetically determined and transmitted by a gene located on the X

Table 5–7 Some Agents Reported to Produce Hemolysis in Patients with G-6-PD Deficiency

Antimalarials	Others
Primaquine	Dimercaprol (BAL)
Pamaquine	Methylene blue
Pentaquine	Naphthalene
Plasmoquine	Phenylhydrazine
Quinocide	Acetylphenhydrazine
Quinacrine (Atabrine)	Probenecid
Quinine (C)	Vitamin K (large doses of water
	soluble analogues)
Sulfonamides	Chloramphenicol (C)
Sulfanilamide	Quinidine (C)
N² Acetylsulfanilamide	Fava beans (C)
Sulfacetamide (Sulamyd)	Chloroquine
Sulfamethoxypyridazine (Kynex, Midicel)	Nalidixic acid (Negram)
Salicylazosulfapyridine (Azulfidine)	Orinase
Sulfisoxazole (Gantrisin)	
Sulfapyridine	Infections
	Respiratory viruses
Nitrofurans	Infectious hepatitis
Nitrofurantoin (Furadantin)	Infectious mononucleosis
Furazolidone (Furoxone)	Bacterial pneumonias
Furaltadone (Altafur)	
Nitrofurazone (Furacin)	Diabetic Acidosis
Antipyretics and Analgesics	
Acetylsalicylic acid (in large doses)	
Acetanilide	
Acetophenetidin (Phenacetin)	
Antipyrine (C)	
Aminopyrine (C)	
p-Aminosalicylic acid	
Sulfones	

(C), to date, only Caucasians.

chromosome. Full expression of the defect therefore occurs more frequently in the hemizygous male ($\overline{X}Y$), because the mutant gene ($\overline{X}$) is not balanced by a normal allele. Complete expression of the defect in the homozygous female (XX) is much less common, but great variability with respect to partial expression of the defect may be seen in the heterozygous female ($\overline{X}X$).

One explanation for the great variability in enzyme levels in the heterozygous female is that only one X chromosome is genetically active in any cell during interphase (Lyon, 1961). Thus, the heterozygous female is in reality a mosaic of G-6-PD deficient and G-6-PD sufficient cells, and the wide range of G-6-PD values in female heterozygotes is a result of the varying proportions of somatic cells containing X chromosomes in which either the normal or the G-6-PD deficient X chromosome has been "inactivated" at an early stage of cell division in the embryo. Evidence for this female G-6-PD mosaicism has been demonstrated in skin cultures by Davidson et al. (1963) and in red blood cells by Beutler and Baluda (1964).

G-6-PD deficiency is widely distributed throughout the world. Among Caucasians, its incidence is highest in groups residing in the Mediterranean area. In some areas of Sardinia, 30 per cent of males are affected (Siniscalco et al., 1961). This deficiency also occurs with great frequency among Sephardic Jews (rare among Ashkenazic Jews), Greeks, and Iranians.

Mongolian groups known to be affected include the Chinese, Malayans, Filipinos, and Indonesians. In the American Black, the incidence of the deficiency is estimated to range from 9 to 13 per cent (Tarlov et al., 1962) in the male and 2 to 3 per cent in the female. In some parts of Africa, the incidence of the deficiency may be close to 25 per cent (Motulsky, 1960). The geographic distribution of the trait closely parallels that found for falciparum malaria, and it is believed that G-6-PD deficiency may provide protection against intracellular invasion by the malarial parasite (Motulsky, 1964). It is suggested that this enzyme deficiency may represent an example of "balanced polymorphism," in which the deleterious effects of the deficiency are balanced by the protection it affords against the severe consequences of malaria.

Genetic Heterogeneity. G-6-PD deficiency is not a homogeneous entity. The differences among ethnic and racial groups may be the result of several mutations occurring at the same gene locus, or they may reflect mutations on the X chromosome in other genes that control the formation and structure of the enzyme.

In general, the heterogeneity of this deficiency is reflected in variations in the degree of enzyme deficiency, differences in the types of drugs necessary to produce hemolysis, differences in the types of cells in the body also affected by the deficiency, differences in susceptibility to neonatal jaundice, and differences in the electrophoretic and catalytic properties of the enzyme among various racial and ethnic groups.

There are two major molecular forms of human glucose-6-phosphate dehydrogenase within red cells (Yoshida, 1967). These molecular variants are under genetic control. The wild type, or common enzyme, has been labeled B^+, and the major variant A^+. These two types can be easily separated by electrophoresis. The molecular difference between these two types appears to be limited to a single amino acid substitution, asparagine in B^+ for aspartic in A^+ (Yoshida, 1967). With rare exception, all Caucasians have the B^+ type, while approximately 18 per cent of American black males have the A^+ enzyme. All Black American males who are hemizygous with respect to G-6-PD deficiency have the A type and are labeled A^-. The enzyme has normal activity per molecule but is easily and irreversibly inactivated both in vitro and in vivo. Young erythrocytes and nucleated red cells, which can synthesize new enzyme molecules, have normal enzyme activity, but this activity declines at an accelerated rate with cell aging (Piomelli et al., 1968). In the Caucasian or B^- type of G-6-PD deficiency the enzyme activity is near zero and even the young cells have greatly diminished activity. The decay of enzyme activity is far more rapid in B^- than in A^-. These molecular differences help to explain the differences in drug sensitivity between blacks and Caucasians with G-6-PD deficiency and the more severe hemolytic process observed in Caucasians when challenged by drugs or infections.

In the black, the deficiency in general is milder than that observed in the Caucasian. In the Caucasian, G-6-PD deficiency has been demonstrated in the leukocytes, saliva, platelets, and liver of the affected subjects, whereas in the Black, the deficiency has been found in the lens of the eye and the platelets. The deficiency in the black, however, is much more generalized because whole body oxidation of glucose-1-C^{14} to $C^{14}O_2$ is below normal (Tarlov et al., 1962).

In the newborn, this genetic heterogeneity has profound clinical implications. There does not appear to be a significantly increased incidence of jaundice in black term infants who are deficient in G-6-PD. In contrast, many instances of jaundice and kernicterus have been observed in Caucasians and Mongolians with G-6-PD deficiency.

Pathogenesis.   The primary defect of the erythrocyte appears to be the deficiency of G-6-PD, the enzyme catalyzing the first step in the pentose phosphate pathway. The metabolic consequences of this deficiency, as well as other metabolic characteristics of the cell deficient in G-6-PD, are listed in Table 5–8.

The activity of G-6-PD in the erythrocytes of the affected black

Table 5-8 Metabolic Characteristics of Erythrocytes of Primaquine-sensitive Black American Males*

Deficient Glucose-6-Phosphate Dehydrogenase Activity; primary metabolic disorder.

Other Abnormalities of the Pentose Phosphate Pathway; impaired NADPH regenerative capacity secondary to a deficiency in G-6-PD activity.
Diminished NADPH and increased NADP content
Diminished responsiveness to redox dyes
Decreased oxygen consumption
Diminished rate of methemoglobin reduction
Diminished pentose formation
Diminished rate of glucose utilization
Decreased rate of dye reduction

Abnormalities Related to the Defective Pentose Phosphate Pathway
Decreased reduced glutathione (GSH) content
Vulnerability of glutathione (GSH) to oxidation
Increased glutathione reductase activity; compensatory, or a reflection of younger RBC population
Increased methemoglobinemia during nitrite administration; insufficient NADPH for methemoglobin reduction
Susceptibility to Heinz body formation in vivo and in vitro; vulnerability of hemoglobin to oxidation
Decreased lipid content

Abnormalities of the Embden-Meyerhof Pathway
Decreased NADH and increased NAD content
Fall in ATP content in vitro with acetylphenylhydrazine; may be secondary to a deficiency of NADH and NADPH.

Decreased Catalase Activity and Further Fall During Drug-induced Hemolysis

Normal Metabolic Characteristics
6-Phosphogluconic dehydrogenase, pentose content, purine nucleoside phosphorylase, transketolase, transaldolase, phosphohexose isomerase, isocitric dehydrogenase, malic dehydrogenase, acetyl cholinesterase, glyceraldehyde-phosphate dehydrogenase, adenosine triphosphate (ATP) content, lactic dehydrogenase, and glutathione peroxidase

*Adapted from Brewer and Tarlov, 1962.

male is approximately 10 to 15 per cent of normal, whereas in many deficient Caucasians the activity is even lower and frequently no G-6-PD activity can be demonstrated.

The mechanism by which G-6-PD deficiency predisposes the cell to hemolysis is not completely understood. In these deficient cells, the capacity to regenerate $NADPH_2$ (TPNH) is limited. This lack of reducing potential makes the cell vulnerable to oxidative denaturation and may result in alterations in hemoglobin, vital cellular enzymes, or constituents of the red cell membrane. It has been suggested that the oxidative denaturation produced by many of the hemolytic agents results from the generation of hydrogen peroxide (Cohen and Hochstein, 1961). The newborn's red cells may already be more vulnerable to damage from hydrogen peroxide because of their lowered levels of glutathione peroxidase and catalase, enzymes necessary for the detoxification of this compound.

Clinical Course of Hemolysis.   In the adult, the clinical course of hemolysis following ingestion of a hemolytic compound has been well described (Dern et al., 1954; Kellermeyer et al., 1961). Following ingestion of a standard dose of 30 mg. of primaquine, the hematocrit usually begins to fall between the second and fourth days and drops to its lowest level by the eighth to twelfth day. Although symptoms are uncommon in this type of experimental situation, transient jaundice may occur. Heinz bodies may be observed during the first few days of the hemolytic episode.

Clinical recovery occurs between the tenth and fortieth days, with reticulocytosis beginning at about the fifth day and reaching a maximum 10 to 20 days after drug ingestion.

More severe hemolysis may be observed if the hemolytic compound is taken in large quantities, if the patient is ill at the time of drug ingestion, or if concurrent liver or renal disease delays detoxification or excretion of the offending compound.

In contrast to the relatively mild hemolytic episode that follows primaquine ingestion is the explosive and sometimes fatal hemolytic reaction that follows ingestion of the fava bean in deficient Caucasians. Mere inhalation from the blossoms of this plant is often sufficient to initiate a severe hemolytic episode. Fava beans, however, have not produced hemolytic anemia in blacks — another example of the genetic heterogeneity of this defect.

G-6-PD Deficiency in the Newborn

Racial Incidence.   In 1960, Panizon called attention to the risks of G-6-PD deficiency in the newborn period when he described 11 cases of severe jaundice in infants from Sardinia in whom there was either a family history of favism and/or glutathione instability of the erythrocytes in either the affected infant or one of the parents. Two of these infants died in the neonatal period, and five survived with severe brain damage believed to be a result of hyperbilirubinemia. In the same year from Singapore, Smith and Vella (1960) reported 13 Chinese infants with kernicterus associated with G-6-PD deficiency, and Weatherall (1960) made similar observations in four infants from the same area.

In Greece, Doxiadis et al. (1961) noted that in one-third of infants requiring exchange transfusions for hyperbilirubinemia no evidence of isoimmunization could be demonstrated. When these infants were more carefully investigated, almost all were found to be deficient in G-6-PD. The association of G-6-PD deficiency with neonatal jaundice has since been reported from Italy (Gaburro et al., 1962), Switzerland (Scharer et al., 1963), Thailand (Flatz et al., 1963), Israel (Szeinberg et al., 1963), Nigeria (Capps et al., 1963), China (Strickland et al., 1963), Hawaii (Jim and Chu, 1963), and Canada (Naiman and Kosoy, 1964).

In surveys performed on black term infants in the United States (Zinkham, 1963; O'Flynn and Hsia, 1963; Wolff et al., 1967), no increased incidence of jaundice has been observed in the G-6-PD deficient groups. In black premature infants, G-6-PD deficiency has been found to be associated with an increased incidence of hyperbilirubinemia and a greater frequency of exchange transfusions (Eshaghpour et al., 1967). The results of these surveys have been thoroughly reviewed by Valaes (1969).

Brown (1966) has observed that, although the average hemoglobin, bilirubin, and reticulocyte count of black term males who were G-6-PD deficient did not differ from their non-deficient counterparts, there was an increased percentage of G-6-PD deficient infants among those with unexplained hyperbilirubinemia. Further investigation revealed that many of these infants were infected, or that their mothers had received drugs, such as long-acting sulfonamides, known to trigger hemolysis. In other instances hypoxia, or acidosis may result in hyperbilirubinemia (Lopez et al., 1971).

Etiology. Although the increased incidence of jaundice noted in the newborn deficient in G-6-PD is apparently the result of hemolysis, in many instances no offending drug or toxin can be incriminated as a precipitating agent. It is apparent that not all, or even the majority, of infants with G-6-PD deficiency develop significant jaundice in the newborn period. Fessas et al. (1962) estimated that approximately 5 per cent of infants with G-6-PD deficiency developed clinically significant jaundice and that these cases often showed a familial pattern. This observed recurrence of severe jaundice in only certain families with infants deficient in G-6-PD has led Fessas et al. (1964)

to speculate that an additional independent genetic factor that determines the appearance of hyperbilirubinemia may be present. This icterogenic factor appears to be more common in certain areas of both Greece and China (Brown and Wong, 1965; Valaes et al., 1969). In these groups the mean peak bilirubin levels achieved by normal newborn infants are higher and thus the combination of this factor with G-6-PD deficiency leads to the development of severe jaundice. This hypothetical factor may alter the internal environment in such a manner as to produce increased red cell destruction, or it may impair temporarily the conjugation of bilirubin, thus making the jaundice manifest.

Clinical Manifestations. In infants with hemolytic disease as a result of G-6-PD deficiency, jaundice, pallor, or signs of kernicterus are the chief physical findings. Hepatosplenomegaly is uncommon and when present should arouse suspicion that a second disease may also be present, such as isoimmunization or infection.

In contrast to the jaundice caused by blood group incompatibilities, jaundice in infants with G-6-PD deficiency usually does not appear during the first 24 hours of life. Doxiadis and Valaes (1964), in reviewing their experience with 135 cases of neonatal G-6-PD deficiency, observed jaundice for the first time on the second day of life in 50 of these infants and on the first day of life in only 12. The maximum bilirubin concentration was generally reached between the third and fifth days of life. Jaundice may not manifest itself until late in the first week of life, with peak levels of bilirubin occurring during the second week. It is in this relatively late jaundice that drugs or moth balls are often found responsible for the hemolytic anemia.

Laboratory Findings. Hyperbilirubinemia, variable degrees of anemia, and morphologic alterations of the red cell are the chief laboratory findings in infants with hemolytic disease due to G-6-PD deficiency.

Bilirubin levels frequently exceed 20 mg./100 ml. on the third to fifth day of life, and values in excess of 50 mg./100 ml. have been observed. Levels in excess of 20 mg./100 ml. can occur in the second week of life with resultant kernicterus.

Hemoglobin values may range from normal to as low as 7 to 8 gm./100 ml. during the first week of life. G-6-PD deficient infants have been found to have lower cord blood hemoglobin values and higher bilirubin levels (Valaes et al., 1969), suggesting that hemolysis may be occurring in utero. Anemia tends to be more profound in infants whose hemolysis is triggered by an exogenous agent. In some cases, both hemoglobin level and reticulocyte count may be normal, again emphasizing that only a small proportion of the red cell population need be destroyed to produce hyperbilirubinemia in the presence of physiologic immaturity of the conjugating and excreting mechanisms of bilirubin in the newborn.

In general, the reticulocyte count is elevated. Morphologic abnormalities on peripheral blood smear consist of a varying number of nucleated red cells, spherocytes, poikilocytes, and crenated and fragmented cells—all findings consistent with hemolytic anemia due to a metabolic derangement of the cells (Fig. 5–7). With supravital staining techniques, red cells containing Heinz bodies can frequently be observed early in the course of the hemolytic episode. Eventually, these cells are cleared by the spleen and thus may not be found. All these morphologic abnormalities disappear when the hemolytic episode has abated.

Although normal newborns have higher levels of red cell G-6-PD than do adults, this difference does not make difficult the diagnosis of G-6-PD deficiency during the newborn period. Glutathione levels are low and glutathione instability is present, but these tests are not as reliable or as meaningful as studies of enzyme activity. Newborns deficient in G-6-PD have markedly reduced levels of enzyme activity that can be detected by screening tests, such as the decolorization test of Motulsky et al. (1961) and the methemoglobin reduction test of Brewer et al. (1962). These screening tests have proved reliable in the detection of the hemizygous male or the homozygous female.

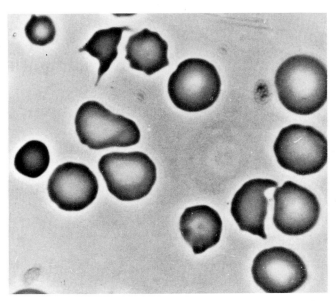

Figure 5–7 Peripheral blood smear from a newborn infant with glucose-6-phosphate dehydrogenase deficiency and a hemolytic anemia induced by moth balls. Note fragmented and distorted erythrocytes with spherocyte on left.

Direct assay of the enzyme by spectrophotometric techniques is often necessary for precise identification of the heterozygous female, and even then the diagnosis may be missed. Zannos-Mariolea and associates (1968) have found that the methemoglobin elution test is more sensitive than enzyme assay in detecting the heterozygous female. This diagnosis can be facilitated in the neonatal period by proving that the female in question must be an obligatory heterozygote by demonstrating the presence of G-6-PD deficiency in her father.

On rare occasions jaundice may be associated with a transient, non-genetically determined deficiency of red cell G-6-PD (Vullo et al., 1961). In our experience this appears to occur in premature infants only and lasts three to five days. Enzyme activity initially is usually decreased to 40 to 60 per cent of normal.

Treatment. The basis for treatment of this condition is simple, but often its application may be difficult. Proper care consists of recognition of the deficient patient who is potentially at risk, avoidance of hemolytic compounds in the care of these infants, careful observation for jaundice, and the treatment of hyperbilirubinemia with exchange transfusions.

In nurseries in which a large percentage of the patients are from ethnic groups susceptible to spontaneous hemolysis in the neonatal period, screening procedures should be introduced to identify the infants at risk. The general incidence of G-6-PD deficiency is listed in Table 5–9.

Potential hemolytic agents (Table 5–7) should not be given to newborns deficient in G-6-PD, and these compounds should also be withheld from the mothers if the child is to be breast fed. Hemo-

Table 5–9   Incidence of Glucose-6-Phosphate
Dehydrogenase Deficiency*

GROUP	INCIDENCE(%)
Ashkenazic Jews (males)	0.4
Sephardic Jews (males)	
Kurds	53.0
Iraq	24.0
Persia	15.0
Yemen	5.0
Arabs	4–8
Sardinians (males)	4–30
Greeks	0.7–3.0
American Negroes (males)	10–14
Chinese (males)	5.5
Filipinos	13.0

*Modified from Marks and Banks, 1965.

lytic anemias have occurred in breast-fed infants of mothers who have ingested fava beans (Emanuel and Schoenfeld, 1961; Taj Eldin, 1971; Kattamis, 1971) or have been exposed to moth balls (Zinkham and Childs, 1958).

In the black infant, there is no apparent danger from the use of naturally occurring vitamin K_1 (Aquamephyton, Konakion), even in doses far in excess of 1.0 mg. (Zinkham, 1963). The water-soluble vitamin K analogues (Synkavite and Hykinone) in large doses can produce hemolysis, but in doses of 1.0 mg. they also appeared to have no jaundice-producing effects in the deficient black. The safe dose for the vitamin K analogues has not been determined for the deficient Caucasian infant. Until more information is available, it is advisable to adhere to the most recent recommendation of the American Academy of Pediatrics (1961) and give the minimum dose (1 mg. intramuscularly to the premature or full-term infant) of the least toxic preparation — vitamin K_1.

Of considerable interest is the observation of Zinkham that the administration of vitamin K_1 or the vitamin K analogue (Synkavite) actually reduced the maximum bilirubin level attained in the black infant deficient in G-6-PD. Zinkham cautions, however: "Until there is conclusive proof that these large doses are necessarily beneficial, no more than 2.0 mg. of vitamin K_1 should be given to these infants."

Following discharge of the deficient infant from the nursery, careful instructions must be given to the parents with respect to exposure to naphthalene. These infants must not be exposed to blankets, bedclothes, or diapers that have been recently removed from storage in moth balls or flakes that contain naphthalene, or exposed to vaporizers containing naphthalene derivatives (Irle, 1965). The parents should also be instructed to bring the child immediately to the hospital if pallor, jaundice, or dark urine is noted.

When hyperbilirubinemia occurs, exchange transfusions should be performed for bilirubin levels in excess of 20 mg./100 ml., even after the first week of life. Kernicterus occurring during the second week of life has been observed in infants with hemolytic anemias from G-6-PD deficiency (Naiman and Kosoy, 1964).

When an infant deficient in G-6-PD is recognized, family studies should be carried out to detect other individuals who may be at risk from the hemolytic consequences of drug therapy.

Prognosis. If hyperbilirubinemia has not resulted in kernicterus, the prognosis for infants deficient in G-6-PD is good. Although these deficient patients will always have red cells with a shorter life span (Brewer et al., 1961), they will not develop anemia or reticulocytosis unless stressed by drugs, infections, or acidosis.

G-6-PD Deficiency as a Cause of a Chronic Hemolytic Anemia. In addition to the common variety of G-6-PD deficiency, which has been estimated to affect 100 million individuals throughout the world, there is another, much rarer form of the disease, which results in a chronic hemolytic anemia of the congenital, nonspherocytic type, even in the absence of drug exposure.

Patients with this type of G-6-PD deficiency have chronic anemia, reticulocytosis, a markedly shortened red cell life span, and spleno-megaly. These patients also become more anemic when given drugs that initiate hemolytic episodes in the common form of G-6-PD de-ficiency. This disturbance is also due to sex-linked characteristics, and it is much more commonly observed in patients of northern Euro-pean stock but has been reported in blacks as well (Grossman et al., 1966).

Individuals with this form of congenital nonspherocytic hemo-lytic anemia may also present in the newborn period with evidence of hemolysis and jaundice (Newton and Bass, 1958; Shahidi and Dia-mond, 1959; Cloutier and Burgert, 1966). A diagnosis of this variety of deficiency can only be arrived at by documenting persistent anemia and reticulocytosis over a period of several months, in the absence of other diseases or known causes of hemolysis.

Other Defects of the Pentose Phosphate Pathway and Disorders of Glutathione Metabolism

The remainder of these defects appear to be uncommon. Because of the paucity of affected individuals it is difficult to establish a clear picture of the anticipated clinical and laboratory findings.

Lausecker and associates (1965) have observed neonatal hyper-bilirubinemia in an infant with red cell 6-phosphogluconic dehydro-genase deficiency. This deficiency may mimic G-6-PD deficiency in its biochemical characteristics. Patients with approximately 50 per cent of normal activity for this enzyme have been found both with evidence of a hemolytic anemia (Scialom et al., 1966) and without this evidence (Brewer and Dern, 1964).

Patients with disturbances in red cell glutathione metabolism have been observed. These disturbances have included deficiencies of glutathione reductase, glutathione peroxidase, glutathione syn-thetase and γ-glutamyl-cysteine synthetase.

As yet, no report of neonatal hemolytic anemia in association with glutathione reductase deficiency has appeared. An extremely varied assortment of hematologic abnormalities has been observed in adults with partial to marked deficiencies of this enzyme (Carson and Frischer, 1966; Waller, 1968). Some patients have been normal while others have had a severe hemolytic process.

Neonatal jaundice and a mild hemolytic anemia have been ob-served in infants who appeared to be heterozygous for a deficiency of glutathione peroxidase (Necheles et al., 1968; Bracci, 1968). This enzyme is generally present in lower than normal quantities during the newborn period. The additional decrease in activity produced by a genetic defect appears to render the cell particularly prone to oxidant-induced injury. Drug-induced hemolysis (Boivin et al., 1970; Steinberg et al., 1970) and a chronic hemolytic anemia (Boivin et al., 1969) have been found in adults with glutathione peroxidase deficiency. The drugs that initiate hemolysis in this disorder appear to be similar to those triggering hemolysis in patients with G-6-PD deficiency.

Glutathione synthetase deficiency, resulting in an inability to synthesize glutathione in the erythrocyte, has been observed in several families (Oort et al., 1962; Boivin et al., 1966; Mohler et al., 1970), although manifestations of this disturbance in the neonatal period have not yet been described. Oort and associates (1962) first observed this defect in a family in which four of 12 siblings suffered from a severe but well compensated hemolytic anemia. Reduced glutathione levels measured 3 to 4 mg./100 ml. of erythrocytes, as contrasted with a normal value greater than 60 mg. The defect has now been shown to result from an inability to synthesize glutathione from its precursors glycine and L-γ-glutamyl-L-cysteine. Another defect in glutathione synthesis, a deficiency of the first enzyme in the pathway, γ-glutamyl-cysteine synthetase, which is responsible for dipeptide synthesis from glutamic acid and cysteine, also results in a hemolytic anemia associated with low red cell glutathione levels (Konrad et al., 1971).

OTHER METABOLIC ABNORMALITIES OF THE RED CELL

In this category, at present, are included red cell adenosine triphosphatase deficiency, adenylate kinase deficiency and galactose-1-phosphate uridyl transferase (galactosemia) deficiency. The precise relationships between the enzyme deficiency and the metabolic disturbance it produces, which results in a shortening of red cell life span, are as yet unclear.

Harvald and associates (1964) and Cotte and co-workers (1968) have reported finding a deficiency of the magnesium-sodium-potassium activated adenosine triphosphatase of red cell membranes in association with a mild hemolytic anemia. The biochemical alteration produced by this deficiency and its mode of inheritance remains obscure. In the reported cases no manifestations of the disease were detected in the neonatal period.

A deficiency of adenylate kinase, the enzyme responsible for the reversible reaction that converts two moles of adenosine diphosphate to one mole each of adenosine triphosphate and adenosine monophosphate, has been observed in three patients with hemolytic anemias (Szeinberg et al., 1969; Boivin et al., 1971). In two of the patients jaundice and anemia were present early in life. This disease appears to be inherited as an autosomal recessive.

Galactosemia, although not generally classified as a primary red cell disorder, may frequently be accompanied by a hemolytic anemia (Hsia, 1961). Jaundice in the newborn period in this disease is not entirely due to the liver damage produced by the ingestion of galactose; it is also a consequence of the increased red cell breakdown. The mechanism by which the deficiency of galactose-1-phosphate uridyl transferase impairs red cell metabolism is still unexplained (Zipursky et al., 1965). In all infants with unexplained hyperbilirubinemia, this inborn error of metabolism should be considered and the urine examined for a non-glucose-reducing substance.

DEFECTS CHARACTERIZED BY ABNORMALITIES OF RED CELL MORPHOLOGY

Hereditary Spherocytosis

Hereditary spherocytosis is characterized by erythrocytes that are spherocytic, abnormally fragile under osmotic stress, and intrinsically defective. The clinical picture is one of a hemolytic process of variable severity that can be corrected by splenectomy.

Inheritance. The defect is believed to be inherited as a mendelian dominant, although in 10 to 25 per cent of cases this may not be demonstrable in either parent (Young, 1955). It affects all races, but from the number of reported cases it seems to be more common in individuals of northern European origin.

Pathogenesis. Although the distinctive features of the red cell in hereditary spherocytosis—their abnormally rapid spheroidal change, their striking increase in osmotic fragility during incubation, their shortened life span, and their marked susceptibility to splenic sequestration—are all well documented, the primary defect in these cells is still unknown.

Glucose metabolism by these cells is unimpaired (Dunn et al., 1963; Jacob and Jandl, 1964). The membrane phospholipids appear normal (DeGier et al., 1961; Phillips and Roome, 1962). Sodium turnover in these cells is greater than normal (Harris and Prankerd, 1953; Bertles, 1957; Jacob and Jandl, 1964), and these cells tend to accumulate more sodium than normal during incubation.

Apparently, a poorly defined primary membrane disturbance in hereditary spherocytosis is present that results in this increased sodium turnover. As a consequence, the red cells consume increased quantities of glucose to provide sufficient ATP to drive the cation pump (Jacob and Jandl, 1964) and maintain sodium equilibrium. When these cells are deprived of glucose, ATP levels decline at an accelerated rate (Mohler, 1964), and the cells rapidly lose their viability (Jacob and Jandl, 1964). That these cells are utilizing increased quantities of glucose to provide energy for cation transport is evidenced by the observation that incubation of these cells with ouabain—an inhibitor of the cation pump—results in decreased glucose consumption and a slowing of the decline in ATP levels (Jacob and Jandl, 1964; Mohler, 1964). These cells must "overwork" to survive, and their "overwork" takes the form of increased cation transport.

It has been proposed by Jacob and Jandl (1964) and Mohler (1965) that during the metabolic stress, believed to occur in the spleen in the form of glucose depletion and a decrease in pH, the cell is no longer capable of "overworking" to compensate for its defective membrane. ATP utilization exceeds ATP generation, the content of ATP falls, the cells become less deformable, osmotic equilibrium cannot be maintained, sodium accumulates, irreversible changes in membrane permeability follow, and ultimately hemolysis occurs.

Clinical Manifestations. Hereditary spherocytosis may first present in the newborn period. In approximately 50 per cent of patients with hereditary spherocytosis, a history of neonatal jaundice may be obtained (Stamey and Diamond, 1957; Burman, 1958). Hyperbilirubinemia may be of sufficient magnitude to result in kernicterus (Roddy, 1954). Pallor and splenomegaly are inconstant findings in the neonate (Trucco and Brown, 1967).

Laboratory Findings and Diagnosis. The anemia is generally mild during the first week of life, and hemoglobin values of less than 10 gm./100 ml. are unusual. The reticulocyte count generally ranges from 5 to 15 per cent, and the serum indirect bilirubin levels may exceed 20 mg./100 ml. On occasion the reticulocyte count may remain in the normal range (Trucco and Brown, 1967).

Examination of the peripheral blood smear usually reveals the characteristic spherocyte. In some infants significant numbers of spherocytes may not be apparent in the peripheral blood until the infant is two to three months of age (Krueger and Burgert, 1966). The spherocyte is significantly smaller in diameter, appears thicker, and takes a more intense stain than does the normal red cell (Fig. 5–8). The normal area of central pallor is missing. The spheroidal nature of these cells can best be appreciated by microscopic examination of a drop of blood diluted with a drop of saline under reduced illumination. In such a wet preparation, the three dimensional nature of the cells is well visualized.

The diagnosis of hereditary spherocytosis is confirmed by family history and laboratory studies performed both on the suspected infant and his parents and siblings.

Because the specific defect is not yet known, no single test is diagnostic, and therefore family studies must supplement the study of the patient. At present, the finding of spherocytosis in a parent must be considered the best diagnostic study.

Hemolytic disease due to ABO incompatibility shares many com-

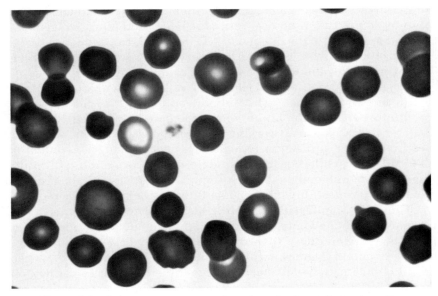

Figure 5-8   Spherocytes appear as densely stained, small circular cells.

mon features with hereditary spherocytosis. In both conditions, spherocytosis, increased red cell osmotic fragility, mild anemia, reticulocytosis, and minimal splenomegaly may be present.

Giant cell hepatitis also has been observed in association with hereditary spherocytosis (Fraga et al., 1968) in the neonatal period. This form of jaundice may confuse or delay the diagnosis of the underlying hematologic abnormality.

Differentiation of ABO Incompatibility. Laboratory studies should include blood typing of the mother and the child and a direct Coombs test on the infant. ABO incompatibility in the presence of spherocytes does not necessarily establish the incompatibility as the cause of hemolytic anemia.

When hereditary spherocytosis is considered as a possible diagnosis, both parents and siblings, in addition to the patient, should have a hemoglobin test, reticulocyte count, careful peripheral blood film inspection, and a red cell osmotic fragility test.

Osmotic fragility tests may be performed on freshly drawn blood or on blood that has been incubated under sterile conditions for 24 hours. On freshly drawn blood, the test may prove normal in 10 to 20 per cent of patients with hereditary spherocytosis, whereas the test is almost always abnormal when performed on an incubated specimen.

If osmotic fragility tests are to be performed on unincubated samples, a control sample from an infant of the same age should be tested simultaneously, because the osmotic fragility of red cells from newborns differs from that of adults in being normally more resistant to osmotic lysis. However, in infants with hereditary spherocytosis, incubated osmotic fragility tests generally give abnormal results, even in comparison to adult norms.

It should be cautioned that erythrocytes in other hemolytic states may demonstrate a similar abnormality in the osmotic fragility test after incubation, so that a positive diagnosis of hereditary spherocytosis cannot be made by this means alone.

The autohemolysis test is generally abnormal in both hereditary spherocytosis and ABO incompatibility. Kostinas and associates (1967) have found that this test may be useful in distinguishing these two conditions. The increased autohemolysis of hereditary spherocytosis was reduced by the addition of glucose to the incubated blood; but glucose had no beneficial effect in infants with hemolytic disease as a result of ABO incompatibility.

If hereditary spherocytosis cannot be differentiated from ABO incompatibility in the newborn period because of a lack of positive family studies, the subsequent course of the disease will distinguish the two entities. The manifestations of hereditary spherocytosis are lifelong, while those of ABO incompatibility are limited to the first few weeks of life.

Mackinney and associates (1962) have evaluated the tests that are of greatest value in ascertaining a diagnosis of hereditary spherocytosis when the disease is already known to be present in one member of a family. They concluded that the diagnosis in additional members of the family can be confirmed or excluded on the basis of four tests — the spherocyte score (the number of spherocytes present in a peripheral blood film examination), the reticulocyte count, and the hemoglobin and bilirubin determinations. They found that these four tests account for 88 per cent of the variability between normals and those patients with hereditary spherocytosis.

Treatment.   The treatment of hereditary spherocytosis in the newborn period is similar to that of other hemolytic anemias. Exchange transfusions may be required to prevent kernicterus (Roddy, 1954), or simple transfusions may be required to correct an anemia that occasionally may become severe during the latter part of the first month of life. Repeated transfusions are rarely needed to maintain adequate hemoglobin levels. It is our opinion that splenectomy, even though it produces a cure and will eventually be required, should not be considered before two to four years of age because of the increased risk of serious infections. In a very rare circumstance, early splenectomy may be necessary to correct severe anemia in which frequent transfusions are needed to maintain a hemoglobin greater than 6 gm./100 ml. and to keep the child free of symptoms.

Hereditary Elliptocytosis

Hereditary elliptocytosis is a disorder or group of disorders characterized by variable numbers of oval and elliptical cells in the peripheral blood (Fig. 5–9). This disease is a rare cause of hemolytic anemia in the newborn period. The incidence of hereditary elliptocytosis is approximately 1 per 2500 in the United States (Wyandt et al., 1941), but only about 12 per cent of individuals with this defect manifest evidence of a hemolytic anemia at any time during their life (Penfold and Lipscomb, 1943).

Inheritance.   The disease appears to be inherited as an autosomal dominant, and only in a few instances has homozygosity for the defect been recorded (Wyandt et al., 1941; Lipton, 1955). In the rare instance when both parents demonstrated elliptocytosis, a relatively severe hemolytic anemia was evident in their presumed homozygous offspring. The anemia, in this situation, can be very marked during the neonatal period (Nielsen and Strunk, 1968). The heterozygous patient may have no sign of hemolysis, or he may demonstrate a compensated or uncompensated hemolytic process. This marked variability in the clinical picture suggests that other defects may be operating to produce disease (Ozer and Mills, 1964).

Clinical and Laboratory Features.   Anemia and jaundice have been observed during the first weeks of life (Wyandt et al., 1941; Dacie et al., 1953; Lipton, 1955; Weiss et al., 1963; Austin and

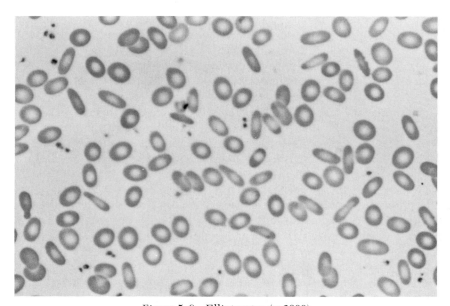

Figure 5–9   Elliptocytes (× 2000).

Desforges, 1969). Although this is rare, a diagnosis can be established only by demonstrating large numbers of elliptical cells in the affected infant as well as in one of the parents. At the present time, no specific biochemical defect has been recognized as characteristic of these cells, and no laboratory test other than the standard hematologic determinations and red cell survival studies is available to separate the patients with the common benign form of the disease from those with a hemolytic process.

Infants who are affected with hereditary elliptocytosis may not show significant numbers of elliptocytes until four to six months of age (Hunter, 1932; Helz and Menten, 1944), although this is not invariably true. The diagnosis in the newborn period may be obscured by the presence of pyknocytes rather than elliptocytes in the peripheral blood of the affected infant (Austin and Desforges, 1969).

It has been our experience that neonates with elliptocytosis may frequently manifest a hemolytic anemia during the first several months of life that gradually disappears by age one year. Apparently, the hemolytic process may be very severe in utero because gallstones have been observed in a three-week-old infant with elliptocytosis (Summerell, 1966). In this child, coexistent toxoplasmosis may have served to accentuate the rate of red cell destruction.

Hereditary Stomatocytosis

An even rarer form of morphologic abnormality associated with a hemolytic anemia is that characterized by red cells in which the central area of pallor is linear rather than circular in "shape" (Fig. 5–10). Because their appearance suggests a mouth-like orifice in the cell, the term "stomatocyte" was selected by Lock and associates (1961) to describe this anomaly. The association of this morphologic abnormality with alterations in red cell function has now been observed in at least six other families (Miller et al., 1965; Meadow, 1967; Zarkowsky et al., 1968; Oski et al., 1969; Miller et al., 1970; Honig et al., 1971).

In these cases of stomatocytosis, jaundice in the newborn period was not evident. It is obvious from the clinical and laboratory studies reported to date that hereditary stomatocytosis is not a single homogeneous entity but a group of disorders, all sharing in common only the morphologic appearance of the red cells. In some patients the hemolytic anemia has been severe (Zarkowsky et al., 1968), while in others the red cell lifespan has been found to be normal (Honig et al., 1971). The osmotic fragility of the erythrocytes has been reported to be both increased and decreased. Nothing is known about the basic biochemical defect in these disorders, although all seem to share some abnormality in membrane cation permeability.

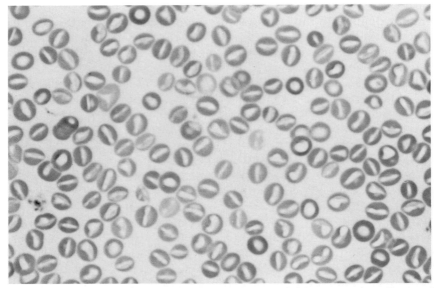

Figure 5–10   Stomatocytes (× 5000). Note the mouth-like area in the cell instead of the normal circular area of central pallor.

Infantile Pyknocytosis

Until more is learned regarding the cause of infantile pyknocytosis, this disorder must be classified in the broad category of hemolytic anemias characterized by abnormalities of red cell morphology. Unlike the other diseases in this category — spherocytosis, elliptocytosis, and stomatocytosis — infantile pyknocytosis is apparently not a hereditary persistent defect of the red cells but is a transient abnormality of the first three months of life.

The Pyknocyte.   Tuffy et al. (1959) applied the term "pyknocyte" to red cells that are distorted, completely irregular in outline, densely stained, and contain multiple spiny projections (Fig. 5–11). These cells are usually much smaller than normal erythrocytes.

Cells of similar appearance ("burr cells") have been described in patients with azotemia, gastric carcinoma (Schwartz and Motto, 1949), and acute acquired hemolytic anemias, such as the "hemolytic anemia — uremia syndrome" (Allison, 1957). The pyknocyte bears a close resemblance to the cells described as acanthocytes in the disorder characterized by a lack of beta lipoprotein. We have also noted cells that are indistinguishable from pyknocytes and acanthocytes in premature infants with hemolytic anemia associated with severe vitamin E deficiency. In all these disorders, the red cell defect is acquired, but the defect is as yet uncharacterized.

A minimal degree of pyknocytosis is seen in all infants during the first three months of life. The degree of pyknocytosis tends to increase during this period, with premature infants having more of these cells than do term infants. Tuffy et al. (1959) found that peripheral blood smears from term infants five to eight weeks of age contained 0.5 to 1.9 per cent pyknocytes, while those from premature infants 1 to 83 days of age contained 0.3 to 5.6 per cent. In contrast, adults never demonstrated more than 0.3 per cent pyknocytes. After three months of age, the number of pyknocytes rapidly declines. Infantile pyknocytosis is felt to be an accentuation of this apparently normal developmental phenomenon. Infants with this disorder may have as many as 50 per cent of their red cells as pyknocytes.

Clinical Manifestations and Laboratory Features. The clinical picture is characterized by jaundice, anemia, reticulocytosis, and often splenomegaly. Although the disease usually manifests itself during the first week of life, jaundice may not appear until the third week, and infants may present with anemia at one month of age.

If the patient does not receive an exchange transfusion, the hemolytic anemia generally progresses to a point of maximum severity at about the third week of life, when the hemoglobin ranges from 4.6 to 9.7 gm./100 ml. The severity of the hemolytic process generally correlates with the number of pyknocytes present. Other than this morphologic abnormality, there is no other consistent laboratory finding. Following exchange transfusions in two infants with pyknocytosis, Ackerman (1969) observed that the donor cells assumed the appearance of pyknocytes. This finding, coupled with

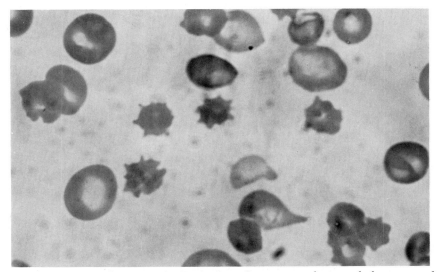

Figure 5–11   Pyknocytosis (× 5000). The pyknocytes are the irregularly contracted cells with the multiple spiny projections.

the report of Keimowitz and Desforges (1965) that both infants' cells and normal donor cells have a shortened survival, strongly suggests that an extracorpuscular factor is responsible for the morphologic alteration and the hemolytic anemia.

Associated Disorders. Tuffy et al. described 11 patients with associated disorders. Zannos-Mariolea and associates (1962) reported on 12 patients, and Ackerman (1969) observed seven infants of Mexican-American origin with this syndrome. One of the patients in the series reported by Tuffy was heterozygous for glucose-6-phosphate dehydrogenase deficiency, while five of the patients in the series of Zannos-Mariolea, all males, were deficient in glucose-6-phosphate dehydrogenase. Most infants with G-6-PD deficiency do not demonstrate significant pyknocytosis, and many of the reported patients with pyknocytosis did not have G-6-PD deficiency, so the exact relationship between these disorders is at present obscure. In all cases, pyknocytosis was absent when the infants were reexamined in later infancy and childhood.

Pyknocytosis is presumably more common than these reports indicate. This implies the need for careful examination of peripheral blood smears in all infants with jaundice and anemia in the first few weeks of life. Severe degrees of hyperbilirubinemia requiring exchange transfusion, and even kernicterus, have occurred in association with infantile pyknocytosis.

Apparently, exogenous factors resulting in an unfavorable red cell environment enhance the normal tendency for the erythrocytes of the newborn infant to form pyknocytes. That this disease occurred in more than one member of a family, had a disproportionately high incidence in the Jewish population in the series of Tuffy et al. (1959), had a low incidence in the black population, and was associated with G-6-PD deficiency in a significant number of the patients reported by Zannos-Mariolea indicates that genetic factors may predispose to the development of pyknocytosis when exogenous factors are present.

Heinz Body Anemia

In 1953, Gasser described the "hemolytic anemia of premature infants with Heinz body formation" as a new syndrome based on his observations of 14 patients. In all cases, doses of vitamin K as high as 50 mg. were given. This disease has since been observed in many premature infants, and also in a full term infant reported by Varadi and Hurworth (1957). At the time these reports were made, glucose-6-phosphate dehydrogenase deficiency was not recognized, and this deficiency therefore remains as a possible predisposing factor in some of the cases.

The Heinz Body. Newborn infants, especially prematures, on exposure to a variety of agents, are particularly susceptible to the development of a hemolytic anemia characterized by Heinz bodies within the erythrocytes. These inclusions appear as refractile irregularly shaped bodies, varying in size from minute particles to those measuring 3 μ, and they are generally situated near the periphery of the cell (Fig. 5–12). They are not visible in the usual blood films stained with Wright's or Giemsa's stain, but they can be demonstrated in wet preparations by phase microscopy or by supravital stains such as methyl violet or brilliant cresyl blue. Heinz bodies are precipitated-denatured globin, the end result of progressive oxidative injury to hemoglobin (Allen et al., 1961). This process occurs normally at a very slow rate as a result of spontaneous aging of hemoglobin within the erythrocyte, and by an acceleration of these changes induced by certain oxidant drugs such as phenylhydrazine, naphthoquinone and its derivatives (menadione, naphthalene), and sodium nitrite.

In the normal adult, naturally occurring Heinz bodies are removed by the spleen and are therefore not seen in the peripheral blood. In the absence of the spleen, as in congenital asplenia or after splenectomy, Heinz bodies may be found in the peripheral blood. A similar situation may exist in the premature infant, in whom increased numbers of Heinz bodies may be seen, in the absence of exposure to agents that increase their production. Recent studies (Acèvedo and Mauer, 1963) suggest an inability of the spleen in prematures to remove Heinz bodies from the circulation.

Pathogenesis. Hemolytic anemia in the newborn associated with Heinz bodies is not a single entity but has many causes. In most cases, a toxic drug has been administered, either in excessive dosage to a normal infant or in normal dosage to an infant with a defect of red cell metabolism impairing the defense against oxidative injury. In this regard, the most vulnerable area of the metabolic pathway is the pentose phosphate shunt (Fig. 5–2), where generation of the essential cofactor $NADPH_2$ takes place. The most common inherited abnormality of this pathway is glucose-6-phosphate dehydrogenase deficiency, which is discussed in detail on page 106. It has been thought that resulting loss of reduced glutathione leads to loss of cellular integrity and hemolysis. More recently, the precise relationship of reduced glutathione to drug-induced hemolysis in such patients has been further elucidated. According to Cohen and Hochstein (1963), the red cell enzyme glutathione peroxidase, utilizing reduced glutathione as substrate, is able to metabolize hydrogen peroxide generated by oxidant drugs, thereby preventing the deleterious effects on hemoglobin, of this compound, which lead to Heinz body formation (Fig. 5–12). Among the hemolytic drugs shown to mediate their oxidative injury via hydrogen peroxide are phenyl-

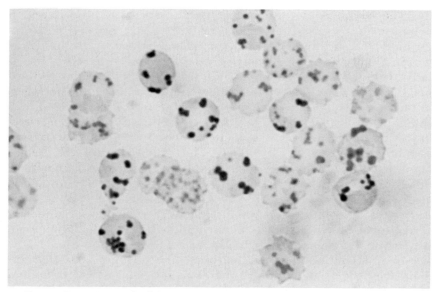

Figure 5–12   Heinz bodies (× 2000). These are small, refractile inclusions that have been stained with supravital dye, brilliant cresyl blue.

hydrazine, primaquine, and menadione (vitamin K₃). Levels of gluta-thione peroxidase in the normal newborn are decreased (Bracci et al., 1965). A transient deficiency of this important enzyme in pre-mature infants makes an attractive explanation for the increased ten-dency to Heinz body formation in prematures, with resultant hemoly-sis and hyperbilirubinemia.

Among the drugs causing Heinz body formation in the newborn, vitamin K₃ (menadione) and its synthetic water-soluble analogues (e.g., Synkavite, Hykinone) are the most important. It has been well documented that excessive doses of these drugs administered to the mother or the infant, especially the premature, result in Heinz body formation, with its attendant hemolytic jaundice and in some cases kernicterus (Sutherland, 1963). Vitamin K₁ does not cause this diffi-culty. In the reported cases, the amounts of vitamin K₃ administered have been in excess of 10 mg. and often as much as 50 to 75 mg. over a period of days. The current recommendation of vitamin K prophy-laxis of hemorrhagic disease in the newborn infant, both full-term and premature, is 1 mg. of vitamin K₁ intramuscularly to the infant at birth (American Academy of Pediatrics, 1961).

Other agents possessing similar aromatic-nitrogen and aromatic-amino chemical structures have been associated with the production of Heinz body anemias. Of particular importance in the newborn are aniline dyes and nitrobenzene derivatives used in the past for marking diapers, skin lotions containing resorcin, and sulfonamides (Gasser, 1959). Many of these drugs also produce methemoglobinemia, although not all methemoglobinemia-producing drugs result in Heinz body formation—for example, nitrates (see p. 169).

Clinical Manifestations.   Gasser characterized the syndrome as one in which jaundice usually begins after the first day and may be prolonged, anemia is progressive during the second to third week, and increased formation of Heinz bodies is noted during the first and second week, preceding the most severe degree of anemia.

Diagnosis.   Gasser noted that reticulocytopenia may be present at the height of the Heinz body formation, and it is then usually followed by an intense reticulocytosis. The infants may demonstrate generalized weakness, feeding problems, and failure to thrive. Splenomegaly is generally not present.

As in many of the other hemolytic conditions, the diagnosis is initially established on morphologic grounds. With use of supravital stains, many Heinz bodies can be observed. In addition, varying degrees of red cell fragmentation and spherocytosis may be observed.

When Heinz bodies are detected, careful inquiry should be made into possible drug exposure. In some cases, the mother may have ingested naphthalene-containing moth balls (Zinkham and Childs, 1957), or the child may have been exposed to diapers stored in naphthalene or marked with dyes that were absorbed through the skin. In all infants with this form of toxic hemolytic anemia, the possibility of glucose-6-phosphate dehydrogenase deficiency should be excluded by methods previously described.

Another form of hemolytic anemia in infancy associated with red cell inclusions has been described (Cathie, 1952; Schmid et al., 1959; Scott et al., 1960; Grimes et al., 1964). This form of congenital Heinz body anemia is not restricted to the newborn period and is associated with a variety of intrinsically unstable hemoglobins (Necheles and Allen, 1970).

Treatment.   Treatment consists of removal of the offending agent and exchange transfusion when necessary for hyperbilirubinemia, or simple transfusion if anemia is progressive and severe.

SUMMARY

As described in Chapter Three, metabolic abnormalities, such as severe acidosis, and infections due to bacteria and viruses may all result in severe hemolytic anemias in the newborn period. The mechanism of red cell damage and destruction in these conditions is as yet poorly understood.

Many causes can be found for hemolytic anemias in the newborn period. Finding marked jaundice generally alerts the physician to the presence of hemolytic disease, while anemia and reticulocytosis are usually uncovered during the laboratory investigation.

In many instances, the cause of the hemolytic anemia is apparent, as in severe respiratory distress or overwhelming sepsis, in which it may be secondary to the microangiopathic process associated with disseminated intravascular coagulation. In other situations careful laboratory investigation is necessary to establish the etiology.

In all infants with anemia or jaundice, an attempt at diagnosis should be made. Diagnosis provides a basis for rational treatment by the physician as well as an accurate prognosis for the anxious parents. An approach to differential diagnosis is presented in Chapter Three. All such attempts at differential diagnosis begin with a carefully determined history and close scrutiny of a well prepared peripheral blood smear.

Chapter Six

DISORDERS OF
HEMOGLOBIN
SYNTHESIS
AND METABOLISM

The major function of the red blood cell is to transport oxygen from the lungs to the tissues. This function is carried out by hemoglobin, which constitutes approximately 95 per cent of the erythrocyte protein. Most of the remaining protein consists of the various enzymes that protect hemoglobin and sustain viability of the erythrocyte.

The erythrocyte of the newborn infant differs from that of the adult in many respects, as outlined in Chapter Five. Differences between the hemoglobins were recognized as early as 1864 by Korber, who showed that the hemoglobin in fetal and cord blood is more resistant to denaturation by alkali than is that in adult blood. Since then, progress in methods of protein isolation and characterization has resulted in the discovery of several characteristics that enable distinguishing between fetal and adult hemoglobin. An appreciation of some of these characteristics and of the factors that affect the concentration of fetal hemoglobin during the newborn period helps in understanding many of the clinical aspects of disturbed hemoglobin synthesis and metabolism at this critical period of infant development.

To approach this problem, a brief outline of adult hemoglobin, its composition, structure, and behavior is of value.

133

ADULT HEMOGLOBIN

Hemoglobin of the normal adult is a protein with a molecular weight of approximately 67,000. It consists of four identical heme (iron-protoporphyrin) groups, each joined to histidine residues of the four polypeptide chains of globin. Each polypeptide chain contains approximately 140 amino acids. Through the intricate folding of these chains, the entire complex forms a three-dimensional structure, the shape of which varies according to whether oxygen is being taken up or released (Perutz, 1964).

From this physicochemical model, three clinically important properties of the hemoglobin molecule may be derived:

1. *Oxygenation.* This results from the reversible combination of oxygen with the ferrous (Fe^{++}) iron of heme, and is the essential transport mechanism of hemoglobin in the respiratory scheme.

2. *Oxidation.* Through loss of electrons, oxyhemoglobin, a red pigment that contains heme iron in the ferrous (Fe^{++}) state, is converted to methemoglobin, a brown pigment that contains heme iron in the ferric (Fe^{+++}) state and is incapable of carrying oxygen. Methemoglobin is therefore of no value in respiration.

3. *Molecular heterogeneity.* Alterations in the amino acid sequence of the polypeptide chains comprising the globin portion of the hemoglobin molecule result in the different normal and abnormal hemoglobins. Each of these hemoglobins consists of two pairs of polypeptide chains, the synthesis of which is under separate genetic control.

In the normal adult, hemoglobin may be separated by electrophoresis at alkaline pH into a major component (A_1), amounting to 95 to 98 per cent, and a slow minor component (A_2), amounting to 2 to 3 per cent (Fig. 6–1). Fetal hemoglobin, as determined chemically, amounts to less than 2 per cent of the total hemoglobin. The polypeptide pairs of these hemoglobins are designated as follows:

HEMOGLOBIN	POLYPEPTIDES
A_1	$\alpha_2\beta_2$
A_2	$\alpha_2\delta_2$
F	$\alpha_2\gamma_2$

The alpha chains of each of the preceding hemoglobins have been shown to be identical (Hunt, 1959; Huehns and Shooter, 1961; Ingram and Stretton, 1962).

In abnormal hemoglobins, a single (rarely two) amino acid substitution takes place, usually in the alpha or beta chain. Depending

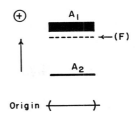

Figure 6–1 Electrophoretic pattern of normal adult hemoglobin at pH 8.6, illustrating the major component (A_1) and the slow minor component (A_2). Hb F, present in amounts less than 2 per cent, migrates slightly behind Hb A.

on the site of this substitution, the altered hemoglobin molecule confers on the erythrocyte one or more of the following handicaps:

1. A *disturbance of cell shape* which may either impede flow (sickling due to formation of intracellular tactoids by Hb S) or be of little more than morphologic interest (target cells of hemoglobins C and E).

2. *Impaired oxygen transport,* resulting in: (a) *cyanosis* (due to methemoglobin of Hb M diseases, or lowered oxygen affinity of hemoglobins such as Hb Kansas), or (b) *polycythemia* (due to increased oxygen affinity of hemoglobins such as Hb Chesapeake).

3. Heinz-body *hemolytic anemia,* due to instability of the hemoglobin (e.g., hemoglobins Zurich, Köln).

The pathophysiology of such hemoglobinopathies has been reviewed by Ranney (1970).

During the newborn period, when fetal hemoglobin predominates, each of the aforementioned characteristics—oxygenation, oxidation, and molecular heterogeneity—assumes its own peculiarities, which are attributable either to the chemical composition of the hemoglobin or to the environment within the newborn's red cell.

FETAL HEMOGLOBIN

The essential property that distinguishes fetal from adult hemoglobin is its resistance to denaturation by alkali. It is this property that forms the basis for most of the chemical methods of estimating the concentration of fetal hemoglobin in blood samples. The most popular of these is the one-minute alkali-denaturation reaction of Singer (1951). By this technique, levels of fetal hemoglobin at birth range from approximately 50 to 85 per cent, fall rapidly to below 10 per cent by four months, and reach the adult level of less than 2 per cent by about three years of age. Spectrophotometric studies of the composition of this small alkali-resistant hemoglobin fraction of normal adults reveal at least five components, only one of which is intact oxyhemoglobin (Falbe-Hansen, 1961). The identity of this component with fetal hemoglobin has not yet been established. In the strictest sense, therefore, it is wise to refer to it as alkali-resistant hemoglobin, with the realization that in situations in which its concentration is increased (over 2 per cent) most of the hemoglobin is in fact fetal in nature.

Hemoglobin Composition of Cord Blood

Cord blood of the normal newborn consists of three electrophoretically distinguishable hemoglobin fractions: Hb F, Hb A, and Hb A_2 (Table 6–1). Fetal hemoglobin predominates, and it has recently been shown by column chromatography to consist of two components, designated F_{II} (80 per cent) and F_I (20 per cent) (Allen et al., 1958). Similar resolution of these two fractions has been obtained by a modified agar gel electrophoresis (Naiman and Gerald, 1963). The major fraction (F_{II}) coincides with the fraction of fetal hemoglobin that is elevated in certain hematologic disorders such as thalassemia major. The minor fraction (F_I) differs chemically from F_{II}. Instead of two identical α chains, one of the chains is acetylated at the N-terminal amino acid (Schroeder et al., 1962). This is the first instance of a hemoglobin that does not contain an identical pair of chains.

The amounts of Hb A_2 in cord blood are lower than in adult blood. Karaklis and Fessas (1963) studied samples of cord blood from 20 newborns and found Hb A_2 values to range from 0 to 0.3 per cent (mean, 0.23 per cent), whereas Minnich et al. (1963) found slightly higher values (ranging from 0 to 1.8 per cent) in a study of cord blood samples from 90 newborns. These differences may be attributable to minor technical variations in the starch block technique and the error inherent in measuring such low concentrations. After birth, levels of Hb A_2 rise steadily to reach the normal adult range (2 to 3 per cent) by about five months of age (Erdem and Aksoy, 1969).

In addition to the three main hemoglobin components previously described, trace amounts of a fast hemoglobin, designated Hb Barts, can be demonstrated in normal newborns. This component consists entirely of γ chains (γ_4) and is described on page 160.

Properties of Fetal Hemoglobin (Hb F)

Amino Acid Composition of Globin. The content and sequence of amino acids in each chain determines the identity of the poly-

Table 6–1   Hemoglobin Composition of Cord Blood

Component	Concentration (%)
F	50–85
A_1	15–40
A_2	<1.8
Barts	<0.5

peptide chains in the globin portion of the hemoglobin molecule. The α chain contains 141 amino acids, whereas the β, γ and δ chains each contain 146 amino acids. The α chains of hemoglobins F, A, and A_2 are identical. It is the γ chain, therefore, that confers chemical specificity and probably also functional specificity to the Hb F molecule. Of the many amino acids present, only isoleucine is unique to the γ chain. Homogeneity of γ chains was presumed in the earlier analysis of Hb F derived from chromatographic separation (Schroeder et al., 1961). However, more recent chemical studies by these workers have shown two types of γ chains, distinguished by the presence of either glycine or alanine in position 136 of the chain; these have been designated γ^G and γ^A respectively (Schroeder et al., 1968; Huisman et al., 1970). This heterogeneity is felt to represent the product of two nonallelic structural genes. The relative proportions of the two chains (ratio of γ^G to γ^A) is 3:1 at birth, and falls steadily during the first five months of life to 2:3, a ratio similar to that found in the Hb F of normal adults (Huisman et al., 1970).

Spectroscopic Characteristics. The absorption spectrum of Hb F differs from that of Hb A in the ultraviolet region, as expected from their distinctive globin compositions. In Hb F the tryptophane fine-structure band occurs at a shorter wavelength (289.8 mμ) compared to that of Hb A (291.0 mμ) (Jope, 1949). This feature is the basis for a sensitive method of estimating Hb F concentration (Beaven et al., 1960).

Solubility. Hb F is more soluble in strong phosphate buffer than Hb A, a fact utilized by Derrien (1958) for isolating Hb F and for studying its heterogeneity.

Oxidation to Methemoglobin. Hb F is oxidized to methemoglobin more easily than Hb A (Betke, 1953). This observation has been confirmed by Martin and Huisman (1963) with purified solutions of Hb F. That the propensity to methemoglobin formation may be a function of the γ chain of Hb F is suggested by the even greater methemoglobin formation rate of Hb Barts, an abnormal hemoglobin of the newborn period consisting only of γ chains (γ_4). The increased susceptibility of the newborn infant to methemoglobinemia is also a result of the decreased activity of the methemoglobin-reducing enzyme system at this age (Ross, 1963).

Oxygen Affinity. Fetal blood has a greater affinity for oxygen than adult blood. An appreciation of the mechanism and physiologic significance of this property requires first an understanding of the normal reaction between hemoglobin and oxygen, as illustrated in the oxygen-hemoglobin equilibrium curve (Fig. 6–2). As blood circulates in the normal lung, the arterial oxygen tension (pO$_2$) rises from 40 mm. Hg to approximately 110 mm. Hg, sufficient to ensure at least 95 per cent saturation of the arterial blood. The shape of the oxygen-

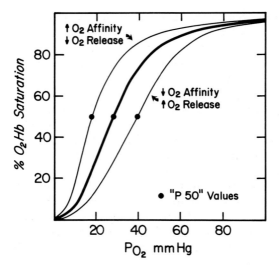

Figure 6–2 The oxygen dissociation curve of normal adult blood. The P_{50}, the oxygen tension at 50 per cent oxygen saturation, is approximately 27 mm. Hg. As the curve shifts to the right, the oxygen affinity of hemoglobin decreases and more oxygen is released at a given oxygen tension. With a shift to the left, the opposite effects are observed. A decrease in pH or an increase in temperature decreases the affinity of hemoglobin for oxygen.

hemoglobin equilibrium curve is such that a further increase in the oxygen tension in the lung results in only a very small increase in the degree of saturation of the blood. The oxygen tension falls as blood travels from the lungs, and oxygen is released from the hemoglobin. In the normal adult when the oxygen tension has fallen to approximately 27 mm. Hg at a pH of 7.4 and a temperature of 37° C., 50 per cent of the oxygen bound to hemoglobin has been released. The P_{50}, the whole blood oxygen tension at a 50 per cent oxygen saturation, would thus be stated as 27 mm. Hg. When the affinity of hemoglobin for oxygen is reduced, more oxygen is released to the tissues at a given oxygen tension. In such situations the oxygen-hemoglobin equilibrium curve is shifted to the right of normal. Alternatively, if the affinity of hemoglobin for oxygen is increased, the oxygen tension must drop to lower than normal before the hemoglobin releases an equivalent amount of oxygen, and thus the equilibrium curve appears shifted to the left.

It has long been recognized that the oxygen affinity of adult hemoglobin in *solution* is considerably greater than that of the intact fresh erythrocyte. This difference suggested that the intact red cell contains a substance or substances that are capable of interacting with hemoglobin and reducing its affinity for oxygen. In 1967, Benesch and Benesch demonstrated that the affinity of a hemoglobin solution for oxygen could be decreased by its interaction with a number of organic phosphates. Of the organic phosphates tested, 2,3-diphosphoglycerate (2,3-DPG) and adenosine triphosphate were most effective in lowering oxygen affinity. The highly charged anion 2,3-DPG was demonstrated by these workers (1968) to bind to deoxyhemoglobin but not to the oxygenated form of the molecule. They found that one mole of 2,3-DPG would bind reversibly to one mole of deoxyhemo-globin tetramer under physiologic conditions of solute concentration and pH. Of the organic phosphates normally found in the human erythrocyte, 2,3-DPG is the one found in largest concentration and thus is quantitatively the most important with respect to modulation of hemoglobin oxygen affinity.

In 1930, Anselmino and Hoffman first observed that the oxygen affinity of human fetal blood was greater than that of maternal blood. The "left-shifted" fetal blood has a P_{50} value that is 6 to 8 mm. Hg lower than that of normal adult blood. In 1953, Allen and associates showed that, although intact fetal cells possess a higher affinity for oxygen than do the red cells of adults, when adult and fetal hemo-globin solutions are dialyzed against the same surrounding solution, the resulting oxygen affinities are identical. This puzzling observation has now been resolved by the finding that deoxy-fetal hemoglobin does not possess the same affinity for 2,3-DPG as does deoxy-adult hemoglobin (Bauer et al., 1968). When either 2,3-DPG or adenosine triphosphate is added to solutions of fetal hemoglobin, the decrease in oxygen affinity produced by these compounds is significantly less than that observed in the adult.

It now appears that the major reason that the blood of the new-born infant possesses an oxygen-hemoglobin equilibrium curve which is shifted to the left of that of the normal adult is the failure of fetal hemoglobin to bind 2,3-DPG to the same degree as does adult hemoglobin.

During the first three months of life, the P_{50} of the full-term infant's blood gradually rises, and by four to six months of age the oxy-gen-hemoglobin equilibrium curve is similar to that of the adult (Delivoria-Papadopoulos et al., 1971). At eight to eleven months of age, the curve in many infants is actually shifted to the right of that of the normal adult (Fig. 6–3).

The percentage of adult hemoglobin and the red cell 2,3-DPG content both influence this change. In this study, Delivoria-Papadopoulos and co-workers, like others, failed to observe a pre-cise correlation between the decrease in the oxygen affinity of the neonate's blood and the progressive decline in the fetal hemo-globin concentration. The P_{50}, in the full-term infant, actually in-creases during the first week of life, while the fetal hemoglobin con-centration remains unchanged. This clearly suggests the influence of other factors. During this first week of life, the level of red cell 2,3-DPG rises sharply and then returns to the initial birth level by the second to third week of life. The position of the oxygen equilib-rium curve, as reflected by the P_{50}, does not directly relate to the red cell concentration of 2,3-DPG. Thus, the change in P_{50} in these in-

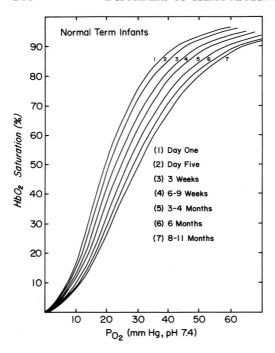

Figure 6–3 Oxygen equilibrium curve of blood from full-term infants at different post-natal ages. The P_{50} on day 1 is 19.4 ± 1.8 mm. Hg and has shifted to 30.3 ± 0.7 at age 11 months. (Normal adult, 27.0 ± 1.1 mm. Hg).

fants does not correlate either with the change in fetal hemoglobin alone or with red cell 2,3-DPG content alone. The progressive decline in oxygen affinity during the first six months of life does correlate precisely with what has been termed "the functioning DPG fraction" (Delivoria-Papadopoulos et al., 1971) or the "effective DPG fraction" (Orzalesi and Hay, 1971). This fraction is derived by multiplication of the total red cell DPG content (millimicromoles per milliliter of red blood cells) by the percentage of adult hemoglobin, and serves to illustrate the fact that both the 2,3-DPG concentration and the adult hemoglobin concentration within the cell, with which the 2,3-DPG primarily interacts, are necessary factors in determining the position of the oxygen equilibrium curve. This relationship helps to explain why infants during the first weeks of life with similar concentrations of fetal and adult hemoglobin may have marked differences in their P_{50}'s. Infants with more adult hemoglobin but less 2,3-DPG may have a P_{50} similar to that of an infant with a high red cell 2,3-DPG content in association with increased quantities of fetal hemoglobin.

The P_{50} in the premature infant is lower than it is in the full-term infant, and the smaller the infant the further left-shifted is the oxygen-hemoglobin equilibrium curve. The curve shifts to the right far more gradually postnatally and appears to reflect total gestational age rather than postnatal age.

It is clear that the increased oxygen affinity of the fetal red cell represents a physiologic advantage in terms of facilitating transfer of oxygen from mother to fetus in utero. After birth, however, fetal hemoglobin may be ill-suited to meet the demands of extrauterine stress because of its inability to respond to hypoxia by significantly increasing its oxygen unloading capacity. Although the infant rapidly rids itself of fetal hemoglobin over the first several months of life, during this period there may be occasions when the infant would fare better with adult blood. The role of exchange transfusions with fresh adult blood in situations of hypoxemia awaits critical evaluation.

Binding of Radioactive Chromium. Chromium-51 labeled sodium chromate is widely used in tagging red cells for survival studies. The chromate ion is bound to hemoglobin, in particular the β chain of the globin moiety (Pearson, 1963). Interpretation of survival studies of the red cells of newborns must take into account the differing globin composition of Hb F and its effect on the affinity for chromate. Several workers have shown an accelerated rate of chromium-51 elution in cord hemoglobin *solutions* when compared with adult hemoglobin solutions (Suderman, 1951; Erlandson, 1958; Kaplan, 1961). From the work of Pearson (1963), it appears that this phenomenon is a consequence of the weaker bond between the chromate ion and the γ chain of fetal hemoglobin in comparison with that between chromate and the β chain of Hb A. More pertinent to in vivo survival studies, however, is the demonstration that with *intact red cells* there is no difference in chromium-51 elution rate between blood from normal infants and adults (Erlandson, 1958; Kaplan, 1961). These findings have been confirmed in vivo by the elegant transfusion studies of Pearson (1966). It is evident, therefore, that fetal hemoglobin does not influence the chromate elution rate of newborn erythrocytes. Reported survival values for such cells remain valid.

Relation to Osmotic Resistance. Erythrocytes of the newborn infant are more resistant to hemolysis in hypotonic saline than those of the adult. Sjolin (1954) showed that this was not related to Hb F concentration. This property may at times make the diagnosis of hereditary spherocytosis in the newborn period difficult (see pp. 28 and 122).

Immunologic Characteristics. Of the various hemoglobins, only Hb F and Hb A_2 have been shown to possess specific antigenicity (Heller et al., 1962). The demonstration of immunologic differences among fetal hemoglobins from normal newborns (McCormick and Walker, 1960) may be explained by the recent demonstration of two chemically different γ chains in Hb F from normal newborns (see p. 137). Another possible source of this apparent immunologic variation is the presence in the antigens of small amounts of the fast minor fetal components or Hb Barts, as suggested by the demonstration of common precipitin bands in the reactions of antisera to Hb F and Hb Barts with their respective antigens (Schneider and Arat, 1964).

Resistance to Acid Elution (Fetal Erythrocyte Staining). When fixed blood smears are immersed in a citrate-phosphate buffer of acid pH (3.3 to 3.4), Hb A is eluted from the erythrocytes, but Hb F is not (Kleihauer et al., 1957). This resistance to acid elution is a specific property of Hb F, not to be confused with its resistance to denaturation by alkali. In blood smears treated in this way and subsequently stained, erythrocytes containing Hb F take up the stain, whereas cells that contain Hb A appear as "ghosts."

Blood smears from normal adults show only rare, faintly staining cells among a sea of ghosts. In smears prepared from the cord blood of newborn infants, most of the erythrocytes are deeply stained, very few ghosts are present, and the remainder of the cells show intermediate degrees of staining (Shepard et al., 1962; Fraser and Raper, 1962). This, plus the fact that the proportion of ghosts was always less than the amount of Hb A determined chemically (by column chromatography), indicates that in newborn erythrocytes Hb F and Hb A are heterogeneously distributed, with a gradient from cells containing almost all Hb F to cells containing almost all Hb A. The only situation in which Hb F is evenly distributed in all erythrocytes is the condition known as "hereditary persistence of high fetal hemoglobin," in which Hb F concentrations of 20 to 30 per cent are present in hematologically normal adults.

Many minor modifications have been incorporated into the acid elution staining technique. A method we have found to be simple and to produce consistent results is described in detail on page 63. This technique has great practical usefulness, both for demonstrating the distribution of Hb F among erythrocytes in hematologic disorders associated with increased amounts of Hb F (e.g., thalassemia major, thalassemia trait, sickle cell anemia, aplastic anemia), and for the detection of small numbers of fetal erythrocytes in the maternal circulation at birth. In the latter situation, the greater sensitivity of this technique compared to the chemical (alkali-denaturation) method for detecting Hb F is of especial value, because it enables detection in the maternal circulation of amounts of fetal blood that might ordinarily be missed by the chemical method. One of the most important applications of this is in the diagnosis of fetomaternal hemorrhage as a cause of neonatal anemia (Zipursky et al., 1959), as discussed in Chapter Three. The ability to detect a relatively minute fetomaternal passage of erythrocytes has also been of great value in the study of the mechanism of isoimmunization in erythroblastosis fetalis, including the influence of various obstetrical procedures, such as amniocentesis and conduct of labor. This subject is discussed in greater detail in Chapter Seven.

That the intense fetal-staining erythrocytes found in the maternal circulation originate from the fetus and not the mother was shown by Borst-Eilers (1961), using a combination of the mixed agglutination reaction and the fetal erythrocyte stain. By this method, it was shown that the fetal-staining cells in the mother possessed a blood group antigen present in the newborn infant but absent on the mother's red cells. Woodrow et al. (1965) have observed in fetal smears from some pregnant women large numbers of cells showing a graded degree of staining. They suggest that such cells may be of maternal origin.

SITE OF SYNTHESIS OF FETAL HEMOGLOBIN

Red cell production in the fetus begins in the liver and spleen, at a time when almost all the circulating hemoglobin is alkali-resistant or fetal in type. At a gestational age of 16 to 20 weeks, the bone marrow starts to produce cells, coincident with the appearance of Hb A in the circulating blood (Fraser and Raper, 1960). This has led to the common assumption that Hb F is produced in the liver and spleen and Hb A is produced later in the bone marrow. That such is not the case is suggested by the in vitro studies of Thomas et al. (1960), who demonstrated synthesis of both fetal and adult hemoglobins in the liver, spleen, and bone marrow taken from a 17 week old fetus. Hb A synthesis was also demonstrated in the liver of a fetus as young as nine weeks. Similar observations were made by Zilliacus and Ottelin (1967) using the acid-elution stain for fetal and adult erythrocytes. It appears, therefore, that the anatomic site of origin does not determine the type of hemoglobin that is produced. Furthermore, the demonstration of varying intensities of fetal erythrocyte staining in cord blood suggests the presence of both Hb F and Hb A in the same cell, an occurrence that is inconsistent with separate organs of synthesis (Fraser and Raper, 1962).

LEVELS OF FETAL HEMOGLOBIN IN THE FETUS AND NEWBORN

Normal Levels at Birth. Since 1951, when Singer and co-workers introduced their one-minute alkali denaturation technique for determining Hb F concentration, numerous workers have studied the cord blood of newborn infants in an attempt to establish normal values for Hb F and to evaluate the effect of various factors on such values. Although a wide range has been found in normal newborns, the results obtained by these various groups have in general been comparable; they are summarized in Table 6–2. The most important factor affecting the Hb F concentration is the gestational age of the infant. The high values of Hb F during intrauterine life (90 to 95 per

Table 6–2   Fetal Hemoglobin Levels in Cord Blood

AUTHOR	YEAR	NO. OF INFANTS	GESTATIONAL AGE	% HB F	METHOD
Chernoff	1952	28	Unselected	50–85	Alkali denaturation
Schulman	1954	36	Premature	81.1 (73–89)	Alkali denaturation
		96	Full-term	71.0 (44–89)	Alkali denaturation
Cook	1957	152	25–44 wks.	90–69°	Alkali denaturation
Gerbie	1959	50	<38 wks.	80.7 (66–92)	Alkali denaturation
		125	38–42 wks.	73.3 (55–92)	Alkali denaturation
		25	>42 wks.	67.6 (42–80)	Alkali denaturation
Kirschbaum	1962	172	26–43 wks.	92.3–77.4°	Column chromatography
Minnich	1962	143	Prem. & Term	77.8 (60–97)	Column chromatography
Armstrong	1963	103	Prem. & Term	74.0 (63–87)	Alkali denaturation
		Same	Prem. & Term	85.5 (79–91)	Column chromatography
Andrews	1965	280	39–41 wks.	79.6 (47–95)	Alkali denaturation

°Mean values

cent) persist until about the thirty-fourth to thirty-sixth weeks of gestation. These values then decrease gradually at a rate of about 3 to 4 per cent per week until 40 weeks, at which time they range from 50 to 85 per cent. Much of the variability found by different groups can be attributed to: (1) decreased sensitivity of this technique at higher Hb F levels; (2) minor technical differences in the method as applied by the various workers; (3) inclusion in groups of full term infants slightly younger and slightly older than 40 weeks gestation. More precise determinations of Hb F concentration by column chromatography have yielded a much narrower range of values and a slightly higher mean value in comparison to those found by the alkali-denaturation technique (Kirschbaum, 1962; Armstrong et al., 1963). The decrease in Hb F concentration as the fetus approaches term has been found to be due not to decreased synthesis of Hb F, but to increased synthesis of Hb A, resulting in a rise in total body hemoglobin *mass* (estimated with blood volume determination) (Brody and Nilsson, 1960).

     Relation to Gestational Age and Birth Weight.   In relating Hb F concentration to prematurity or postmaturity, gestational age rather than birth weight should be employed. The greater validity of gestational age as an index is to be expected, because replacement of Hb F by Hb A is essentially a maturational process that is not of necessity connected with body growth. This is illustrated by the finding of identical Hb F concentrations in twins of differing birth weights (Salzberger, 1956; Andrews and Falkner, 1968). Although most workers have found significant differences in Hb F concentration between groups of premature, term, and postmature infants (Schulman et al., 1954; Walker and Turnbull, 1955; Cottom, 1955; Abrahamov et al., 1956; Gerbie et al., 1959; Cotter and Prystowsky, 1963), the wide range of values among infants of a particular age prevents accurate prediction of gestational age from Hb F concentration in an individual infant. The best correlation has been found by Brody (1960), who showed that when the ratio of Hb F concentration to birth weight (in kg.) was charted against gestational age, reasonably good linearity and minimal scatter was obtained, as indicated by a correlation coefficient of 0.77 and a 95 per cent confidence range of ± 18.3 days. The greatest practical value of such an estimation might seem to be in determining whether an underweight newborn is truly premature or is suffering from intrauterine growth retardation (Gellis, 1965). However, the validity of such a prediction is lessened by the recent observations of Bard and co-workers (1970), who showed that small-for-gestational-age newborns had *higher* levels of Hb F than normal infants of the same gestational age. Actual *rates* of Hb F synthesis in such infants were also higher, and with increasing gestational age declined at a slower rate than was observed in the infants whose weight was appropriate for their age.

Effect of Intrauterine Anoxia.   *Acute* anoxia arising from complications during labor does not alter the Hb F concentration in the cord blood of the newborn (Bromberg et al., 1956). The same authors found that *chronic* intrauterine anoxia, on the other hand, due to maternal conditions, such as cardiac failure, severe asthma, and severe anemia, resulted in increased levels of Hb F in the newborn. They attributed this to a delay in synthesis of Hb A. In vitro studies by Thomas et al. (1959) using the liver from a 17 week old fetus demonstrated also that decreasing oxygen concentrations induced a relative increase in the proportion of Hb F compared to Hb A. The failure of intrauterine hypoxia of relatively short duration to produce an increased concentration of Hb F was confirmed in a study of 28 infants, who showed meconium staining of the skin, nails, and umbilical cord at birth (Cook et al., 1957).

Effect of Maternal Diabetes.   Gerbie et al. (1959) studied the newborn infants of six diabetic women whose pregnancies were terminated between the thirty-fifth and thirty-eighth weeks of gestation; they found a lower average Hb F concentration (74.1 per cent) compared to that of infants of similar gestational age (80.7 per cent). Further observations on such infants are needed before significance can be given this finding.

Effect of Maternal Toxemia.   Neumayer (1966) could find no difference between the cord fetal hemoglobin concentrations of infants of toxemic mothers and infants of healthy mothers.

Effect of Erythroblastosis Fetalis.   Jonxis, in 1948, found increased amounts of Hb A in newborns with erythroblastosis; he attributed this to preferential destruction of erythrocytes containing Hb F. Contrary to this interpretation, Mollison (1943) found that when Rh-erythroblastotic infants were transfused with adult Rh-positive blood, there was indiscriminate destruction of the infant's and the donor adult erythrocytes. Neither Schulman and Smith (1954) nor Brody and Engström (1960) could show that the increase in proportion of Hb A was associated with an increased absolute concentration of this pigment compared to that in a control group of full-term newborns. However, when the erythroblastotic newborns were matched with normal newborns of *similar gestational age*, as in a more recent study by Oppé and Fraser (1962), a significant increase in the absolute concentration of Hb A could be demonstrated. From this observation, they concluded that the lower Hb F concentrations in erythroblastosis fetalis are due to the effects of random hemolysis and blood regeneration occurring at a time when there is a normal increase in the synthesis of Hb A. Following exchange transfusion in erythroblastotic newborns, a rise in Hb F concentration can be demonstrated, indicating postnatal synthesis of this fraction (Baar, 1948; Schulman and Smith, 1954). Comparison of Hb F concentrations before and immediately after exchange transfusion has been used to estimate the efficiency of blood exchange (Bromberg et al., 1955; Maggioni, 1959).

Effect of Genetic Disorders.   Infants with Down's syndrome (G trisomy) have lower levels of fetal hemoglobin at birth and through the first two months of life (Wilson et al., 1968). Infants with Trisomy 13 (D_1) have increased levels at birth, with a slower rate of decline during the first year of life (see p. 150).

Postnatal Decline.   The Hb F of intrauterine life is almost completely replaced by Hb A during the first three years of life. These changes in composition of hemoglobin during development of the embryo, fetus, and child are depicted in Figure 6–4. Although most of the decline in Hb F concentration is due to increasing Hb A synthesis, appreciable amounts of Hb F continue to be synthesized during the first few months of life (Garby et al., 1962). The relative rates of synthesis of Hb F and Hb A in the first three months of life were studied by Garby and co-workers with a technique involving incorporation of intravenously administered radioactive iron[59] into the two hemoglobins. At birth 50 to 65 per cent of hemoglobin *synthesis* is of the fetal type; this declines to approximately 5 per cent by three months of age. During this period, the actual *concentration* of Hb F in the circulating blood is somewhat higher, owing to the presence of erythrocytes that have been released into the circulation at an earlier time when Hb F synthesis was more active. The decline of Hb F concentration is gradual during the first weeks of life. Coincident with recovery of the bone marrow from the transient postnatal depression

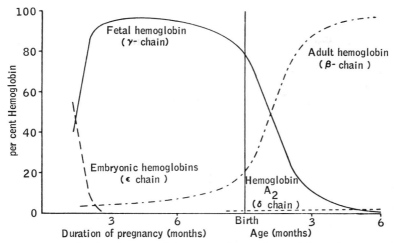

Figure 6–4 The developmental changes in human hemoglobins. (From Huehns, E. R., and Shooter, E. M.: *Journal of Medical Genetics*, 2:48, 1965.)

and increased synthesis of Hb A, there is a more rapid decline in Hb F concentration at about two months of age, terminating in levels of about 10 to 15 per cent by four months of age. After this, there is a gradual decline to adult levels of less than 2 per cent by three years of age. These changes are depicted in Figure 6–5 (Garby et al., 1962).

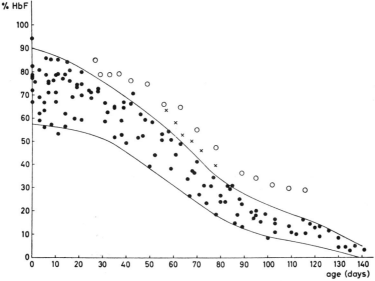

Figure 6–5 Declining concentration of fetal hemoglobin after birth. The region between the curved lines contains 120 observations made on 17 normal infants. (From Garby, L., Sjölin, S., and Vuille, J. C.: *Acta Paediatrica*, 51:245, 1962.)

The rate of postnatal decline of Hb F concentration is not affected by persistent anoxia due to cyanotic congenital heart disease (Farrar and Blomfield, 1963). However, it is delayed in certain hematologic disorders of early life associated with either impairment of Hb A synthesis (thalassemia major, sickle cell anemia, congenital hypoplastic anemia, Fanconi's anemia) or hemolysis (some cases of hereditary spherocytosis). Extramedullary hematopoiesis secondary to marrow obliteration in osteopetrosis (marble bone disease) does not usually result in the persistence of elevated Hb F concentrations (Beaven et al., 1960).

The change from Hb F to Hb A reflects a biochemical change from gamma to beta chain synthesis during the first few months of life (Fig. 6–4). The mechanism regulating this change is primarily genetic, in which an operator gene turns off the structural gene controlling gamma chain synthesis, while it turns on the structural gene controlling beta chain synthesis. A mutation of this operator gene is believed to underlie the condition of "hereditary persistence of high fetal hemoglobin," in which Hb F levels of 20 to 30 per cent are found after childhood in the absence of anemia or abnormal red cell morphology. The exact nature of the physiologic mechanism governing this change in the normal infant is not yet known. An opposite situation, precocious synthesis of adult hemoglobin, has been described in association with a syndrome of congenital anomalies and reciprocal C/D chromosomal translocation (Weller et al., 1966). This infant at 24 days of age showed a Hb F concentration of only 9 per cent.

EMBRYONIC HEMOGLOBIN

The existence of a distinctive *embryonic hemoglobin* that precedes the formation of Hb F during early embryonic development was first suggested by Drescher and Künzer (1954). Its initial characterization was based on the finding of an alkali-denaturation rate intermediate between that of Hb F and Hb A. On electrophoresis, this embryonic hemoglobin migrates slightly slower than Hb F, as shown by Halbrecht et al. (1958) in 9 of 15 embryos between 10 and 20 weeks gestation. Other workers, studying fetuses older than 10 weeks gestation, were unable to confirm the presence of this hemoglobin (Butler et al., 1960; Matsuda et al., 1960). This question appears to have been resolved by the recent report of Huehns et al. (1964), who showed by sensitive electrophoretic techniques, that an embryonic hemoglobin was present in all of 12 embryos smaller than 8.5 cm. in crown-rump length (corresponding to a gestation age of approximately 12 weeks), but in none of 10 specimens larger than this. The embryonic hemoglobin was named Gower 2, and it migrated slower than Hb A_2, the slow minor fraction of normal adult blood (Fig. 6–6). The concentration of Hb Gower 2 was greatest in the youngest embryos (at levels of 10 to 15 per cent) and decreased with age. Accompanying Hb Gower 2 was a slightly faster component, which has been called Gower 1. Subsequent study (Hecht et al., 1966) of even younger embryos (5 to 6 weeks' gestation; less than 2.5 cm. in length) has shown that Hb Gower 1 is the major hemoglobin of early embryonic life, exceeding in concentration that of Hb Gower 2 and Hb F. Preliminary analysis suggests that the globin of Hb Gower 2 consists of two α chains and two chains differing from the previously described β, γ and δ chains. These have been designated "epsilon" (ϵ) chains, and the globin is therefore represented as $\alpha_2\epsilon_2$. Hb Gower 1 appears to consist only of ϵ chains, resembling the previously described tetramers of the β chains (β_4, or Hb H) and of the γ chains (γ_4, or Hb Barts). In the same young embryos, the minor Hb A-like component has been shown to be a different hemoglobin, lacking α chains, and instead composed of two γ chains and two unknown chains, possibly ϵ in type (Hecht et al., 1967). This hemoglobin was found in concentrations of 0.5 to 2 per cent in a number of newborns with multiple anomalies, and in two normal newborns in a concentration of less than 0.2 per cent. It was designated Hb Portland 1 and appears to be a normal embryonic hemoglobin. In a recent study of 9 to 18 week fetuses, true Hb A was found, accounting for 8 to 14 per cent of the total hemoglobin *synthesized* (Hollenberg et al., 1971); the actual *concentration* of Hb A is about 5 per cent (Walker and Turnbull, 1955).

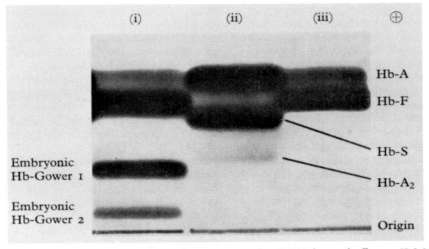

Figure 6–6 Starch gel electrophoresis in a *tris = EDTA*–borate buffer at pH 8.6: hemolysate from 3.5 cm. (crown = rump) human embryo (*i*); HbA + S marker (ii); and normal cord blood (III). (From Huehns, E. R., and Shooter, E. M.: *Journal of Medical Genetics*, 2:48, 1965.)

The prenatal development of the four major types of human hemoglobins may be summarized as follows (see Fig. 6–4):

Gower 1 ———→ Gower 2 ———→ F ———→ A

(ϵ_4) $(\alpha_2\epsilon_2)$ $(\alpha_2\gamma_2)$ $(\alpha_2\beta_2)$

The intracellular demonstration of embryonic hemoglobin has been accomplished by Kleihauer and co-workers (1967). When the acid-elution test (p. 63) is performed at a pH of 2.9 instead of the usual pH of 3.3 to 3.4, embryonic hemoglobin is even more resistant to elution than is fetal hemoglobin.

Occurrence in Trisomy 13 (D_1) in the Newborn Period

Infants born with this rare syndrome of multiple congenital anomalies associated with an extra 13 (D_1) chromosome have been shown to have various abnormalities of hemoglobin composition. Huehns et al. (1964) first demonstrated trace amounts (less than 1 per cent) of Hb Gower 2 and increased amounts of Hb Barts at birth; both of these components disappear by about one month of age. Hb Portland 1, a normal minor embryonic hemoglobin, has also been found in increased concentrations in four newborns with trisomy 13 (Hecht et al., 1967); it was found also in two other newborns with different chromosomal-anomaly syndromes. Fetal hemoglobin concentrations are usually increased at birth and fall postnatally at a slower rate than normal (Walzer et al., 1966; Wilson et al., 1967). In a 27-month-old child studied by Powars et al. (1964), the Hb F level was 34 per cent. Low levels of Hb A_2 and the enzyme carbonic anhydrase have also been seen in such infants at birth (Walzer et al., 1966). The latter observations seen to support the suggestion of Huehns that the elevations in embryonic and fetal hemoglobins represent specific retardation of the normal maturational change (disappearance) seen with these hemoglobins. Signs of nuclear immaturity in the neutrophils are also seen in infants with trisomy 13 and are discussed in Chapter 10 (p. 331).

Hemoglobin abnormalities similar to those described above have also been described in infants with trisomy 13 associated with D/D translocation (Walzer et al., 1966; Pinkerton and Cohen, 1967).

An earlier report by Halbrecht et al. (1959) of an "embryonic" hemoglobin in two full-term newborns with multiple congenital malformations may be a further example of this association. Chromosome analysis of these infants was not given.

Trisomy of the the 17–18 (E) group or of chromosome 21 (Down's syndrome) is not associated with the presence of these embryonic hemoglobins (Huehns et al., 1964).

DISORDERS OF HEMOGLOBIN SYNTHESIS

Abnormalities of hemoglobin synthesis may be divided into two broad groups—disorders of heme synthesis or disorders of globin synthesis—depending on the portion of the hemoglobin molecule that is affected (Table 6–3).

Disorders of Heme Synthesis

Because the heme moiety consists of an iron-protoporphyrin complex, defects in the synthesis of protoporphyrin, such as congenital erythropoietic porphyria, may be included here. This is a rare condition characterized by a vesicular skin eruption, hemolytic anemia, splenomegaly, red urine, and reddish discoloration of the teeth. Of 45 cases collected from the literature by Goldberg and Rimington (1962), 14 showed some manifestation at birth, usually red staining of the diapers by the porphyrin compounds in the urine and meconium. Hemolytic anemia and the skin eruption usually appear later, after the neonatal period. These authors cite one case in which the condition probably existed in utero, and the infant died four hours after birth. Red urine due to porphyrins may also occur in normal newly born infants of mothers with porphyria. In this situation, however, the phenomenon of "passive porphyria" disappears after one or two days (James et al., 1961).

Increased amounts of the various heme precursors have been found in red cells of the normal newborn, in proportion to their younger cell age (Fikentscher et al., 1969).

Disorders of Globin Synthesis

Two types may occur: *qualitative disorders* (hemoglobinopathies), in which an amino acid substitution in one of the polypeptide chains results in the production of an abnormal hemoglobin; and

Table 6–3   Inherited Disorders of Hemoglobin Synthesis

HEME	GLOBIN
Congenital erythropoietic porphyria	Qualitative (hemoglobinopathies; e.g., Hb S, C, M, etc.)
	Quantitative (thalassemia syndromes, e.g., α and β thalassemia)

quantitative disorders (thalassemia syndromes), in which there is a decreased *rate* of synthesis of one of the normal polypeptide chains.

Although disorders of globin synthesis usually present after the first few months of life, sufficient evidence has accrued from electrophoretic studies of cord blood in various populations to indicate that important hemoglobin abnormalities may be detected during the newborn period.

HEMOGLOBINOPATHIES

Occurrence in the Neonatal Period.   It has long been recognized that sickle cell disease, one of the commonest of the hemoglobinopathies, rarely presents clinically until after the first few months of life. In such infants followed from birth, the percentage of sickle cells and of Hb S was low initially and gradually increased to adult levels by about four to six months of life (Haggard and Schneider, 1961; Minnich et al., 1962). A similar trend is seen in infants with Hb C, another hemoglobinopathy involving the β polypeptide chain.

Until recently, it was widely thought that the paucity of manifestations of sickle cell disease in the newborn period was a result of a protective effect of the high concentration of Hb F acting to prevent sickling. A more plausible explanation, however, may be found by examining the polypeptide chains of the normally occurring hemoglobins during this period of transition. The replacement of Hb F $(\alpha_2\gamma_2)$ by Hb A $(\alpha_2\beta_2)$ represents a switch from γ to β polypeptide production, as discussed earlier (Fig. 6–4). Thus, hemoglobinopathies involving the β chain, such as Hb S and Hb C, would not be manifest at birth. With increasing β chain synthesis in the first few months of life, however, sufficient concentrations of the abnormal β chain variant would soon be reached in the erythrocyte, so that the accompanying clinical and hematologic consequences of the abnormal hemoglobin would be manifest. Alpha chain variants on the other hand would be present at birth not only in the form corresponding to Hb A, but also as a fetal form because identical α chains occur in Hb F and Hb A. In such cases, four major hemoglobin fractions can be demonstrated in cord blood: the normal Hb A, Hb F and the α chain variants of

Table 6–4   Hemoglobinopathies in the Newborn

SITE OF DEFECT	EXAMPLES	USUAL AGE OF ONSET
α Chain	Hb D$_\alpha$ I	Birth
β Chain	Hb S, C, E	After 3 months
γ Chain	Hb F$_{\text{Alexandra,}}$	Birth
	F$_{\text{Aegina,}}$ F$_{\text{Roma,}}$	Birth
	F$_{\text{Texas}}$	Birth

each of these components. Variants of the γ chain are the other possible sources of abnormal fetal hemoglobins at birth. A number of these have been described and are summarized in Tables 6–4 and 6–7.

Hb Barts, a fast hemoglobin composed of four normal γ chains (γ_4) results from a deficiency of α chain synthesis and will therefore be considered under α thalassemia (p. 160).

HEMOGLOBINOPATHIES INVOLVING THE β CHAIN

Numerous abnormal hemoglobins resulting from an amino acid substitution in the β chain have been described. The most important of these is Hb S, which results in the sickling phenomenon. Because of the infrequency of the others (C, D, E, etc.) and the paucity of their hematologic manifestations, further discussion is limited to Hb S. An excellent review of the neonatal development of these hemoglobinopathies may be found in the paper by Minnich et al. (1962).

Sickle Cell Disease

This disease is an inherited disorder of hemoglobin synthesis, limited almost exclusively to Negroes, and characterized by erythrocytes that assume a sickle shape under conditions of diminished oxygen tension. The heterozygous form results in the asymptomatic sickle cell trait found in approximately 8 per cent of Negroes in the United States. The homozygous form, sickle cell anemia, is a clinical disorder of variable severity, consisting of a chronic hemolytic anemia, sickling-vascular thromboses with resultant painful crisis and tissue infarction, hepatosplenomegaly, and jaundice.

Age of Onset.   Although almost 50 per cent of cases of sickle cell anemia are diagnosed in the first two years of life, only a handful of cases have had their onset in the neonatal period. Of 54 patients reviewed by Haggard and Schneider (1961), none had symptoms prior to three months of age. Booker et al. (1964) reported two infants with onset of symptoms at three months of age from a group of 18 patients with sickle cell anemia who were diagnosed under two years of age. Porter and Thurman (1963) combined their experience from two university hospitals in the southern United States and collected 64 cases diagnosed before one year of age; three of these infants presented in the first month of life. Another four individual case reports account for a total of seven infants with sickle cell anemia whose symptoms began in the first month of life (Cohen et al., 1947; Frazier and Rice, 1950; Heldrich, 1951; Leikin and McCoo, 1958).

Clinical Manifestations.   The pertinent clinical and hematologic data on the cases mentioned in the previous paragraph is summarized

Table 6–5   Reports of Sickle Cell Anemia with Onset
of Symptoms in the Neonatal Period

CASE NO.	AUTHOR	YEAR	AGE (DAYS) Onset	AGE (DAYS) Admission	JAUNDICE	ASSOCIATED ILLNESS	HEPATO-SPLENOMEGALY
1	Cohen,	1947	29	30	+	Otitis media	0
2	Frazier,	1950	3	19	(+)	Anoxia	0
3	Heldrich,	1951	1	1	(+)	0	0
4	Leikin,	1958	23	24	(+)	0	+
5	Porter,	1963	17	23	+	"Colic"	+
6	Porter,	1963	18	19	0	Pneumonia	+
7	Porter,	1963	1	15	(+)	Hemorrhagic disease of newborn	0

+ = Present
0 = Absent
– = Not stated

in Table 6–5. Jaundice was present in six of the seven infants; in four
of these it was the presenting symptom. The jaundice was associated
with hemolytic anemia in each of the cases. In two of the patients, an
associated blood group (ABO) incompatibility was a possible cause
of the jaundice. Infection appears to have triggered the hemolysis in
two patients, as is frequently observed in this age group (Porter and
Thurman, 1963). Three of the seven infants died. Neonatal (giant cell)
hepatitis and early cirrhosis were found at autopsy in one infant, an
interesting association described previously in young infants with
hemolytic disease due to other causes such as blood group incompatibility (Craig, 1950), hereditary spherocytosis (Bain et al., 1957),
and glucose-6-phosphate dehydrogenase deficiency (Naiman and
Kosoy, 1964).

Diagnosis.   Although it is apparent that sickle cell anemia presents only rarely in the newborn period, it should be considered a
possible cause of unexplained or prolonged jaundice in Negro newborns. The diagnosis may not be easy to confirm at this age, however,
as illustrated in two of the patients reported by Porter with negative
sickle cell preparations when first seen. In this situation, if sickle
cell anemia is suspected, repeated testing of the infant and of both
parents should be carried out. A negative sickle cell preparation on
the mother's blood is sufficient to exclude this diagnosis. A positive
sickle cell preparation on the infant should be followed by an electrophoretic analysis of the hemoglobin pattern. The distinction between
sickle cell trait (AS) and sickle cell anemia (SS) may be difficult because of the large amount of Hb F present at this age, obscuring the
region of Hb A on the electrophoretic pattern. However, if Hb A can
be demonstrated (with refined techniques, such as starch or agar gel
electrophoresis), the diagnosis of sickle cell anemia can be excluded.
The possibility of antenatal diagnosis of sickle cell anemia from fetal
erythrocytes obtained by amniocentesis is suggested in the recent
studies of Hollenberger et al. (1971). Their demonstration of Hb A

Table 6–5   Reports of Sickle Cell Anemia with Onset
of Symptoms in the Neonatal Period (*Continued*)

Sickle Prep.	Hb (gm./100 ml.)	Reticulocytes (%)	Serum Bilirubin (mg./100 ml.)	Blood Group Incompatibility	Outcome
Pos.	11.5→5.5	–	–	No	Died
Pos.	11.5	–	7.5	–	Alive
Pos.	13.3	–	13.3	B–0	Alive
Pos.	7.0	6.8	°°D=10.8/T=19.4	No	Died
°Neg.	6.8	–	°°D=0.8/T=2.8	–	Alive
Pos.	7.8	3.8	0.9	–	Died
°Neg.	6.2	–	D=8.4/T=23.5	A–0	Alive

(+) = Presenting symptom
° = Later positive
°° = Direct/total

synthesis in the mid-trimester fetus may pave the way for detecting Hb S and distinguishing the fetus with sickle cell anemia.

The postnatal fall in hemoglobin concentration was observed in a prospective study of 19 Congolese newborns with sickle cell anemia identified at birth during the course of a study of cord blood by van Baelen and co-workers (1969) (Fig. 6–7). Anemia was present at birth in one infant and was definite by one month of age in the majority. The decline in hemoglobin concentrations leveled off at around 7 gm./100 ml. by nine months of age.

Treatment.   Treatment of the infant who presents with sickle cell anemia during the first few weeks of life is similar to that of the older infant. Because infection in the reported cases seems to be a precipitating factor, a careful search for an etiologic organism followed by appropriate antibiotic therapy is essential. Blood transfusion may be necessary for the hemolytic anemia at this time, although it is rarely necessary in older children with this disease.

Sickling in the Newborn.   The incidence of positive sickle cell preparations among Negro newborns in the United States has been studied by several workers. The results are summarized in Table 6–6. Aside from the lower figures obtained by Scott et al. (1948), the frequency of positive sickle cell preparations is approximately the same as that found in adult Negro populations—8 to 10 per cent. Statistically, almost all these cases represent sickle cell trait. Only in the study of Minnich et al. (1962) were serial hematologic examinations carried out to confirm this development. The percentage of erythrocytes that can be induced to sickle is much less in newborns, varying from as low as 0.5 per cent to as high as 40 per cent, according to the various studies. Differences in technique among these workers probably account for the wide range of results. The most sensitive method in use at present employs a reducing agent such as sodium metabisulfite to accelerate sickling. Because of the slower rate of sickling and

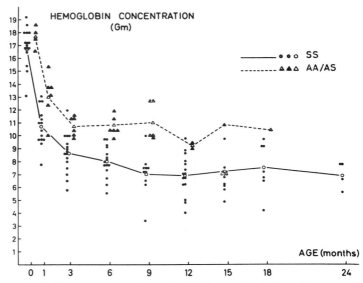

Figure 6–7   Development of anemia in infants with sickle cell anemia (SS) diagnosed at birth. The evolution of the mean hemoglobin value of SS is compared with that of control infants (AS and AA). (From van Baelen et al., Ann. Soc. belge Méd. trop. *49*:157, 1969).

the smaller percentage of cells that can sickle in newborns, it is recommended that sickle cell preparations in such bloods be sealed with paraffin and observed for at least three to four hours before discarding as negative. In the study carried out by Minnich et al. (1962), the actual concentration of Hb S was determined in those infants with positive sickle cell preparations. The amount of Hb S in the cord bloods varied from 1.7 to 8.5 per cent, with a mean of 4.2 per cent. No correlation was found between the concentration of Hb S in cord blood and

Table 6–6   Incidence of Sickling in Negro Newborns

| | | | Positive Sickle Prep. | |
| | | | *(%) Sickle Cells* | |
Author and Year	No. of Cases Studied	*Frequency (%)*	Mean	Range
Scott, 1948	262	3.4	–	0.5–40
Watson, 1948	226	8.4	11.0	0.5–29.5
Schneider, 1955	84	8.3	–	3–15
Minnich, 1962	449	10.5	5.1	0.9–13.0

the actual per cent of red blood cells that could be sickled. Serial values obtained in five of these infants with sickle cell trait showed a parallel increase in Hb A and Hb S, reaching levels comparable to those found in adults with sickle cell trait within three to eight months.

Danger of Exchange Transfusion with Sickle Cell Trait Blood. Fatal intravascular sickling in the newborn has been reported in an icteric white premature infant who received an exchange transfusion with blood from a donor with sickle cell trait (Veiga and Vaithanathan, 1963). The infant died five days later, following a period of hypoxia and dehydration. Autopsy revealed generalized intravascular sickling with focal infarcts in the brain. Although this is a very rare occurrence, it indicates the need to perform a sickle cell preparation on Negro donor blood that is being cross-matched for exchange transfusion in newborns. Blood from donors with sickle cell trait, although safe for ordinary transfusion in adults, should not be used for exchange transfusion or given to infants with hypoxia such as is seen in respiratory distress syndrome.

Fetal Hemoglobinopathies

Abnormal fetal hemoglobins may result from an alteration in the chemical structure of either the α chain or the γ chain. Several examples of the α chain type have been described; in each case the total alkali-resistant hemoglobin consisted of not only the normal Hb F but also the abnormal Hb F. These fetal variants have usually been detected in cord bloods, either during the course of family studies of adults with α chain hemoglobinopathies or in the course of screening large numbers of cord bloods for abnormal hemoglobins. In most cases, there were no associated clinical or hematologic abnormalities such as jaundice or anemia. The infants inherited the abnormal α chain from one of the parents, who showed the adult form of the abnormal hemoglobin. As the infant grew older and the γ chains were replaced by β chains, both types of Hb F were replaced by their corresponding adult hemoglobins. The main significance of these observations lies in their indication of identity of the genes controlling synthesis of the α chains of Hb F and Hb A.

Hb F variants resulting from an abnormal γ chain are exceedingly rare. Because they are not associated with any hematologic disturbances and they are limited to the period of γ chain synthesis, they are detected only during the course of screening large numbers of cord bloods by electrophoretic methods. A number of such hemoglobin variants have been described and are listed in Table 6–7. Their electrophoretic mobilities are shown in Figure 6–8. The concentration of these hemoglobins in cord blood is approximately 10

Table 6–7   Gamma Chain Hb F Variants

Authors	Year	Hb F Variant	Source	Amino Acid Substitution
Fessas et al.	1959	Alexandra	Greece	12 Thre → Lys°
Fessas et al.	1961	Aegina	Greece	—
Silvestroni and Bianco	1963	Roma	Italy	—
Schneider and Jones	1964	Texas I	Black	5 Glu → Lys°°
Larkin et al.	1968	Texas II	Britain	6 Glu → Lys°°
Huisman et al.	1965	Warren°°°	Black	—
Schneider et al.	1966	Houston°°°	Black	—
Sacker et al.	1967	Hull	Britain	121 Glu → Lys
Gauchi et al.	1969	Malta	Malta	117 His → Arg

Amino acid substitutions (number refers to position in gamma chain) determined later by Loukopoulos et al. (1969)° and by Jenkins et al. (1967).°°
°°°These variants may be identical.

to 20 per cent of the total hemoglobin. Each of these variants shares the other characteristics of Hb F, such as resistance to denaturation by alkali, ultraviolet spectral pattern, cathodal mobility on agar gel electrophoresis, and gradual disappearance during the first few months of life.

Hb Barts is a fast hemoglobin found in cord blood, sharing many of the previously mentioned properties of Hb F. Hb Barts is a tetramer consisting of four normal γ chains (designated γ₄), resulting from a relative deficiency of α chain synthesis, and it is therefore discussed in the section under α thalassemia (p. 160). Other tetramer hemoglobins occurring in the newborn but involving abnormal β chains

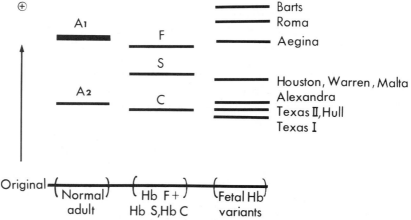

Figure 6–8 Relative mobilities on starch gel electrophoresis of Hb F variants at pH 8.6 (right), compared to hemoglobins of normal adult and common variants (Hb S and Hb C).

such as those found in Hb S and Hb C are also discussed in that section.

Thalassemia Syndromes

The thalassemia syndromes are a group of inherited disorders of hemoglobin synthesis in which there is a specific impairment of production of one of the polypeptide chains of globin. This results in a hypochromic microcytic anemia of varying severity, associated with alterations in the composition and types of the hemoglobin within the erythrocyte. Depending on the type of chain defect, the disorders may be classified as α thalassemia (including Hb H and Hb Barts) or β thalassemia. β thalassemia is the usual form seen in Mediterranean persons, in either the heterozygous state as thalassemia minor manifesting typically with mild anemia and increased Hb A_2 levels, or the homozygous state as thalassemia major (or Cooley's anemia) manifesting with severe anemia requiring frequent blood transfusions, hepatosplenomegaly, and high levels of Hb F. Other less common forms of thalassemia have been described, including Hb Lepore (a hemoglobin with S-like mobility resulting from fusion of portions of the β chain and the δ chain) and δ thalassemia (resulting in decreased synthesis of Hb A_2).

Occurrence in the Newborn Period. α thalassemia manifests mainly at birth, when Hb F is the major fraction that contains α chains. As Hb F is replaced by Hb A in the first few months of life, increasing β chain synthesis takes place; the manifestations of β thalassemia therefore becoming increasingly evident.

Significance of Hb Barts in Cord Blood. Hb Barts is a tetramer consisting of γ chains (γ_4) but no α chains (Hunt and Lehmann, 1959). It was first described at St. Bartholomew's Hospital in London, England, in an infant whose red cell morphology resembled that seen in thalassemia (Ager and Lehmann, 1958). Since then it has been reported not only in other newborns with a mild hemolytic anemia, but also in minute amounts in normal cord blood (Fessas and Mastrokalos, 1959). It is generally felt that Hb Barts results from defective synthesis of α chains, the relative excess of γ chains polymerizing to form the γ_4 tetramer. In the case of the normal newborn in which only trace amounts (< 1.0 per cent) of Hb Barts are found (Weatherall, 1963), there may actually be a slight excess in production of γ chains. Because γ chains are thought to compete less effectively for α chains than do the β chains, the free γ_2 subunits polymerize to form the γ_4 molecule of Hb Barts. Where an inherited defect of α chain synthesis also exists, relatively large amounts (5 to 25 per cent) of Hb Barts result, often associated with abnormal red cell morphology and hemolytic anemia (Weatherall, 1963; Horton et al., 1962). It is this second group on which we now focus our attention.

Alpha Thalassemia in the Newborn—Barts Hemoglobinopathy

Alpha thalassemia is an inherited disorder in which impaired synthesis of α chains during the neonatal period results in the formation of a γ chain tetramer known as Hb Barts. Although the genetic aspects of this condition are not fully understood, there appear to be two main types: heterozygous and homozygous.

Heterozygous. Such newborns are usually clinically and hematologically normal, with Hb Barts being detected during a survey of cord bloods by electrophoresis. In some cases, however, the infant may present with a hemolytic anemia of mild to moderate degree, associated with reticulocytosis and abnormal red cell morphology consisting of target cells, hypochromia, and microcytosis. Hb Barts, initially present in concentrations of 5 to 25 per cent, gradually disappears over the first three to four months of life (parallel with the decrease in Hb F concentration), after which the infant appears normal except for the minimal hematologic signs of α thalassemia trait (p. 161). Family studies in such cases have shown signs of α thalassemia trait in one (or both) of the parents.

Homozygous. Nearly 100 cases of homozygous α thalassemia have now been reported (Lie-Injo, 1962; Pootrakul et al., 1967; Todd et al., 1967; Thumasathit et al., 1968; Lie-Injo et al., 1968). Most have occurred in the Far East, among infants of Chinese, Indonesian and Malaysian backgrounds, as expected from the relatively high incidence of α thalassemia trait in these populations. Although the majority of the reported infants were stillborn at gestational ages ranging from 28 to 38 weeks, a number were born alive but died from one to 70 minutes after birth (Kan et al., 1967; Thumasathit et al., 1968). The clinical picture is uniformly that of severe hydrops fetalis (without evidence of isoimmunization), ascites, and gross hepatomegaly with only minimal splenomegaly. The latter finding contrasts with that in hydrops fetalis due to blood group incompatibility, in which the degree of splenomegaly parallels the degree of hepatomegaly. Marked pallor due to severe hemolytic anemia occurred in these infants, who did not live long enough to develop jaundice. On electrophoresis, all the hemoglobin was composed of Hb Barts. Cases in which both parents could be studied gave evidence of α thalassemia trait.

Incidence. Heterozygous α thalassemia, diagnosed by the presence of increased levels of Hb Barts in cord blood, has been found in a number of racial and ethnic groups throughout the world. In contrast to β thalassemia, which is found mainly in Mediterranean persons, α thalassemia occurs with greatest frequency in Orientals and Negroes. Studies among Negro newborns in Baltimore and St. Louis reveal incidences of 2.1 and 7.1 per cent respectively (Weatherall, 1963; Minnich et al., 1962), which is somewhat less than the figures obtained in similar studies in Africa (9.3 to 17.9 per cent). Among Orientals, the incidence varies from about 3 per cent in Chinese to 6 per cent in Indonesians and Malaysians (see Table 6–8). Cases of hydrops fetalis due to homozygous α thalassemia have been reported mainly among Orientals to date. In view of the relatively high incidence of α thalassemia trait among Negroes, the absence of reports of newborns with hydrops suggests that α thalassemia in this group differs from that described in other races. To date, the only cases reported from the United States and Canada involved a Filipino infant (Pearson et al., 1965) and three Chinese infants (Nathan et al., 1966; Kan et al., 1967). A Greek Cypriot infant with this condition was reported from England by Diamond et al. (1965).

Laboratory Findings. Heterozygous Form. The usual hematologic findings consist of a mild degree of hypochromia, microcytosis, and occasional target cells, with little or no anemia. Among 46 Thai infants detected during a survey of cord bloods for Barts hemoglobin (Pootrakul et al., 1967), the mean hemoglobin concentration was 14.2 gm./100 ml., slightly but significantly lower than that of the control group, and the range of two standard deviations extended from 10.6 to 17.8 gm./100 ml. Reticulocyte counts and levels of alkali-

Table 6–8   Incidence of Increased Levels of Hb Barts in Cord Blood

Source	Author and Year	No. Studied	Hb (%) Barts
Far East			
Thailand	Tuchinda, 1959	415	5.2
	Pootrakul, 1967	1100	6.2
	Na-Nakorn, 1970	287	30.7
Singapore	Vella, 1959	1962	3.3 (Chinese)
		555	0.4 (Indonesian)
Djakarta	Eng, 1959	633	3.3 (Chinese)
		480	0.4 (Indonesian)
Hong Kong	Todd, 1969	500	3.0 (Chinese)
Mediterranean			
Italy	Silvestrone, 1962	3556	0.3
Sardinia	DeLuca, 1968	200	6.0
Africa			
Nigeria	Hendrickse, 1960	140	10.7
Sudan	Ventruto, 1963	64	9.3
Senegal	Oudart, 1968	345	1.75
Congo	van Baelen, 1969	636	17.9
United States (Negroes)			
St. Louis	Minnich, 1962	449	7.1
Baltimore	Weatherall, 1963	900	2.1
Galveston	Schneider, 1971	7018	4.3

resistant hemoglobin did not differ significantly from the controls. Similar findings were obtained by Todd et al. (1969) among 15 Chinese newborns with this condition. In addition, these authors noted a decrease in osmotic fragility, due to the presence of thin, hypochromic erythrocytes. The diagnosis is made by the finding of Hb Barts on electrophoresis. At alkaline pH, this hemoglobin migrates as a fast hemoglobin, between Hb A and Hb H. Definite identification and separation from other fast hemoglobin variants can be made better by electrophoresis at pH 7.0. In such a case, only Hb Barts and Hb H migrate toward the anode, the former slightly slower than the latter. Trace amounts of Hb Barts may be found in normal cord bloods. Levels in excess of 1 per cent are felt to indicate the existence of α thalassemia (Na-Nakorn et al., 1969). In such infants, the levels of Hb Barts average around 6.5 per cent and may range as high as 10 to 15 per cent (Pootrakul et al., 1967; Todd et al., 1969). The genetic implication of the amount of Hb Barts in an individual infant will be discussed below. In most cases in the newborn period, a small amount of Hb H (β_4) accompanies Hb Barts. This is further evidence of a common deficiency of α chain synthesis as the mechanism for the formation of these two hemoglobin tetramers. The concentration of Hb Barts gradually decreases after birth, in parallel with the normal postnatal decrease in Hb F concentration. By the time the infant is three to four months of age, Hb Barts is usually no longer detectable. From this age on, the child seems to be normal except for the minimal hematologic signs of α thalassemia trait, including mild anemia (hemoglobin, 9 to 11 gm./100 ml.), slight hypochromia, microcytosis and target cells on blood smear, decreased osmotic fragility, and normal levels of Hb A_2 and Hb F. Family studies usually reveal similar findings in one of the parents. Such persons with α thalassemia trait may show small inclusions in a few of the red cells upon incubation of whole blood with brilliant cresyl blue. (Fessas, 1961).

Homozygous Form.   Based on combined data from 43 hydropic infants reported from the Far East by Lie-Injo (1962), Todd et al. (1967) and Thumasathit et al. (1968), a fairly uniform hematologic picture emerges. Severe hemolytic anemia is evidenced by hemoglobin concentrations varying between 3 and 11 gm./100 ml., reticulocyte counts of 10 to 20 per cent, and extreme erythroblastosis, with as many as 1000 to 2000 nucleated red cells per 100 white cells. Serum bilirubin levels were only slightly increased (highest 2.9 mg./100 ml.). Morphologic abnormalities were striking and consisted of marked hypochromia, poikilocytosis, and target cells. Such abnormalities in the presence of a negative Coombs test exclude erythroblastosis due to blood group incompatibility, the other major cause of neonatal hydrops. Unstained wet preparations may show sickling after a few hours at room temperature (in the absence of Hb S). Upon incubation with brilliant cresyl blue, intracellular crystals may develop, owing to precipitation of the unstable Hb Barts within the erythrocyte. Such inclusions are probably the same as those described in similarly treated samples of blood from persons with Hb H, another form of α thalassemia. Hemoglobin electrophoresis reveals almost 100 per cent Hb Barts, with small amounts of an unidentified component migrating between Hb A and Hb H.* Specialized techniques indicate that Hb F and Hb A are entirely absent (Todd et al., 1967; Kan et al., 1968). The lowered values for alkali-resistant hemoglobin (35 to 75 per cent, compared to 90 to 95 per cent expected in infants of comparable gestational age) are explained entirely, therefore, on the basis of an intermediate degree of alkali-resistance of Hb Barts.

Pathogenesis. In the heterozygous form, partial deficiency of α chain synthesis results in a mild thalassemia-like condition at birth characterized by variable depression of Hb F ($\alpha_2\gamma_2$) synthesis, the excess γ chains combining to form the γ_4 tetramer of Hb Barts. In the homozygous form, marked depression of α chain synthesis results in almost complete replacement of Hb F by Hb Barts. The recent observation by Horton et al. (1962) that the oxygen dissociation curve of Hb Barts lacks the sigmoidal shape of normal Hb F and Hb A, thereby resulting in impaired release of oxygen to the tissues at low tensions, is of help in explaining the occurrence in these infants of hydrops fetalis in the presence of a degree of anemia that is less than that usually seen in hydrops associated with blood group incompatibility (Fig. 6–9). Heart failure leading to generalized hydrops in α

---

*Todd et al. have identified this component as Hb Portland I, a hybrid hemoglobin lacking α chains (see p. 149).

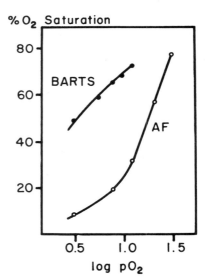

Figure 6–9 Oxygen dissociation curves of hemoglobin components of cord blood. Hb Barts and the Hb A and Hb F mixture (abscissa refers to the logarithm of the oxygen tension). (From Horton, B. F., et al.: *Blood,* 20:302, 1962.)

thalassemia, therefore, is a consequence of anoxia due both to anemia and to a poorly functioning hemoglobin.

Genetic Variants of α Thalassemia. Aside from the dosage differences described above (heterozygous and homozygous states), variations in expression of this gene in Blacks (see p. 161) and the peculiar genetic status of individuals with Hb H disease have suggested the possibility of different forms of the α thalassemia gene. Hemoglobin H disease appears best explained by the interaction of two α thalassemia genes of differing severity, one typical of that seen in the parents of the hydropic infants described above (severe—"α thalassemia$_1$") and another showing no hematologic abnormality (mild—"α thalassemia$_2$"). Support for this hypothesis is derived from a study of newborn offspring of families in which one parent had Hb H disease (Na-Nakorn et al., 1969). Hb Barts was found in 30 of 31 infants studied, with its concentration segregating into two groups, either 1 to 2 per cent (α thal$_2$) or 5 to 6 per cent (α thal$_1$). Four newborns who had Hb Barts concentrations in the range of 24 to 29 per cent (Pootrakul et al., 1967) appear to represent cases of Hb H disease (α thal$_1$, α thal$_2$). This relationship is summarized in Table 6–9. From the absence of case reports of hydrops due to α thalassemia among Negroes, one might infer that the gene in this racial group is of the milder variety, and therefore associated with very low concentrations of Hb Barts in the cord blood of heterozygous infants. However, the studies of Minnich et al. (1962) and Weatherall (1963) show Hb Barts concentrations varying from 2 to 13 per cent. Application of more precise techniques for quantitating α chain synthesis (Kan, Schwartz and Nathan, 1968) in the study of newborn heterozygotes for α thalassemia may help resolve some of these genetic variations.

Treatment. In most cases of heterozygous α thalassemia in the newborn, no treatment is necessary. If anemia should occur and persist, transfusion with packed cells may be required. This decision should be tempered by the knowledge that the natural course of this condition is one of gradual improvement by three to four months of life. Infants with homozygous α thalassemia usually die in utero because of severe hydrops fetalis, the stillbirth occurring soon afterward. It is conceivable that, if this condition could be anticipated early in

Table 6–9   Genetic Variants of α Thalassemia

Approx. Concentration of Hb Barts (%) (cord blood)	Genotype	Phenotype
1–2	α thal$_2$	"Silent carrier"
5–6	α thal$_1$	Mild anemia (trait)
26	α thal$_1$, α thal$_2$	Hb H disease
80–100	α thal$_1$, α thal$_1$	Hydrops fetalis

gestation, intrauterine intraperitoneal transfusions might be considered. However, one would expect that such a child, even if it survived, would be left with a condition resembling severe thalassemia major, which itself is usually fatal.

Prognosis. Infants with heterozygous α thalassemia, as they lose their Hb Barts in the first few months of life, are left with the signs of α thalassemia trait, which persists throughout life. The degree of this abnormality varies greatly among different individuals.

Combination of α Thalassemia with Abnormal Hemoglobins

In a Negro family studied by Huisman (1960), a normal mother and a father with combined sickle cell trait and α thalassemia trait produced an infant whose cord blood showed, in addition to Hb F and Hb A, two abnormal hemoglobins. One of these was Hb S, present in a concentration of 0.8 per cent (compared to approximately 6.5 per cent Hb S in the average newborn with sickle cell trait). The other, a fast hemoglobin migrating like Hb Barts, consisted entirely of the β chains of Hb S. The latter tetramer, (β^{S}_{4}) was called Hb Augusta I. Its concentration decreased from 3.2 per cent at birth to 2.1 per cent at 45 days of age, concurrent with an increase of Hb S to 1.9 per cent. These observations are consistent with the hypothesis that deficiency of α chain synthesis resulted in the lower concentration of Hb S $(\alpha^{A}_{2}\beta^{S}_{2})$ with the excess β chains of sickle hemoglobin combining to form the tetramer β^{S}_{4}. Another infant in this report by Huisman showed a comparable situation, resulting in a tetramer of the β chains of Hb C (β^{C}_{4}); this was called Hb Augusta II.

Beta Thalassemia in the Newborn (Cooley's Anemia Thalassemia, or Mediterranean Anemia)

Beta thalassemia is an inherited disorder in which impaired synthesis of β chains results in an anemia that becomes increasingly prominent in the first few months after birth. It occurs in heterozygous and homozygous forms, usually designated thalassemia minor or trait and thalassemia major, respectively. Thalassemia minor is usually manifested as a mild hypochromic microcytic anemia unassociated with clinical symptoms. Thalassemia major, in its fully manifest state, consists of severe anemia requiring frequent blood transfusions and displaying marked hepatosplenomegaly, bony changes due to marrow hyperplasia, stunting of physical growth, and progressive hemosiderosis. Marked elevation of Hb F concentration characterizes this homozygous form of the disorder.

Because β chain synthesis is normally low at birth, as reflected by the low concentration of Hb A $(\alpha_2\beta_2)$, in relation to Hb F $(\alpha_2\gamma_2)$, a hereditary defect in synthesis of β chains would not be expected to affect total hemoglobin concentration until after the first few months of life when Hb A becomes the predominant fraction. Therefore, the clinical symptoms due to anemia, such as pallor, irritability, and poor feeding, would become increasingly evident during this period.

Incidence.   Beta thalassemia occurs mainly in persons from the Mediterranean countries, including Greece, Italy, Sardinia, and Turkey. The incidence of the heterozygous form varies approximately from 1 to 10 per cent in different localities of these countries.

Clinical Manifestations in the Neonatal Period.   Although most children with thalassemia major are diagnosed by the end of the first year of life, the earliest onset of symptoms is usually not until two to three months of age, for the reasons just given. In an infant followed from birth by us (we were alerted by this condition in an older sibling), significant pallor and anemia (Hb 8.5 gm./100 ml.) were first evident at seven weeks of age. Listlessness, irritability, and poor feeding became evident over the next few weeks, in association with a decrease in hemoglobin concentration to 5.2 gm./100 ml. by 12 weeks of age. At this time, the liver and spleen were first noted to be enlarged, both palpable 2 cm. below the costal margins. Following blood transfusion, the course of the disease in this child was that of typical thalassemia major in its fully manifest state. A similar sequence of events was described in two infants reported from Cyprus by Banton (1951) and in three infants observed in New York by Erlandson and Hilgartner (1959).

Laboratory Findings.   THALASSEMIA TRAIT.   At birth, target cells and slight hypochromia may be seen on careful examination of the blood smear. Hb A_2 levels, which are usually increased in adults with classic β thalassemia trait, have not been adequately studied in newborns with this condition. The normal newborn shows very low levels of Hb A_2 (p. 136). Hb F concentration, usually normal or only slightly increased in adults with thalassemia trait, shows no significant alteration during the newborn period.

THALASSEMIA MAJOR.   This condition can be diagnosed with reasonable certainty within the first two months of life. Although significant anemia may not be evident until two to three months of age or later, careful hematologic examination and serial measurement of Hb F concentration from birth can help to establish an early diagnosis. Morphologic abnormalities, such as target cells, hypochromia, and poikilocytosis, may be present to a minor but definite degree at birth. These changes become increasingly prominent with age, and by two to three months of life they are accompanied by increased numbers of nucleated red cells in the peripheral blood. The most important early laboratory sign of thalassemia major is an increased concentration of Hb F. In comparison with the range of normal values at a given age during the first few months of life, (see Fig. 6–5), the values in infants who are in the stage of development of thalassemia major are definitely increased (Erlandson and Hilgartner, 1959; Mollica, 1962). Furthermore, the rate of fall of Hb F concentration is much slower than in normals or in thalassemia heterozygotes. Serial values are therefore of great help in early diagnosis of the homozygote. The development of these abnormalities is depicted in Figure 6–10.

Recent advances leading to the direct measurement of rates of synthesis of the various polypeptide chains of hemoglobin have enabled diagnosis of both the heterozygous and homozygous forms of thalassemia at the time of birth. In a newborn infant who did not show the typical hematologic findings of thalassemia trait until four months of age, Kan and Nathan (1968) demonstrated an approximately half-normal incorporation of C^{14}-labeled leucine into beta chains (indicative of reduced beta chain synthesis). Gaburro and associates (1970), using H^3 (tritium)-labeled amino acids, demonstrated complete absence of beta chain synthesis in two infants who were later

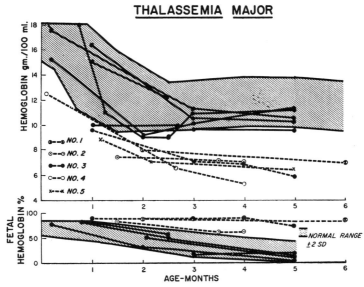

Figure 6–10 Progression of hematologic findings in thalassemia major in five infants followed from birth. Interrupted lines represent patients and solid lines represent normal or heterozygous infants. (From Erlandson, M. E., and Hilgartner, M.: *Journal of Pediatrics, 54:*566, 1959.)

shown to have thalassemia major. Although at present the complexity of these techniques limits their application to certain specialized centers, their ultimate value may be more evident with the development of improved methods of treatment such as bone marrow transplantation, the success of which may depend on application at a very early age.

Treatment. As soon as significant anemia develops, a program of periodic blood transfusions should be initiated. In uncomplicated typical thalassemia major, this usually does not occur until at least three to four months of age and often later.

Prognosis. Although there is wide variation in the severity of this disease, in its typical form it is usually fatal by late childhood or adolescence.

Gamma and Beta Thalassemia in the Newborn

Kan and co-workers (1972) described a newborn who presented at one day of age with jaundice, hepatosplenomegaly, and a severe hemolytic anemia characterized by hypochromia and target cells. Other causes of hypochromia and hemolysis were excluded. Hemoglobin F level was slightly reduced (52 per cent).

Beta thalassemia trait was suggested by the finding in the father and several of his relatives (all of English extraction) of hypochromic, microcytic erythrocytes associated with evidence of impaired β chain synthesis (using C^{14}-labeled leucine). In the infant, the rate of synthesis of *both* β and γ chains was reduced. Follow-up study over the first five months of life showed a gradual subsidence of the anemia. The defect in β chain synthesis persisted whereas γ chain synthesis fell even further, parallel to that expected in the normal infant during this period. Of interest was a history of neonatal jaundice among several of the affected relatives, a few of whom also received blood transfusions.

Combined γ and β thalassemia must now be added to homozygous α thalassemia as disorders of hemoglobin synthesis that may present at birth with a picture resembling erythroblastosis fetalis. The possibility that isolated depression of synthesis of γ chains (γ thalassemia) may cause milder degrees of transient neonatal anemia has been suggested recently by Stamatoyannopoulos (1971). If the mutation affects the gene regulating synthesis of γ^G chains, the anemia would be expected to be more severe than if it affected the gene for γ^A chains, since the former represent 75 per cent of the fetal hemoglobin present at birth and the latter only 25 per cent. Reduced concentrations of fetal hemoglobin in an anemic newborn might provide the clue to further biochemical investigations in pursuit of this diagnosis.

METHEMOGLOBINEMIA

Methemoglobinemia is characterized by a diffuse slate gray cyanosis resulting from excessive amounts of methemoglobin in the erythrocytes. This disorder occurs particularly in the newborn period and should be considered along with cardiac and pulmonary disorders in the differential diagnosis of all infants with cyanosis. The main causes of methemoglobinemia are: exposure to certain oxidizing agents and drugs, deficiency of one of the enzymes necessary for reduction of methemoglobin, and the presence of an abnormal methemoglobin, and the presence of an abnormal methemoglobin resistant to reduction (so-called hemoglobin M diseases).

Pathogenesis. Methemoglobin is the oxidized derivative of hemoglobin, in which the iron of the heme groups is changed from the usual ferrous (Fe^{++}) to the ferric (Fe^{+++}) state. As a consequence, the iron is no longer able to form a complex with oxygen, and methemoglobin is therefore unable to function in oxygen transport.

In the normal person, small amounts of methemoglobin are being continually formed. The concentration in the blood, however, is maintained below approximately 1 per cent by certain physiologic mechanisms. The most important of these is methemoglobin reductase, or diaphorase, and its cofactor reduced nicotinamide adenine dinucleotide ($NADH_2$).* Another enzymatic pathway is provided by the reduced nicotinamide adenine dinucleotide phosphate ($NADPH_2$)-dependent methemoglobin reductase. The source of $NADH_2$ and $NADPH_2$ is discussed in Chapter Five (p. 91). This latter enzyme system is stimulated by methylene blue, thus providing in patients with a deficiency of the $NADH_2$-dependent diaphorase an effective means of reducing methemoglobin. Other agents, such as ascorbic acid, glutathione, and ergothioneine, may act directly to reduce methemoglobin. The relationship of these various factors regulating formation and reduction of methemoglobin is illustrated in Figure 6–11.

Increased amounts of methemoglobin may occur as a result of an increased formation of methemoglobin and an impaired reduction of methemoglobin.

INCREASED FORMATION OF METHEMOGLOBIN. Increased amounts of methemoglobin may be formed because of exposure to drugs or toxic agents that oxidize hemoglobin directly, such as nitrates (from contaminated well water), sodium nitrate, bismuth subnitrate, benzocaine, and aniline dyes. Although contaminated well water has accounted for most instances of methemoglobinemia from drinking water, the possibility that tap water from municipal sources may also

---

*Alternate terms for $NADH_2$ and $NADPH_2$ are reduced diphosphopyridine nucleotide (DPNH) and reduced triphosphopyridine nucleotide (TPNH).

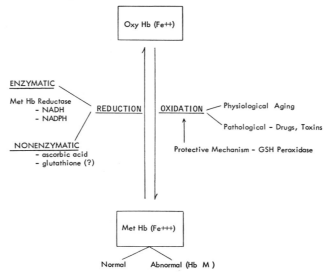

Figure 6–11   Pathogenesis of methemoglobinemia.

cause this problem should not be overlooked, especially when no other offending agent is evident (Vigil et al., 1965; Aussannaire et al., 1968). Administration of methemoglobinemia-producing agents to the mother prior to delivery should also be suspected when the cyanosis is present at birth; the use of prilocaine, a local anesthetic for obstetric analgesia, is a notable example of this (Climie et al., 1967). A list of agents to which the newborn may be exposed is given in Table 6–10. It is important to recognize that the newborn infant is unusually susceptible to the development of methemoglobinemia on exposure to such agents. This is well illustrated by the infant who develops methemoglobinemia from ingestion of an artificial formula

Table 6–10   Agents That May Cause Methemoglobinemia in the Newborn

Agent	Source
Nitrates ($\longrightarrow$ nitrites)	Well water (contaminated)
	Bismuth subnitrate (antidiarrheal)
Nitrites (ethyl)	Sweet spirit of nitre
Aniline derivatives	Diaper marking dyes
	Disinfectants (e.g., TCC, or trichlorocarbanilide)
	Benzocaine (skin applications)
Resorcin	Skin applications
Acetophenetidin	Analgesic compounds
Prilocaine	Local obstetrical analgesic
Sulfonamides (older)	Sulfanilamide, sulfathiazole, sulfapyridine

made from well water containing large quantities of nitrates, although older members of the family drinking the same water remain unaffected. This peculiar handicap of the newborn is transient and probably reflects two biochemical abnormalities. (1) There is increased sensitivity of fetal erythrocytes to oxidizing agents causing formation of fetal methemoglobin (Betke et al., 1956). Martin and Huisman (1963) showed this to be a function of the γ chain of Hb F. (2) There is decreased activity of the $NADH_2$-dependent methemoglobin diaphorase. Ross (1963) showed that the level of this enzyme in cord blood erythrocytes was reduced to approximately 60 per cent of that in the erythrocytes of normal adults. Even greater reduction in activity was found in prematures compared to that in term infants. Bartos and Desforges (1966) have shown that this low enzyme activity persists through the first four months of life, the age beyond which the incidence of well water methemoglobinemia declines strikingly. In this condition, the nitrates of well water are reduced to nitrites by coliform bacteria in the upper gastrointestinal tract, and it is the absorbed nitrite that causes formation of methemoglobin. Earlier studies by Cornblath and Hartmann (1948) suggested that the susceptibility of the newborn to this type of methemoglobinemia is related to decreased gastric acidity, permitting growth of such nitrate-reducing bacteria. This view no longer seems tenable in view of the more recent demonstration of the aforementioned defects in the erythrocyte, which would explain the sensitivity of the newborn to methemoglobinemia resulting not only from nitrates but also from other agents.

Impaired Reduction of Methemoglobin. This may result from a deficiency of $NADH_2$-dependent methemoglobin diaphorase (reductase), which may be transient as in the normal newborn, or permanent as in the condition known as congenital or hereditary methemoglobinemia. This is transmitted by an autosomal recessive gene. Affected homozygotes are cyanotic from birth and show almost complete lack of enzyme activity, whereas heterozygotes are generally not cyanotic, have intermediate degrees of enzyme deficiency, and show normal levels of methemoglobin (Scott, 1960). About seven cases of this type of hereditary methemoglobinemia have been diagnosed during the newborn period, cyanosis usually being evident at the time of delivery (Nurse, 1960; Lees and Jolly, 1957; and Dine, 1956). In two unusual reports, transient neonatal cyanosis was present in infants *heterozygous* for the enzyme deficiency (Harper et al., 1968; Lo et al., 1970).

Reduction of methemoglobin is also impaired by the presence of an abnormal methemoglobin resistant to reduction by the normal enzymatic mechanism. The group of abnormal hemoglobins with this property are collectively designated hemoglobin M diseases or hemoglobinopathy M. As in the other hemoglobinopathies, there is a single amino acid substitution in the globin moiety, but in this case the location of the substitution is near the heme groups so that the new amino acid forms a stable complex with the oxidized (ferric) heme, preventing its reduction to the ferrous form. Such a substitution may occur at one of several positions in the α or the β chains of the globin moiety, thus explaining the large number of chemically different hemoglobins M (Gerald and Efron, 1963). At birth, however, synthesis of α chains predominates over synthesis of β chains. Therefore, it is only the M hemoglobins of the α chain type that are associated with *congenital* cyanosis, owing to the presence of the fetal form of the abnormal methemoglobin (Farmer et al., 1964). The onset of cyanosis in Hb M of the β chain type is usually at around two to four months of age. In contrast with hereditary methemoglobinemia due to enzyme deficiency, the Hb M diseases are inherited by an autosomal dominant mode of transmission.

Clinical Manifestations. Methemoglobinemia presents with generalized cyanosis, with maximal intensity in the buccal mucous membranes, lips, nose, cheeks, fingers, and toes. The cyanosis has been described as dusky, slate gray, brownish, or violet. The characteristic feature is the absence of respiratory distress except when very high levels of methemoglobin are reached. The onset of cyanosis without dyspnea in a previously pink infant suggests acquired methemoglobinemia due to toxins or drugs, whereas cyanosis from birth favors one of the hereditary conditions previously mentioned, or an agent received via the mother prior to delivery.

The main problems in differential diagnosis are congenital cardiac conditions, associated with right-to-left shunt (e.g., transposition of the great vessels or tetralogy of Fallot) and severe pulmonary disorders. The absence of respiratory distress, pulmonary râles, and cardiac murmurs will usually exclude these disorders. A normal chest x-ray and electrocardiogram are of further help. A simple, rapid bedside test for methemoglobinemia has been described by Harley and Cellermajer (1970). This "red-brown" screening test consists of collecting drops of capillary blood from the infant's heel and from a normal adult control on a piece of Whatman No. 1 filter paper. The paper is waved gently in the air for about 30 seconds to oxygenate the blood. If the infant's blood appears chocolate brown in comparison to the red blood of the control, one may predict a methemoglobin level of greater than ten per cent. Since levels less than this do not usually produce detectable cyanosis, the sensitivity of this test renders it clinically useful, especially when the need for treatment may be urgent.

Laboratory Diagnosis.   Blood from such infants is brown in the test tube and does not turn red on shaking with air, as described above. The presence of methemoglobin may be confirmed spectro-scopically by demonstrating the characteristic absorption peak at 634 mμ, which disappears on addition of cyanide. Based on this prop-erty, various methods of determining the precise concentration of methemoglobin are available, the most popular of which is that described by Evelyn and Malloy (1938). In normal adults, methemo-globin levels average 0.82 per cent of the total hemoglobin, with a range of 0 to 1.9 per cent. Kravitz et al. (1956) found slightly higher levels in newborn infants during the first week of life. In prematures, a mean value of 2.3 per cent was found (range 0.08 to 4.4 per cent), compared to a mean of 1.5 per cent in term infants (range 0.0 to 2.8 per cent). Surprisingly, levels in cord blood were the same as in nor-mal adults, a finding that has since been confirmed by Betke (1964). Workers in Finland (Pihlaja et al., 1968), comparing blood samples of term newborns in the first 24 hours of life with samples obtained at 4 to 7 days of age, were unable to detect either an elevation in methemoglobin level or a difference between the levels at the two age periods. These divergent findings may be attributable to inac-curacies of the method of determination at this low range, and to possible environmental variations, such as the nitrate content of the drinking water.

Levels of methemoglobin in newborns with cyanosis due to methemoglobinemia generally exceed 10 per cent of the total hemo-globin, and they may be as high as 60 to 70 per cent in severely af-fected infants. Once an elevated methemoglobin concentration is found, its cause must be sought, beginning with a careful examination of the infant's environment for possible toxic agents (listed in Table 6–10). If the cyanosis occurs in a hospital nursery and other infants are affected, careful scrutiny of the hospital procedures for suspicious aniline-containing materials is imperative (Fisch et al., 1963). If this search is negative, assay of the infant's erythrocytes for activity of the enzyme $NADH_2$-dependent methemoglobin diaphorase (reduc-tase) should be carried out. In infants with methemoglobinemia due to a hereditary deficiency of this enzyme, activity is usually not demon-strable and therefore is easily distinguished from normal newborns, who show definite although reduced activity. This form of hereditary methemoglobinemia, along with acquired methemoglobinemia due to drugs and toxins, responds within one to two hours to injection of methylene blue in a dose of 1 to 2 mg./kg., intravenously. Recurrence of methemoglobinemia in the absence of re-exposure to toxins sug-gests hereditary methemoglobinemia due to enzyme deficiency. Methemoglobinemia persisting in spite of methylene blue adminis-tration is suggestive of an abnormal methemoglobin M. In this case, careful analysis of the absorption spectrum of a solution of the whole hemoglobin (or preferably of the electrophoretically purified hemoglobin M) usually reveals an abnormal spectrum, with the peak at 634 mμ displaced to the 600 mμ region of the spectrum. Hemoglobin electrophoresis in starch gel or starch block at pH 7.0 with the hemoglobin oxidized to methemoglobin by potassium ferricyanide will reveal the abnormal methemoglobin migrating less cathodally than normal methemoglobin A (Gerald, 1958).

The preceding diagnostic procedures are summarized in Table 6–11.

With methemoglobinemia caused by certain toxic agents such as the aniline derivative TCC (Table 6–10), a severe hemolytic anemia with jaundice may also occur (Quie et al., 1962).

Treatment. In a newborn with cyanosis suspected of being a result of methemoglobinemia, a single intravenous dose of methylene blue (1 to 2 mg./kg. as a 1 per cent solution in normal saline) is indicated. Subsequent therapy depends on the response to this trial dose, and the results of the other investigations just discussed. A favorable response consists of the disappearance of cyanosis and a sharp drop in methemoglobin level to normal limits within 60 minutes. Thus, in acquired methemoglobinemia, once the offending agent is recognized and removed, further treatment with methylene blue is usually not necessary. In hereditary methemoglobinemia due to enzyme deficiency, continued therapy is required. Although this is most effectively accomplished by methylene blue orally, the staining of non-disposable diapers due to the excretion of methylene blue in the urine may present a problem. In this case, ascorbic acid in large doses of 300 to 400 mg. orally per day may be tried.

Table 6–11   Investigation of a Newborn with
Methemoglobinemic Cyanosis

| | TYPE OF DISORDER | | |
| PROCEDURE | *Hereditary* | | *Acquired* |
	Enzyme Deficiency	*Hb M°*	
History			
Familial cyanosis	0	+	0
Presence at birth	+	+°	0
Toxic agents	0	0	+
Laboratory Findings			
Absorption spectrum of methemoglobin	Normal	Abnormal	Normal
NADH-methemoglobin reductase activity	↓ ↓ or 0	Normal	Normal
Hemoglobin electrophoresis (ph 7.0)	Normal	Hb M	Normal

°Only if defect is in alpha chain, resulting in a fetal methemoglobin M ($\alpha^{M}_{2}\gamma^{A}_{2}$).

Excessive doses of methylene blue in the treatment of methemoglobinemia in the newborn may damage the erythrocytes producing a hemolytic anemia of moderate severity (Goluboff and Wheaton, 1961). In the two cases reported by these authors, this complication resulted from failure to appreciate that the concentration of methylene blue in their preparation was 5 per cent rather than the usual 1 per cent. Although a dose of 0.5 to 1 cc. of 1 per cent solution of methylene blue is a safe dose, it is perhaps wiser to calculate the dose of methylene blue in the terms of milligrams as described previously and to administer this as a 1 per cent solution.

SULFHEMOGLOBINEMIA

Sulfhemoglobin is a derivative of hemoglobin resulting from exposure to certain oxidizing agents or to hydrogen sulfide. Its precise chemical nature and mode of production are not known. The absorption spectrum is characterized by a peak at 618 mμ which does *not* disappear with cyanide, in contrast to the 634 mμ peak of methemoglobin, which does disappear with cyanide.

In concentration greater than 0.5 gm./100 ml., cyanosis is clinically evident. Miller (1957) reported an infant with persistent cyanosis from birth who had increased sulfhemoglobin levels. The presence of cyanosis and sulfhemoglobinemia in the father and several other family members suggested a diagnosis of congenital sulfhemoglobinemia. However, the dominant inheritance in this family and the proximity of the sulfhemoglobin peak to that seen in some of the hemoglobin M diseases raise the question that this may in fact be a form of hemoglobin M disease (Gerald, 1965).

Chapter Seven

ERYTHROBLASTOSIS FETALIS

In the expanding list of conditions capable of causing hemolytic disease in the newborn, the condition due to blood group incompatibility still remains the most common and most important in terms of potential severity. Since the first unifying concept of the clinical syndromes previously known as icterus gravis neonatorum, congenital anemia of the newborn, and hydrops fetalis (Diamond et al., 1932), our knowledge and understanding of this condition have expanded considerably. The etiologic role of blood group incompatibility, first discovered in the Rh system by Levine in 1940; the development of the antiglobulin test for detection of antibody-coated red cells by Coombs in 1946; and the use of exchange transfusions by Diamond et al. (1947) in the treatment of the affected infant all represent major milestones in the unfolding history of erythroblastosis fetalis. As a consequence of these and other contributions, what was once a major cause of neonatal mortality and later neurologic handicap has now become a condition amenable to rational, effective treatment in the majority of cases, resulting in a normal healthy infant. The classic monograph by Allen and Diamond in 1957 reviews erythroblastosis fetalis in great depth and clarity, and is a basic prerequisite to an understanding of the problem of this disorder and the important advances that have occurred in recent years.

The purpose of this chapter is not to repeat what has already been well written nor to attempt to review the voluminous literature on this condition, but it is to summarize the present status and concepts of pathogenesis, diagnosis, and management, stressing recent advances and their relevance to prevention and amelioration of disease in the

176

newborn. Hopefully, proper application of such concepts, in particular the administration of anti-D gamma globulin to future Rh-negative mothers, will sufficiently diminish the incidence and severity of hemolytic disease of the newborn to render much of this chapter of largely historical interest by the end of this decade.

PATHOGENESIS

Fetal red cells, possessing an antigen lacking in those of the mother, cross the placenta into the maternal circulation, where they stimulate production of antibodies. These antibodies return to the fetal circulation, attach to the antigenic site on the surface of the red cell, and lead to eventual destruction of the cell. This hemolytic process takes place in utero and results in marked compensatory overproduction of young nucleated red cells in the fetal erythropoietic sites — thus the term erythroblastosis fetalis. Because compensation is usually not complete, varying degrees of anemia may develop in utero. Hyperbilirubinemia does not often become a problem until after birth, because bilirubin is removed by the placenta and taken into the maternal circulation.

Blood Group Incompatibility

ABO incompatibility accounts for approximately two-thirds of cases of hemolytic disease and Rh incompatibility for almost one-third (Allen and Diamond, 1957). The remainder, about 2 per cent, involves the minor blood factors — c, E, Kell and others.

In terms of severity, hemolytic disease due to Rh (D) incompatibility is by far the most important and therefore occupies the major portion of the subsequent discussion.

Effect of ABO Incompatibility on Rh Sensitization. Levine in 1943 noted a deficiency of ABO incompatible matings among the parents of infants with Rh hemolytic disease. He suggested that ABO incompatibility affords protection against Rh sensitization because such fetal red cells are destroyed by the anti-A or anti-B in the maternal circulation before sensitization to Rh can take place.

This protection is not absolute. Gunson in 1957 reported several cases of combined ABO and Rh incompatibility. In 1964 Donohue and Wake reviewed the ABO status in 438 families in which Rh sensitization had occurred, and they found nine families in which ABO incompatibility was present. It appears, therefore, that the protective effect is not an all-or-none phenomenon, implying that in some cases ABO incompatible red cells survive sufficiently long in the maternal circulation to stimulate production of antibodies to the Rh

factor. Vos (1965) obtained quantitative data to support this. In studying a large unselected group of Rh-sensitized mothers, he found that
the incidence of ABO incompatibility varied inversely with the
maternal Rh antibody titer at term. In mothers with low antibody
titers, the incidence of ABO incompatibility was the same as in the
normal population. In those with very high titers, a much lower incidence of ABO incompatibility was found. He suggested that the low
figures reported by many workers that formed the basis for the concept of the protective effect of ABO incompatibility were probably
a function of the bias introduced by selection of cases based on severity of previously affected infants.

Entry of Fetal Red Cells into the
Maternal Circulation

Although Levine et al. in 1941 postulated transfer of fetal red cells
across the placenta as the mechanism of maternal sensitization to Rh,
it was not until 13 years later that direct evidence for such transfer
became available. Chown (1954) used the technique of differential
agglutination to demonstrate small quantities of fetal cells in the
maternal blood in the first well documented case of neonatal anemia
due to fetomaternal transfusion. In both his case and in a similar one
reported by Gunson (1957) Rh antibodies appeared in the maternal
blood soon afterward. However, hemorrhage of this magnitude is
infrequent and unlikely to be the usual circumstance leading to Rh
sensitization. Much smaller hemorrhages (as little as 0.004 ml.) are
relatively common and may be detected by the acid elution technique
for staining erythrocytes containing Hb F (Chapter Three, p. 63).
With this method, Cohen et al. (1964) found fetal erythrocytes appearing by the third month of gestation and occurring in as many
as 50 per cent of ABO compatible mothers at term. In a later study
of ABO incompatible mothers at term, Cohen and Zuelzer (1967)
observed such transplacental hemorrhages (TPH) in only 20 per cent
of the mothers. Zipursky et al. (1963) made similar observations, but
because they included ABO incompatible pregnancies, the incidence
of fetal cells was only 15.8 per cent (in such pregnancies it is expected
that many ABO incompatible red cells would be destroyed by the
natural anti-A or anti-B as soon as they entered the maternal circulation). The volume of fetal blood in the maternal circulation was
estimated to be only 0.1 to 0.2 ml. in most of the cases, and this amount
was felt to be insufficient to produce primary sensitization. Based on
repeated injection studies of Rh-positive cord blood into adult Rh-
negative recipients, antibodies developed only after a total volume
of about 1.0 ml. was given. Zipursky and co-workers postulate the
mechanism of sensitization in pregnancy to consist of a primary

stimulus because of transfer of 0.5 ml. or more of fetal blood, antibodies usually appearing only after "booster" stimuli of smaller transfusions (of the order of 0.1 to 0.2 ml. of fetal blood) in subsequent
pregnancies. The importance of transplacental hemorrhage in the
pathogenesis of Rh sensitization has been since confirmed by several
groups. Sullivan and co-workers (1967) found antibodies within three
months of delivery in 20 per cent of Rh-negative women with TPH at
delivery, compared to only 3.7 per cent in those without TPH at
delivery. Comparable figures were obtained (14.3 and 3.0 per cent,
respectively) in a larger series studied by Zipursky and Israels (1967).
These workers noted, however, that *among women who became sensitized*, the majority had either no evidence of TPH after delivery or
had amounts considered insignificant (less than 0.1 ml.). They concluded that, in such women, sensitization must have resulted from an
antigenic stimulus prior to labor or perhaps as a result of a "small,"
frequently undetectable, hemorrhage during labor. On this basis,
they raised the question of the need for antenatal administration of
anti-D gamma globulin and have since pursued such a study.

Estimates of the incidence of sensitization in studies such as
those cited above have generally been based on the detection of Rh
antibodies 3 to 6 months after delivery. That this may underestimate
the true incidence of sensitization is borne out by the more recent
data of Woodward and Donohue (1968) and Ascari et al. (1969).
These workers showed that after an ABO-compatible pregnancy in
an Rh-negative mother delivering an Rh-positive infant, Rh antibodies
appeared by six months postpartum in about 7 to 8 per cent of cases
and at the end of a subsequent Rh-positive pregnancy in another 7
to 8 per cent. Woodward and Donohue's data suggested that the larger
stimuli of fetal cells are more likely to result in overt antibody formation, while the smaller stimuli are more likely to prime, with antibodies not being detected until a second stimulus occurs during the
next pregnancy. The observation by Bowman et al. (1969) that antibodies may occasionally develop during the first pregnancy and be
initially detectable (by sensitive papainized cell techniques) only
transiently in the few days after delivery may account for some of
the women who are wrongly classified as unsensitized when studied
several months postpartum. Such women probably account for the
majority of failures of the anti-D gamma globulin.

The fact remains that one of the major factors in the development
of maternal sensitization by Rh is the volume of fetal cells reaching
the maternal circulation at the time of the primary stimulus. The influence of various obstetrical factors on this volume of fetomaternal
transfusion assumes great importance in any efforts directed at mini-
mizing or preventing Rh sensitization of the mother.

Obstetrical Influences.   The early data on this are conflicting and probably reflect minor differences in obstetrical techniques and in the methods used to demonstrate transfer of fetal cells into the maternal blood stream. In a large-scale population analysis in Birmingham, England, by Knox (1968), the main obstetrical determinants were toxemia, cesarean section, breech delivery and a very short interval between the sensitizing and subsequent pregnancy. A study by Montague and Krevans (1968) revealed that about one-third of women undergoing cesarean section show evidence of TPH. In these women, more important than the procedure itself was the association with active labor and obstetrical complications such as breech delivery, twin pregnancy, transverse lie, adherent placenta, placenta previa, and abruptio placentae. Such variables may explain the conflicting observations on the role of cesarean section made previously by Zipursky et al. (1963) and Cohen et al. (1964). Other factors reported to favor increased TPH include manual removal of the placenta (Zipursky et al., 1963; Queenan et al., 1964) and external cephalic version (Pollack, 1968). If the latter procedure is deemed advisable in order to reduce the risk of TPH associated with breech extraction, it would seem wise to administer anti-D gamma globulin to the mother shortly afterward. (The safety of antenatal administration of this material has been demonstrated by Zipursky and Israels, 1967.) Post-term pregnancies, surprisingly, have not been associated with increased size of fetomaternal bleeding (Pollack and Montague, 1968).

The technique of amniocentesis is being used with increasing frequency in following Rh-sensitized women and might be expected to result in placental injury with increased transplacental passage of fetal red cells. In 13 women studied by Zipursky et al. (1963), this procedure was unsuccessful in four because of entry of the needle into the placenta, resulting in aspiration of fetal blood. Transplacental hemorrhage occurred in all four, with estimated losses of 10 to 50 ml. of fetal blood. Significant rises in the titer of anti-D occurred in two of the three Rh-negative women who delivered Rh-positive infants. Similar observations were made by Queenan and Adams (1964). In a study of 74 women undergoing amniocentesis, Woowang et al. (1967) demonstrated fetomaternal hemorrhages varying from 0.5 ml. to 58 ml. in 10.8 per cent of the women. When the group was further analyzed according to whether the amniocentesis was performed with ease or difficulty, it was found that all of the hemorrhages occurred in the latter group, in a frequency of 32 per cent. Similar findings were obtained by Peddle (1968), who, in addition, showed a rise in maternal antibody titers in over half of those with a TPH exceeding 0.1 ml. It should be noted that in each of these studies transplacental hemorrhage occurred predominantly in cases in which amniocentesis was associated with aspiration of fetal blood and presumably injury to the placenta. That such hemorrhage may aggravate maternal sensitization and present a danger to future infants seems clear. Fair-weather et al. (1963) studied a large series of patients and were unable to show that amniocentesis, in their hands, induces either a rise in antibody titer or increased severity of the disease in that or subsequent pregnancies. They did not estimate the number of fetal cells in the maternal blood. Jennison and Walker (1963) underscored these observations and implied that the difference in conclusions between these two studies may reflect differences in the degree of placental damage occurring with amniocentesis as performed by the two groups of workers.

Abortion is associated with an increased incidence of transplacental hemorrhage. This is particularly so for therapeutic abortion, regardless of the technique employed (Matthews and Matthews, 1969; Voigt and Britt, 1969; Queenan et al., 1971). Conflicting results have been obtained in studies of spontaneous abortion—positive results by Litwak and co-workers (1970) and negative results by Katz (1969) and Matthews and Matthews (1969). In each situation, the volume of hemorrhage has usually been rather small, of the order of 0.2 ml. or less. Such amounts are generally considered insufficient to cause primary immunization. However, the margin of safety is small and the present availability of the anti-D gamma globulin is sufficiently great that its administration is recommended following all abortions occurring after 7 to 8 weeks' gestation. Support for this comes from observations such as those of Jorgenson (1969), who found that 3 of 30 unsensitized Rh-negative women developed antibodies during the year after an abortion.

Production of Rh Antibody by the Mother

Because the Rh antigens of the fetus are well developed as early as six weeks of gestation (Chown, 1955), entry of such cells into the maternal circulation may represent a potent stimulus to antibody production at any time during pregnancy. The ability of an Rh-negative recipient of Rh-positive blood to respond by producing antibodies is not a universal one; about 10 per cent of such transfusions are never associated with antibody production (Allen and Diamond, 1957). In a more recent study, Mollison and co-workers (1970) injected Rh-positive erythrocytes into 34 Rh-negative subjects. Using sensitive serologic and erythrokinetic indices of sensitization, they demonstrated two types of Rh-negative subjects: those who were sensitized after a single injection (about 50 per cent) and the remainder, who could not be sensitized even after multiple injections. Other factors that limit the incidence of maternal sensitization include Rh heterozygosity of the father, associated ABO incompatibility, and avoidance of obstetrical factors that might injure the placental barrier. The

Table 7–1   Approximate Chances of Eventual Sensitization
to Rh by Pregnancy Alone, in the Rh-negative Wives
of Rh-positive Men*

HUSBAND'S ZYGOSITY FOR RH	ABO COMPATIBILITY OF HUSBAND		ABO TYPE OF HUSBAND UNKNOWN
	INCOMPATIBLE (%)	COMPATIBLE (%)	
Heterozygous	1	3	2
Homozygous	4–5	11	9
Zygosity unknown	2–3	7–8	5

*From Allen, F. H., Jr., and Diamond, L. K.: *Erythroblastosis Fetalis*. Boston, Little, Brown and Co., 1957.

chances of eventual Rh sensitization by pregnancy are given in Table 7–1.

More recent data by Woodward and Donohue (1968) and Ascari et al. (1969) showed that the incidence of Rh sensitization after the first ABO-compatible pregnancy is best assessed by the determination of maternal antibodies at the end of the *second* Rh-positive pregnancy. By this method, the incidence of Rh sensitization is approximately 17 per cent, twice that which would have been estimated from data obtained only after the first pregnancy.

It has been suggested by Taylor (1967) that the Rh type of the *mother* of an Rh-negative woman may influence the likelihood of her being sensitized by pregnancy. An increased incidence of Rh-positive grandmothers among mothers of affected children suggested the possibility of primary sensitization occurring in utero, from transfer of Rh-positive red cells to the Rh-negative fetus. The conclusions of this study are open to question, based on objections to the sampling methodology used in selecting the controls (Gardner, 1967).

Anti-Rh antibodies of the saline-reacting variety are 19S (IgM) gammaglobulins, do not cross the placenta, and are therefore not of direct significance in relation to hemolytic disease in the fetus. Incomplete anti-Rh, on the other hand, is predominantly a 7S (IgG) antibody and is able to cross the placenta and damage fetal red cells. This type of antibody is usually detected by its reaction with albumin-suspended or enzyme-treated red cells or by the indirect Coombs test. Recently, Dodd and Wilkinson (1964) demonstrated small amounts of incomplete anti-Rh in the IgA and IgM fractions of the immunoglobulins. This may explain some of the discrepancy observed between the amount of anti-Rh in the mother's serum and the amount in the infant's serum. Although it generally is true that the higher the titer of incomplete anti-Rh, the greater the severity of hemolytic disease, this correlation does not always hold (Mollison, 1961).

Transfer of Antibodies Across the Placenta to the Fetus

The major factors determining transfer of antibodies across the placenta are the size and configuration of the antibody molecule. For Rh, only the incomplete (albumin-reacting or indirect Coombs-reacting) antibodies cross the placenta. In ABO incompatibility, in which the mother is usually group O and the infant group A or B, it is only the "immune" (IgG) anti-A or anti-B that cross the placenta and not the naturally occurring (IgM) anti-A or anti-B (Abelson and Rawson, 1961). In utero, such isohemagglutinins may be found as early as the 13th to 14th week of gestation (Toivanen and Hirvonen, 1969). These workers also showed that in the sera of term newborns, a small proportion contain anti-A or anti-B differing from that present in maternal serum; presumably these antibodies were synthesized by the fetus itself. Other incomplete antibodies in this category are those of the Kell, Duffy, and Kidd systems. An exception to this rule is the reported appearance of IgM cold agglutinins, both normal and immune, in cord blood. In this infant, mild hemolytic disease developed (Eskin and Frumin, 1963).

Antibodies in the fetus may be demonstrated in the serum by the indirect Coombs test or, more commonly, on the infant's red cells by the direct Coombs test. A positive direct Coombs test has been found in a fetus as young as six weeks, indicating that antibody may cross the placenta very early in pregnancy.

Reaction of Antibody with Fetal Red Cells to Produce Hemolysis

Although a variety of abnormalities have been found in sensitized fetal red cells, the precise mechanism of their destruction is not known. Among these abnormalities are:

1. Appearance of spherocytes (only in ABO incompatibility).
2. Decrease in oxygen-carrying capacity (Abrahamov and Diamond, 1969).
3. Decrease in glucose utilization (Abrahamov and Diamond, 1960).
4. Increased osmotic fragility (Spiess and Wolf, 1963).
5. Increased phosphate uptake (Greenwalt et al., 1962).
6. Decreased acetylcholinesterase activity—in ABO incompatibility (Kaplan et al., 1964).
7. Increased carboxyhemoglobin levels—a nonspecific index of hemolysis and hemoglobin degradation (Oski and Altman, 1962).
8. Lower Hb F concentration (Chapter Six, p. 145).
9. Decreased ATP synthesis (Schrier et al., 1968).

The absence of free hemoglobin in the serum of infants with hemolytic disease suggests that the hemolysis is occurring extravascularly (Allen and Diamond, 1957). Destruction probably takes place mainly in the spleen, as suggested by the work of Jandl et al. (1957). In this study, chromium-51 labeled red cells sensitized in vitro with incomplete Rh antibody were injected and the radioactivity shown to localize predominantly over the spleen.

The main consequences of destruction of the infant's red cells are anemia and hyperbilirubinemia. The rate of destruction of anti-D coated red cells is dependent on factors in addition to the amount of anti-D on the red cell, as suggested by the poor correlation found between the latter and cord hemoglobin and bilirubin levels (Hughes-Jones et al., 1967). Such factors include the efficiency of the particular antibody in promoting phagocytosis and the capacity of the reticuloendothelial system to remove coated cells (mainly dependent on the degree of saturation with red cells). Other factors that influence the degree of anemia and hyperbilirubinemia are discussed below.

Anemia. The degree of anemia depends on the ability of the fetal erythropoietic cells to keep pace with the hemolytic process. Thus, in mild cases the cord hemoglobin concentration may be normal or only slightly decreased. In severe cases, it is markedly decreased, occasionally as low as 3.0 gm./100 ml., with accompanying signs of hydrops fetalis due to congestive failure.

Hyperbilirubinemia. Degradation of hemoglobin released from the destroyed red cells results in the formation of large amounts of free (indirect-reacting) bilirubin. The chief importance of bilirubin lies in its relationship to the development of kernicterus. Although significant correlation has been established between serum indirect bilirubin levels and the incidence of kernicterus (Hsia et al., 1952), it is actually the amount of bilirubin that enters the nervous tissue that determines whether brain damage will ensue. Therefore, factors that influence the distribution of bilirubin between serum and tissues are as important as the total amount of bilirubin in the body. At this point, a brief review of bilirubin metabolism in the newborn is in order.

BILIRUBIN METABOLISM IN THE FETUS AND NEWBORN

Since Van den Bergh in 1913 characterized bilirubin as direct (water-soluble, early-reacting) and indirect (water-insoluble, lipid-soluble, late-reacting), our knowledge of bilirubin metabolism and its relation to neonatal jaundice has made significant gains. The recent literature contains several excellent reviews (Brown, 1962; Odell, 1967; Gartner and Arias, 1969).

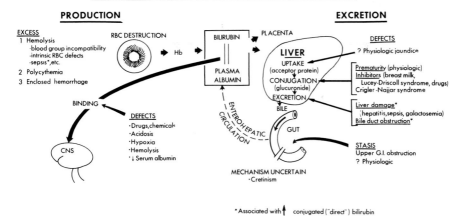

Figure 7-1   Pathophysiology of neonatal hyperbilirubinemia.

The metabolic pathway of bilirubin may be considered in several phases: production, transport in plasma, hepatic uptake, conjugation and excretion, and placental excretion. This pathway and its disturbances leading to hyperbilirubinemia in the newborn are illustrated in Figure 7-1.

Production of Bilirubin

Bilirubin is formed mainly from the catabolism of hemoglobin by the reticuloendothelial system, approximately 35 mg. of bilirubin resulting from 1 gm. of hemoglobin. Increased breakdown of hemoglobin due to accelerated hemolysis is the major (but not the only) factor in the hyperbilirubinemia of hemolytic disease due to blood group incompatibility. This type of bilirubin is free or indirect-reacting and is the form that may cause brain damage and kernicterus. Increased amounts of direct-reacting bilirubin may also be found in some infants and are probably due to liver damage.

Transport in Plasma

Bilirubin, both direct and indirect, is transported in the plasma bound to albumin in a molar ratio of 2:1. The ability of albumin to bind bilirubin is the major determinant of the distribution of bilirubin between the vascular compartment and the tissues. Because it is the *tissue* concentration of bilirubin that is crucial in relation to kernicterus, the binding capacity of serum albumin is of great importance.

The subject of bilirubin binding and distribution has been reviewed by Diamond (1969) and Odell (1970). Factors that influence the bilirubin binding capacity are:

1. Total serum albumin concentration.

2. Presence of other organic ions that bind to albumin, displacing bilirubin (the latter include drugs — such as sulfonamides, salicylates, heparin, caffeine, and sodium benzoate — nonesterified fatty acids, and hematin released during hemolysis). Antibiotics (penicillin and semi-synthetic derivatives, kanamycin) commonly used to treat neonatal infections do not, in therapeutic concentrations, interfere with bilirubin binding capacity (Cohen et al., 1971).

3. Hydrogen ion concentration, increases of which (as in acidosis) result in impaired bilirubin binding (Odell, 1959).

The clinical implications of these properites are especially evident in two situations in the neonatal period. The first occurs in the premature infant who, because of a lower serum albumin concentration and a tendency to acidosis (associated with anoxia and respiratory distress), may be at greater risk from displacement of bilirubin into the tissues. The second is the infant with hyperbilirubinemia due to hemolytic disease in whom hematin displaces bilirubin from the binding sites on albumin. This results in higher tissue bilirubin concentrations than might be found in an infant with comparable serum bilirubin levels unassociated with hemolysis.

Attempts to estimate the bilirubin binding capacity of the serum of icteric newborns seem to be important in evaluating the potential cellular toxicity of a given serum concentration of bilirubin. Waters and Porter (1961) have developed such an assay based on the observation that phenolsulfonphthalein is bound to serum in direct proportion to the albumin concentration, and in inverse proportion to the concentration of bilirubin and other substances that are bound to albumin. Other methods of estimating bilirubin binding capacity have been developed, including HABA [2-(4'-hydroxybenzeneazo) benzoic acid] binding (Johnson and Boggs, 1970), Sephadex filtration (Bratlid and Fog, 1970) and the salicylate saturation index of Odell et al. (1969). The value and limitations of such tests are discussed on page 199.

A small but significant amount of unconjugated bilirubin is bound by erythrocytes, probably because of its solubility in the lipid of the membrane (Watson, 1962; Oski and Naiman, 1963). This property is lost when erythrocytes are coated with Rh antibody, and its restoration may constitute one of the fringe benefits of exchange transfusion in hemolytic disease due to blood group incompatibility.

Platelets have been shown to bind bilirubin, with resultant dysfunction (Suvansri et al., 1969).

Hepatic Uptake and Conjugation and
Excretion of Bilirubin

Uptake. Recently, two proteins, designated Y and Z, which bind bilirubin and other organic anions, have been isolated from the liver-cell cytoplasm in a number of mammalian species. It has been suggested that these "acceptor" proteins (especially Y) are important mediators in the hepatic uptake of bilirubin from the plasma (Levi et al., 1970). The demonstration by these workers of a relative deficiency of Y protein in newborn Rhesus monkeys in association with elevated serum bilirubin concentrations has suggested its possible importance in the genesis of "physiologic" hyperbilirubinemia. The role of acceptor proteins in hepatic uptake of bilirubin by the newborn infant has not yet been studied.

Conjugation. Direct-reacting bilirubin consists of bilirubin conjugated largely with glucuronic acid (Billing and Lathe, 1956), and to a lesser extent with sulfate. These reactions are illustrated in Figure 7–2. The conjugation reaction takes place in the microsomes of the liver and is dependent on glucuronyl transferase.

The liver of the normal newborn and particularly that of the premature infant has been shown to have relatively less activity of glucuronyl transferase at birth and in the first few weeks of life than does the normal adult (Brown and Zuelzer, 1958). Since then, conflicting observations on the activity of this enzyme in newborns have been obtained by several workers. Strebel and Odell (1969) found normal activity whereas Gartner and Lane (1971) found reduced activity. Whether variations in methodology or in animal species studied account for these different observations is not clear. A possible explanation was offered recently by Bakken (1969, 1970). Observing that conjugated bilirubin in newborns appears only after the prior accumulation of unconjugated bilirubin (either in the mother or fetus), he showed that glucuronyl transferase is normally present in newborns but requires the presence of unconjugated bilirubin for its activation. The accumulation of unconjugated bilirubin in the first

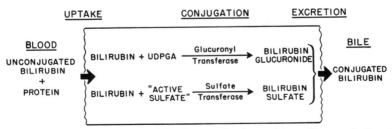

Figure 7–2 Metabolism of bilirubin in the liver. (From Cracco, J. B., et al.: *Proceedings of the Staff Meetings of the Mayo Clinic,* 40:868, 1965.)

few days after birth therefore could be interpreted to reflect not so much a deficiency of transferase but the time necessary for its substrate to reach a concentration sufficient for its activation. That this delay in conjugation is the major rate-limiting factor in the hepatic passage of bilirubin is suggested by the studies of Gartner and Lane (1971) in newborn Rhesus monkeys. This handicap is one of the reasons why minimal degrees of hemolysis in the newborn period may result in pronounced degrees of hyperbilirubinemia, even without much decrease in hemoglobin. Individual variations in bilirubin conjugating capacity probably account for some of the variation in jaundice among different erythroblastotic infants with comparable degrees of hemolysis.

Excretion of Bilirubin.   Bilirubin, rendered soluble by conjugation with glucuronic acid (or sulfate), is excreted into the bile canaliculus and eventually via the bile ducts to the intestine. A defect in the ability of the fetal liver to excrete conjugated bilirubin has been found recently in the guinea pig (Schenker et al., 1964). These workers speculate that the increased amounts of direct-reacting (conjugated) bilirubin occasionally seen in severe erythroblastosis (so-called "inspissated bile syndrome") may result from a lag in maturation of the liver's excretory capacity over its conjugative capacity. Bakken and Fog (1967) have suggested that, just as the accumulation of unconjugated bilirubin acts as a trigger for the conjugating mechanism, so does conjugated bilirubin act for the excretion mechanism. Data on the hepatic excretory capacity of the human infant are not yet available.

Conjugated bilirubin is excreted as bile into the small intestine where it is hydrolyzed back to bilirubin by the beta-glucuronidase activity within the intestine. Reabsorption of such bilirubin (enterohepatic circulation) may contribute to neonatal hyperbilirubinemia as suggested by its occurrence among infants with bile stasis due to upper gastrointestinal obstruction, and its prevention by the oral administration of agents which adsorb or bind bilirubin, such as charcoal or agar (Poland and Odell, 1971).

Placental Excretion of Bilirubin

Schenker et al. (1964) have shown in pregnant guinea pigs that carbon-14 labeled bilirubin injected into the fetal circulation is largely cleared into the maternal circulation. This mode of excretion occurred mainly with unconjugated bilirubin and only to a minimal extent with the conjugated fraction. Because labeled albumin did not cross the placenta, it was felt that during the process of placental transfer bilirubin dissociated from its usual complex with albumin. Similar observations obtained with pregnant monkeys suggest that placental excretion of bilirubin probably occurs in the human also (Lester et al., 1963).

The placental excretion of bilirubin seems to account for the virtual absence of significant elevation in serum bilirubin levels of cord blood from erythroblastotic infants, and for the rapid increases that occur during the first 24 hours after birth.

CLINICAL MANIFESTATIONS

The main signs of hemolytic disease in the newborn infant are jaundice, pallor, and enlargement of the liver and spleen. Birth weight does not differ from that of normal infants of comparable gestational age (Kitchen, 1970; Vidyasagar, 1971).

Jaundice. Jaundice is generally absent at birth, for reasons previously mentioned. In some infants, however, cord bilirubin levels as high as 8 mg./100 ml. may be found in the absence of jaundice. Allen and Diamond (1957) suggest that exposure to light may be necessary for the development of skin jaundice following birth. Supporting this supposition, they cite the interesting observation of Hirsch (1913) that areas of the skin of a jaundiced infant that are covered with adhesive tape remain free of jaundice.

Jaundice usually becomes evident during the first 24 hours after birth (often by four to five hours of age), reaches a peak by the third or fourth day of life, and then gradually subsides. Detection of early jaundice is important and requires proper lighting—either daylight or a white fluorescent lamp. Pressure over the forehead of the infant to blanch the skin capillaries facilitates observation of the yellow tinge in the skin.

Although there are many causes of neonatal jaundice, onset in the first 24 hours of life is almost always indicative of hemolytic disease. When jaundice is not detected until after this time, other conditions must also be considered (Table 7–2 and Fig. 7–1). The commonest of these is so-called *physiologic jaundice,* due to a number of possible factors, as discussed earlier. This, however, is a diagnosis of exclusion made in an otherwise well newborn with no blood group incompatibility. Hemolysis associated with *sepsis* (bacterial, viral, or protozoal) is an important cause that often must be sought by vigorous diagnostic efforts. *Inherited defects of the red cell,* such as hereditary spherocytosis and enzyme-deficiency hemolytic anemia (most commonly glucose-6-phosphate dehydrogenase and pyruvate kinase deficiencies), frequently become evident in the newborn period with jaundice that may be of sufficient severity to cause kernicterus. In a newborn infant with *"enclosed" hemorrhage,* such as a large cephalhematoma or extensive cutaneous purpura, absorption of bilirubin

Table 7–2 Causes of Jaundice During the First Week of Life

Hemolytic diseases
  Erythroblastosis fetalis; Rh or ABO incompatibility, etc.
  Inherited red cell defects:
    Hereditary spherocytosis
    Enzyme deficiencies (± drugs):
      glucose-6-phosphate dehydrogenase, pyruvate kinase, etc.
  Drugs and toxins: vitamin K_3 (excessive doses), naphthalene (moth balls)

Infections
  Bacterial: sepsis, congenital syphilis
  Viral: cytomegalic inclusion disease, disseminated
    herpes simplex, congenital rubella syndrome
  Protozoal: congenital toxoplasmosis

Enclosed hemorrhage

Metabolic disorders
  Galactosemia
  Crigler-Najjar syndrome
  Breast milk jaundice (Newman and Gross, 1963)
  Transient familial neonatal hyperbilirubinemia (Lucey et al., 1960;
    Arias et al., 1965)
  Cretinism

Neonatal (giant-cell) hepatitis

Physiologic jaundice

---

from degraded hemoglobin may result in a moderate degree of jaundice in the first few days of life (Rausen and Diamond, 1961). A similar mechanism probably underlies the hyperbilirubinemia seen in newborns with melena (Nelson, 1965; Egan et al., 1969) and renal vein thrombosis (Walters and Holder, 1966). Jaundice associated with vomiting following the introduction of milk feedings raises suspicion of *galactosemia*, which should be excluded by testing for reducing substances in the urine. Upper gastrointestinal obstruction should also be considered in such infants.

The severity of erythroblastosis fetalis reflects both the severity of the hemolytic process and the impairment of bilirubin-conjugating capacity of the newborn's liver. Exaggeration of the latter in the premature infant presents an additional handicap that must be taken into consideration in the decision about exchange transfusion in such infants.

Occasionally, prolonged jaundice associated with elevation of the direct-reacting bilirubin fraction occurs—the so-called "inspissated bile syndrome." This poor term describes a pathological condition that rarely exists. Such a bilirubin pattern may also be seen early in the course of the disease (often in cord blood), when it usually correlates with the severity of the hemolytic process. The mechanism of the apparent obstruction has not been well elucidated from the study of postmortem cases (Harris et al., 1962). These authors suggest a functional defect in the ability of the liver to excrete conjugated bilirubin as the basis for the accumulation of the direct fraction in the blood. The experimental work of Schenker et al. (1964) in guinea pigs showing that conjugated bilirubin was less efficiently excreted by the placenta than was unconjugated bilirubin might support this. Other workers have shown definite histopathologic abnormalities in the liver at autopsy, varying from necrosis and giant-cell reaction (Dunn, 1963) to overt fibrosis (Craig, 1950; Cornblath et al., 1955).

Kernicterus. With increasing jaundice and elevation of the serum indirect bilirubin levels above 20 mg./100 ml., kernicterus may develop. That kernicterus usually becomes manifest during the first five days of life in erythroblastotic infants is merely a reflection of the fact that serum bilirubins are highest during this time and they generally subside afterwards. However, excessive bilirubinemia at *any time in the first few weeks of life* (and occasionally later in cases of the Crigler-Najjar syndrome) may cause kernicterus, a fact that is often not appreciated in arriving at a decision regarding exchange transfusion.

The clinical manifestations of kernicterus have been well reviewed by Vaughan et al. (1950) and Van Praagh (1961). The earliest signs of kernicterus are increasing lethargy, hypotonia, and poor feeding (due to loss of the sucking reflex). These are followed by opisthotonos as evidenced by retraction of the head, extension of the arms and pronation of the wrists, and then generalized spasticity and irregular respirations. Terminally, there may be oozing of bloody froth from the nose and pharynx due to pulmonary hemorrhage. Milder cases survive and may be left with the postkernicteric syndrome, consisting of high-frequency nerve deafness, athetoid cerebral palsy, and dental enamel dysplasia (Perlstein, 1960). In such infants, lessening of spasticity usually occurs about the end of the first week of life and may suggest (wrongly) that kernicterus has not developed (Van Praagh, 1961). Even among infants with no apparent abnormalities during the newborn period, long term follow-up may show subtle neurologic abnormalities, psychologic difficulty or sensorineural hearing loss (Johnston et al., 1967; Hyman et al., 1969). (Since most of the infants in both of these studies received streptomycin prophylaxis after exchange transfusion, it is possible that this may have contributed to the hearing loss observed on follow-up.) All of the above abnormalities occurred more frequently among infants with low birth weights, higher bilirubin levels or other neonatal complications associated with hypoxia or acidosis. A more recent study by Odell et al. (1970) showed that late evidence of central nervous system damage in such infants correlated better with tests of serum bilirubin binding capacity than with serum bilirubin levels, an observation that fits with the increased incidence of neurologic problems noted above among small sick newborns (whose binding capacity would be expected to be decreased).

Anemia.   The degree of anemia reflects the capacity of the infant's erythropoietic mass to respond to the deficit of red cells resulting from the hemolytic process. The majority of erythroblastotic infants show only mild anemia with little or no pallor. With increasing severity of the anemia, pallor becomes marked and is associated with signs of congestive heart failure. Such infants are either stillborn or born alive with massive generalized edema, ascites, pleural effusions, petechiae, tachycardia, weak heart sounds, and marked hepatosplenomegaly—the picture of hydrops fetalis. Survival beyond a few hours is unusual.

Hydrops fetalis is not always a result of blood group incompatibility. It has been described in association with homozygous α thalassemia (see p. 160), chronic fetomaternal transfusion (Weisert and Marstrander, 1960), congenital syphilis, and maternal hydramnios (Dyggve, 1960). In maternal hydramnios, the mechanism of the hydrops was not clear. A list of causes of hydrops fetalis has been compiled by Driscoll (1966) and is shown in Table 7–3.

"Late" anemia may develop in erythroblastotic infants under two sets of circumstances. In one, the infant does not become sufficiently jaundiced in the initial neonatal period to require exchange transfusion. After the second week of life, however, a progressive decrease in hemoglobin concentration may occur, resulting in severe, often fatal anemia. This possibility should be anticipated when the maternal anti-Rh titer is high. The other, more common situation is that occurring after exchange transfusion; it consists of a gradual decrease in hemoglobin concentration to levels as low as 5 to 6 gm./100 ml. at around four to six weeks of life. This anemia is not well explained, although decreased red cell production is probably an important factor, as reflected in low reticulocyte counts. In almost all cases, this anemia abates spontaneously by about eight weeks of age (see also p. 218).

Hepatosplenomegaly.   Like anemia and jaundice, hepatosplenomegaly varies with the severity of the disease—from no enlargement to massive enlargement in hydrops fetalis. When massive enlargement develops, the presence of ascites may render palpation of the liver and spleen difficult.

Hemorrhage.   Petechiae and purpuric spots may occur in infants with severe anemia because of associated thrombocytopenia and perhaps anoxic injury to the capillaries. It is a bad prognostic sign. In severely affected and fatal cases, intracranial and pulmonary hemorrhage are common findings. Among such infants there is, in addition

Table 7-3 Causes of Hydrops Fetalis*

A. *Severe chronic anemia in utero*
  1. Erythroblastosis fetalis
  2. Homozygous alpha-thalassemia
  3. Chronic fetomaternal transfusion or twin-to-twin transfusion

B. *Cardiac failure*
  1. Severe congenital heart disease
  2. Premature closure of foramen ovale
  3. Large A–V malformation (hemangioma) (Daniel and
     Cassady, 1968)

C. *Hypoproteinemia*
  1. Renal disease
     a. Congenital nephrosis
     b. Renal vein thrombosis
  2. Congenital hepatitis

D. *Infections* (intrauterine)
  1. Syphilis
  2. Toxoplasmosis
  3. Cytomegalovirus

E. *Miscellaneous*
  1. Maternal diabetes mellitus
  2. Parabiotic syndrome (multiple pregnancy)
  3. Sublethal umbilical or chorionic vein thrombosis
  4. Fetal neuroblastomatosis
  5. Chagas disease
  6. Achondroplasia
  7. Cystic adenomatoid malformation of the lung
  8. Pulmonary lymphangiectasia
  9. Dysmaturity
  10. Cardiopulmonary hypoplasia with bilateral hydrothorax

---

*From Driscoll, 1966.

to thrombocytopenia, a complex disturbance of coagulation that in most instances suggests disseminated intravascular coagulation (Chessells and Wigglesworth, 1971). In a few infants studied by these workers, there were also deficiencies of the vitamin-K-dependent coagulation factors, suggesting impaired synthesis due to hepatic dysfunction; a similar observation was made in two hydropic infants studied by Hathaway (1970).

Maternal Complications. In mothers bearing severely affected fetuses, there is an increased incidence of polyhydramnios and pre-eclamptic toxemia. Also, a syndrome appearing between 28 and 30 weeks of gestation and characterized by the sudden onset of gross dependent edema of the legs in the absence of other signs of toxemia has been described (Cohen, 1960; Beazley, 1965). After intrauterine death has occurred, absorption of placental thromboplastin may result in afibrinogenemia and hemorrhages (due to disseminated intravascular coagulation).

LABORATORY FINDINGS

Hematologic Abnormalities

Decreased hemoglobin concentration, increased reticulocyte count, and increased numbers of nucleated red blood cells in the peripheral blood are the main findings. These reflect the severity of the hemolytic process and the degree of marrow compensation.

Hemoglobin Concentration. Determinations carried out in cord venous blood most accurately indicate the severity of the hemolytic process. Comparing hemoglobin determinations from cord blood and heel-prick in erythroblastotic (and normal) newborns, Moe (1967) found substantially higher values in the heel-prick (capillary) blood; in fact, one-third of the infants requiring exchange transfusion had normal hemoglobins by the capillary method.

The degree of anemia (and also hypoxemia and acidosis) can be evaluated early in labor from samples of fetal blood obtained by scalp puncture. By this method, Hobel (1970) found excellent correlation with hemoglobin levels in cord blood (obtained 90 minutes later on the average). In the infant suspected of being severely affected, the advance data so obtained may be helpful in prompt and aggressive management immediately after birth. Further experience with this technique is necessary before it can be generally recommended.

Values below 14 gm./100 ml. in cord blood are considered abnormal. Although the degree of anemia usually indicates the severity of the disease, normal hemoglobin levels may occur with severe jaundice. Presumably, this indicates effective marrow compensation, which leads to an increased number of red cells available for destruction and bilirubin formation. In hydrops fetalis, the hemoglobin concentration may be as low as 3 to 5 gm./100 ml.

Repeat determinations of hemoglobin concentration after the initial one are of little value in assessing the need for either the initial or repeat exchange transfusions. However, in the Coombs-positive infant who does not become sufficiently jaundiced to require exchange transfusion, hemoglobin determinations should be followed once or twice weekly in the first month after discharge from the hospital because of the risk of severe (often fatal) anemia during this period.

Reticulocyte Count. This is increased above 6 per cent and may be as high as 30 to 40 per cent.

Nucleated Red Blood Cells. Concentrations greater than 10 per 100 white blood cells are usual. In severe cases, extremely high counts may be obtained.

The peripheral blood smear reveals, in addition, marked polychromasia and anisocytosis, which reflect the presence of young red cells. Spherocytes are seen only in ABO incompatibility.

Platelet Count. In infants with severe anemia and also following exchange transfusion, the platelet count may be decreased (see Chapter Nine).

Hypoglycemia

Hyperplasia of the pancreatic islets is a well recognized finding among infants dying of erythroblastosis fetalis. Only recently, however, has the occurrence of hypoglycemia been documented in newborns with this condition (Hazeltine, 1967; Barrett and Oliver, 1968). In a prospective study of 16 consecutive infants with moderate to severe erythroblastosis, Barrett and Oliver observed symptomatic hypoglycemia after exchange transfusion in 5 infants; 2 of the 5 were also hypoglycemic before the exchange. The lowest blood glucose levels were reached around 1 to 2 hours after completion of the exchange. In these infants, increased serum insulin levels accompanied the hypoglycemia.

The mechanism of the hyperinsulinism has been studied by Steinke and associates (1967). Based on the finding of inhibition of insulin activity by hemolysates in vitro, they suggested that products of hemolysis also inactivate circulating insulin, thus stimulating compensatory hyperplasia of beta cells and increased production of insulin. Further stimulation of insulin synthesis due to the glucose present in the ACD-anticoagulated donor blood probably accounts for the subsequent drop in blood glucose levels during the few hours after completion of the exchange transfusion (Schiff et al., 1971a). Although use of heparinized blood might seem preferable to avert this complication, the absence of glucose in this additive might deny possible benefit to those infants who are already hypoglycemic before the exchange transfusion (Schiff et al., 1971).

To protect erythroblastotic infants from the deleterious effects of hypoglycemia, determination of blood glucose should be included in the initial evaluation and after exchange, a screening blood glucose test such as the Dextrostix* should be carried out about two hours later. If the diagnosis of hypoglycemia is established, it should be treated promptly with intravenous hypertonic glucose.

In view of the recent report of delayed hypoglycemia appearing in two siblings 7 and 25 months after births complicated by severe erythroblastosis, further follow-up studies of such infants seem indicated (Danks, 1969).

---

*Dextrostix Reagent Strips, Ames Co., Elkhart, Indiana.

Serologic Abnormalities

The essential findings consist of Rh(D)-negative maternal red cells and maternal serum that contains antibodies to the Rh(D)-positive red cells of the infant. The Rh(D)-positive cells of the infant are coated with antibody, resulting in a positive direct Coombs test.

Maternal Rh sensitization and hemolytic disease in the newborn are rare in first pregnancies. When they occur, there is usually (but not always) a history of previous abortion, blood transfusions or intramuscular injection of blood. Because 30 years have now lapsed since recognition of the importance of the Rh factor in blood transfusion, the generation of Rh-negative females exposed to Rh-positive blood during infancy and childhood can be expected to disappear shortly from future obstetric populations. Sensitization by fetal red cells during pregnancy will then represent the sole mechanism of production of hemolytic disease of the newborn.

Antibodies to the Rh factor are usually classified according to the medium in which they react with the red cells. The three main types are saline, albumin, and indirect Coombs-reacting. The last two are termed incomplete (IgG) antibodies. Because saline antibodies are 19S (IgM) globulins, they do not cross the placenta and their titer in the mother is of no prognostic significance. Most data on the relation of maternal antibody titer to outcome of pregnancy have been collected for the albumin (7S or IgG) antibodies (Allen et al., 1954). In essence, these workers found a significantly higher incidence of stillbirths and hydrops fetalis in infants born of mothers with albumin titers greater than 1:64 compared to those with titers less than 1:64. Antibody titers obtained by the indirect Coombs method are usually about two- to three-fold higher than those in albumin.

Antibodies are usually evident about six to eight weeks after the first sensitizing pregnancy, presumably reflecting the antigenic stimulus of fetal red cells entering the maternal circulation near term and during labor. Such antibodies, usually IgM, are demonstrable in saline or by the more sensitive techniques using enzyme-treated red cells. Their titer remains low during subsequent pregnancies until the booster stimulus of further fetal red cells entering during the third trimester results in a second rise, this time predominantly of the IgG class and demonstrable by albumin or indirect Coombs techniques. If the antibody response is of sufficient magnitude, the fetus will develop hemolytic disease. Because of this, it has been found that the most informative antibody titers consist of a baseline value obtained around 16 weeks gestation, with a second value at 28 to 32 weeks of gestation and subsequent values at intervals of one to four weeks, depending on the rate of rise in titer. Once the maternal indirect Coombs antibody titer has reached 1:64 or greater, its predictive value is limited, and subsequent monitoring of the degree of fetal hemolysis is best obtained by estimation of the pigment concentration in amniotic fluid (p. 202).

Procedures for the identification of antibodies and their measurement in pregnant Rh-negative women are summarized in Figure 7–3.

Although, as discussed above, hemolytic disease in the newborn is rare in first pregnancies, the incidence of maternal Rh sensitization is not as rare as was originally believed. Using a sensitive enzyme technique, Bowman and co-workers (1969) demonstrated weak (IgM) Rh antibodies within three days of delivery in 5 of 210 primigravidae (2.4 per cent). In two women (one of whom received anti-D gamma globulin) followed through a second pregnancy, the antibody was no longer detectable six months after the first nor in the second trimester of the second pregnancy. During the third trimester, however, it became detectable by the usual IgG techniques in both women and

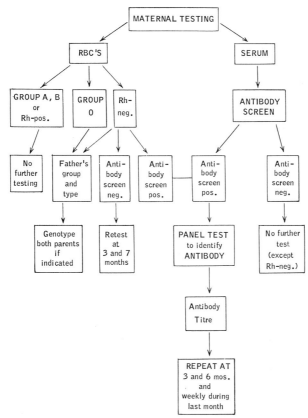

Figure 7–3 Serologic study of a pregnant Rh-negative woman. (From Humes, J. J., and Harmeling, J. G., 1965.)

the infants were born with positive direct Coombs tests. These observations indicate that fetomaternal transfusion and maternal sensitization can occur antenatally and that such events may go undetected and account for subsequent failures of the anti-D gamma globulin.

Except when maternal antibodies are present in low titer, the red blood cells of Rh-positive infants give a direct positive Coombs test, indicating the presence of gamma globulin on the red cell surface. Occasionally, this coating is sufficiently heavy to block the Rh antigenic sites, causing a false negative result for Rh typing (the so-called "blocked D"). In such cases, it can be presumed that the infant is Rh-positive if the direct Coombs test is sufficiently strong. Another situation associated with negative Rh typing of an affected infant's red cells was described by Cohen et al. (1970). In an infant requiring six intrauterine transfusions, the development of Rh reactivity was delayed for five months. Neither the "blocking" phenomenon nor dilution with Rh-negative donor erythrocytes could be proved. It was their opinion that persistence of maternal Rh antibody in the infant's serum resulted in specific suppression of development of Rh antigens.

Rarely, infants with hemolytic disease may show a false negative direct Coombs test. Caviles et al. (1964) found six such infants among 237 cases seen over a two year period. They attributed this to an atypical antibody that was absorbed only by *enzyme-treated* red cells. In a later study by Weiner and Wingham (1966), 10 similar infants were found in a group of 733 Rh-immunized mothers. In 7 of the 10 infants, the presence of antibody coating their erythrocytes was demonstrated by elution tests. In none of the cases was the antibody shown to be atypical. The rather low titers of Rh antibody among mothers of these infants resulting in "light" coating of infant erythrocytes was felt to be the basis for the observed discrepancy in serologic findings.

Serum Bilirubin Levels

Levels of bilirubin in cord blood are closely related to severity of the disease and mortality rate (Mollison, 1961). Values above 4 mg./100 ml. are uncommon, but when present, suggest severe disease. From birth onward, the rate of rise in serum bilirubin reflects both the rate of production (from hemolysis) and the rate of maturation of the liver enzyme system necessary for conjugation and excretion of bilirubin. Van den Bergh fractionation reveals the proportion of total bilirubin level that is conjugated (direct-reacting); the remainder, or indirect-reacting fraction, is the one of importance in terms of potential brain damage. Recent studies by Odell and co-workers (1970) have shown that the risk of neurologic impairment correlates better with the *duration* of serum bilirubin levels in excess of 15 mg. per 100 ml. than with *peak* serum bilirubin level. Elevated direct-reacting bilirubin may be seen either at birth in a severely affected infant or in a less severely affected infant who shows prolonged jaundice lasting more than one week.

In a severely affected infant, peak bilirubin levels are usually reached by the third day of life and may be as high as 40 to 50 mg./100 ml. With levels above 20 mg./100 ml., the risk of kernicterus becomes increasingly great. The most frequently quoted figures are those of Hsia et al. (1952), who showed that kernicterus occurred in 18 per cent of infants with serum bilirubin levels between 16 and 30 mg./ 100 ml., and in 50 per cent of those in whom levels above 30 mg./100 ml. were seen. Because *peak* bilirubin values were not obtained, the incidence of kernicterus may have been slightly exaggerated in the lower bilirubin group.* Of equal or greater importance in regard to the neurotoxicity of a given level of bilirubin are factors that influence its binding to serum albumin, such as hypoproteinemia, acidosis, and the use of competing drugs and chemicals (see p. 186). Evaluation of the risks of kernicterus should also take into consideration the less obvious late neurologic, psychologic, and auditory sequelae (Hyman et al., 1969) that may occur at lower levels of bilirubin than those mentioned above.

In following bilirubin levels in erythroblastotic newborns, methodology is of great importance. Micromethods are desirable and require the collection of heel-prick blood with minimal hemolysis. A variety of such methods for determining bilirubin concentration is available, most of which are based either on azo dye coupling or on direct spectrophotometry. Aside from details of technique, the most important single variable in the results of bilirubin determinations among different laboratories is the bilirubin standard employed. To minimize such variation and allow comparison of criteria for exchange transfusion and follow-up neurological status among various centers, the Committee on Fetus and Newborn of the American Academy of Pediatrics has adopted specific recommendations for the preparation of a uniform and stable bilirubin standard (1963). These should certainly be adopted by any hospital that must treat jaundiced newborns.

A graph of serum (indirect) bilirubin levels plotted against the infant's age is helpful in decisions concerning exchange transfusion. Examples of such a guide are those prepared by Allen and Diamond (Fig. 7–4).

Bilirubin Binding Capacity of Serum Albumin

Indirect-reacting bilirubin in serum is bound to albumin; only the amount that is unbound is toxic to the central nervous system.

---

*Coincident with the clinical onset of kernicterus, serum bilirubin levels may actually *fall* (Ackerman et al., 1971).

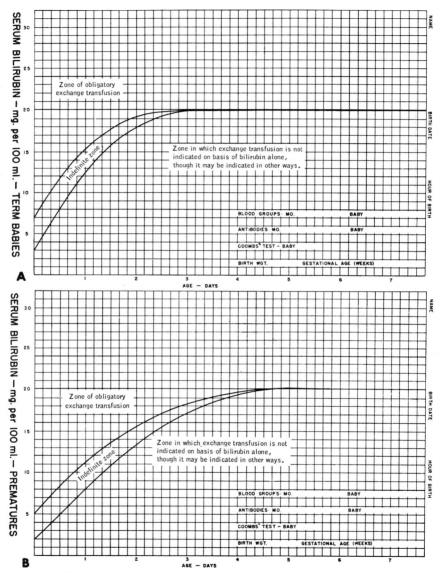

Figure 7–4 **A,** Bilirubin chart for term newborns. **B,** Bilirubin chart for premature newborns. (Courtesy of Dr. Louis K. Diamond and the Blood Grouping Laboratory, Boston.)

Estimation of the binding capacity of albumin may therefore provide valuable information on the potential toxicity of a given serum bilirubin concentration.

Blondheim (1955) showed that the amount of phenolsulfonphthalein (PSP) bound by serum was related to the albumin concentration. This amount was reduced in jaundiced serum, presumably because the bilirubin tied up the binding sites on the albumin molecule. Using this principle, Waters and Porter (1961) developed a technique employing the PSP-binding capacity as a measure of the ability of serum albumin to bind further bilirubin. In cord serum from erythroblastotic newborns, they found a significant decrease in PSP-binding capacity compared to that in serum from normal newborns. They also demonstrated an inverse relationship between serum bilirubin levels and PSP-binding capacity in erythroblastotic infants, and they used this to determine the need for exchange transfusion (1964). Preliminary data on neurologic status (during the neonatal period) suggest that in infants with bilirubin levels above 20 mg./100 ml. brain damage occurred only in those with low PSP-binding capacities (Waters, 1967). However, a subsequent study by Lucey et al. (1967) of 93 newborn infants from Greece with serum bilirubin levels ranging from 20 to 52 mg. per 100 ml. failed to show a reduction in PSP-binding capacity among infants with bilirubin levels in the higher ranges. Particularly disturbing was the finding of normal PSP-binding in 8 of 11 infants with established kernicterus. The reason for the discrepancy between these results and those of Waters is not clear. The larger number of more severely jaundiced infants in the study of Lucey et al. certainly lends weight to the significance of their observations. The fact that sera in their kernicteric infants were obtained several days after the onset of clinical manifestations raises the question of whether PSP-binding determinations may have actually been lower when kernicterus first developed.* Credence to such a possibility is derived from limited observations by Johnson and Boggs (1971) showing that bilirubin binding may be low at this time and may rise subsequently. For the present, however, one must conclude that the data of Lucey et al. and the impracticality of this test (requiring a dialysis time of 2 hours) render it of little use in evaluating the need for exchange transfusion in hyperbilirubinemic infants.

A number of other methods of estimating bilirubin binding capacity have since been developed. Among these are the Sephadex gel filtration method (Kaufmann et al., 1969), the HABA [2-(4'-hydroxybenzeneazo) benzoic acid] binding method (Porter and Waters, 1966; Johnson and Boggs, 1970) and the salicylate saturation method of Odell et al. (1969). To be useful, any such test should satisfy certain prerequisites: 1. it should require micro-samples (20 to 50 lambda) of serum; 2. it should be rapid and sufficiently simple to be

---

*The finding of Ackerman et al. (1971) that serum bilirubin levels may *fall* with the onset of kernicterus suggests a possible explanation for these conflicting observations.

performed with ease and accuracy by the usual night laboratory personnel; and 3. it should correlate well with the risk of late neurologic, psychologic and audiologic impairment. Of the above cited methods, those of Odell et al. and Johnson and Boggs seem to best fit these criteria for acceptance. Further experience with these and other methods as they are used in other laboratories seems necessary before any firm recommendations of their ultimate value can be made.

Addition of fresh human albumin to blood used for exchange transfusion has been shown to produce a significant increase in bilirubin binding capacity (Waters and Porter, 1964; Wood et al., 1970).

Amniotic Fluid Examination

Amniotic fluid, normally clear and colorless, acquires a yellow pigmentation in cases of severe hemolytic disease. This pigment has been identified as bilirubin (Brazie et al., 1966) and arises from the fetus through breakdown of red cells by Rh antibody. Unconjugated bilirubin formed in the fetus is transferred across partitioning membranes into the amniotic fluid (and maternal plasma), where it is bound by albumin (Cherry et al., 1970). With increasing severity of fetal hemolysis, there is a corresponding increase in the amniotic fluid concentrations of both bilirubin and albumin. The amount of bile pigment has been shown to reflect more accurately the degree of fetal affliction than does the maternal antibody titer (Bevis, 1956). The maternal antibody titer, coupled with the history of previous pregnancies, has been relied on in the past to guide the physician in the management of the sensitized mother and her unborn infant. Unfortunately, this information does not always predict accurately the outcome of the pregnancy, hydropic or stillborn infants occasionally being born of mothers with low, stationary, or falling titers. This has prompted several workers to study the amniotic fluid in an attempt to correlate the pigment concentration with the condition of the fetus at birth.

The concentration of bilirubin pigments is generally measured by spectrophotometry of amniotic fluid over the range from about 350 to 700 mμ. Normal amniotic fluid, when plotted on a logarithmic scale, describes a straight line, but when pigment is present a bulge appears around 450 mμ. This can be measured and is usually referred to as the optical density (O.D.) rise of the 450 mμ peak (Fig. 7-5).

Liley (1961), studying 101 Rh-sensitized pregnancies, found a significant correlation between the magnitude of this O.D. rise and the severity of the anemia at birth as indicated by the cord blood hemoglobin concentration (Fig. 7-6). Correlation with cord bilirubin concentration was poor, as might be expected, because this is influenced by extraneous factors such as placental and hepatic excretory

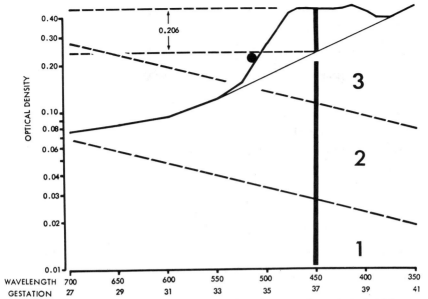

Figure 7–5 Example of optical density (O.D.) curve of amniotic fluid from an isoimmunized woman. The O.D. rise at 450 mμ is measured from the point where a tangent joining 550 mμ with 365 mμ intersects 450 mμ. The value of 0.206 obtained here falls into zone 3 in relation to the gestational age of 34.5 weeks. (From Bowman, J. M., and Pollock, J. M.: *Pediatrics*, 35:815, 1965.)

Figure 7–6 Relation between cord hemoglobin levels and the size of the 450 mμ peak recorded within one week. (From Liley, A. W.: *American Journal of Obstetrics & Gynecology*, 82:1359, 1961.)

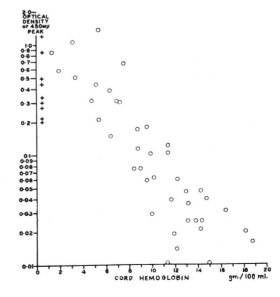

function. In a later publication, Liley (1963) summarized his observations on almost 400 patients studied at various stages of pregnancy after 28 weeks, and he was able to correlate the O.D. rise at a given gestational week with fetal outcome (Figs. 7–7 and 7–8). In Figure 7–7, the O.D. rise was roughly divided into three zones that indicated the degree of fetal affliction:

3. Severe disease, impending fetal death.

2. Indeterminate disease.

1. Rh-negative infant or mildly affected Rh-positive infant.

Because the O.D. rise, even with constant degrees of hemolysis, tends to fall with advancing gestation, repeat samples at two to three week intervals are necessary to follow the progression of the hemolytic process; stationary or rising O.D. values indicate worsening hemolysis. Such information is of great importance in determining the need for and optimal timing of premature induction of labor (with or without preliminary intrauterine intraperitoneal blood transfusions).

Subsequent experience with amniotic fluid examinations in other centers has revealed a number of instances of incorrect predictions based on readings from single samples. It is now generally agreed that predictions should be based on the *trend* of readings from two to three specimens separated by one to two week intervals. *A high*

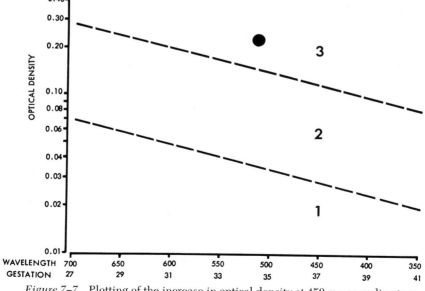

Figure 7–7   Plotting of the increase in optical density at 450 mμ according to gestational age, and zoning of the increase in optical density according to Liley's data. **Zone 3,** Severe disease; impending fetal death. **Zone 2,** Indeterminate disease. **Zone 1,** Rh-negative infant or mildly affected Rh-positive infant. (From Bowman, J. M., and Pollock, J. M.: *Pediatrics,* 35:815, 1965.)

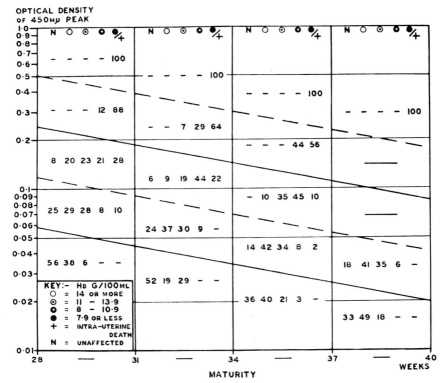

Figure 7–8 Percentage probability of the various grades of fetal affliction for the 450 mµ peak size in a single specimen. Maturity is in brackets of three weeks. (From Liley, A. W.: *American Journal of Obstetrics & Gynecology,* 86:485, 1963.)

reading that remains flat or rises is strong evidence pointing to the likelihood of intrauterine or neonatal death. A *line that is falling* suggests a live infant who is likely to survive. These conclusions are well illustrated in Figures 7–9, 7–10 and 7–11. A number of other methods of studying amniotic fluid have been employed by various workers. Included are direct measurements of bilirubin concentration (Gambino and Freda, 1966; Brazie et al., 1969) and estimates of antibody content of amniotic fluid (Dalton, 1970). A discussion of the relative merits of these various methods of amniotic fluid examination is beyond the scope of this book and may be found by consulting recent reviews (Liley, 1968; Walker, 1970). Additional efforts have been made to circumvent the need to relate amniotic fluid bilirubin content to gestational age. Cherry et al. (1965) showed that the ratio of pigment concentration (O.D.$_{450}$ to O.D.$_{600}$) to total protein concentration of amniotic fluid remained fairly constant through the later stages of pregnancy. The predictive value of this method has not been verified by other workers (Queenan, 1967). Muller-Eberhard

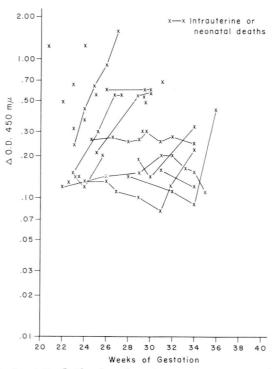

Figure 7–9 Amniotic fluid values from intrauterine or neonatal deaths. Values are recorded as deviation from normal in optical density at 450 millimicrons. Serial values are connected by lines. (From Queenan, 1967.)

and Bashore (1970) pursued this further and have shown that the ratio of bilirubin concentration (chemical) to *albumin* in amniotic fluid was a more accurate indicator of the degree of fetal hemolysis than Liley's spectrophotometric determination. However, they made most of their comparisons only on single samples of amniotic fluid, thus raising some questions of the real advantage of the additional chemical determinations over the Liley determinations on *two or more* amniotic fluids.

The technical details of collection, preparation, and spectro-photometric examination of amniotic fluid have been reviewed by Liley (1961, 1963, and 1965), Bowman (1965), and Queenan (1967). Amniocentesis is usually performed in the first sensitized pregnancy, when the maternal anti-D titer (indirect Coombs) exceeds 1:32. In such pregnancies, the procedure is usually deferred until around 28 to 29 weeks' gestation. In later pregnancies in which there is a history of a previous affected infant or stillbirth, amniotic fluid examinations are usually initiated around 10 weeks before the time in gestation at which the previous pregnancy ended.

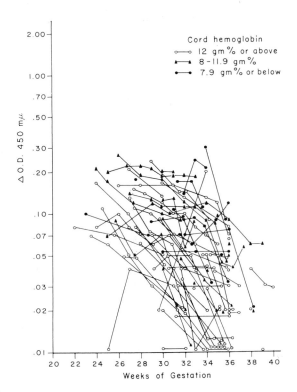

Figure 7-10 Amniotic fluid values from surviving infants, with or without exchange transfusions. Note definite downward trend of values. (From Queenan, 1967.)

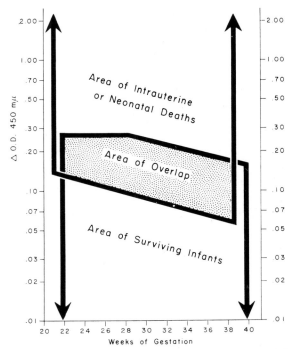

Figure 7-11 Representation of the distribution of amniotic fluid values in Figures 7-9 and 7-10. Note area of overlapping values.

207

In experienced hands, this procedure is generally agreed to be safe. Reported complications are rare. They include hemoperitoneum, accidental hemorrhage, fetal exsanguination, and infection. Careful localization of the placenta, usually obtainable by palpation of the fetal parts, is important to avoid trauma with subsequent transfer of fetal cells into the maternal circulation. This has been shown to aggravate antibody production in the mother (Zipursky et al., 1963; Peddle, 1968). For this reason, amniocentesis should not be carried out on unsensitized mothers. Occasionally, placental localization requires isotopic methods, using chromium-51 labeled red cells or iodine-131 labeled human serum albumin.

Sources of Error.   Important sources of error in measurement of amniotic fluid pigment concentration include the following:

CONTAMINATION WITH MECONIUM OR VERNIX CASEOSA.   This causes turbidity interfering with the optical density readings. Routine centrifugation and filtration of all amniotic fluid specimens removes most of this turbidity. If it persists, dilution with distilled water may be necessary.

CONTAMINATION WITH FETAL BLOOD.   The fetal origin of such blood may be confirmed by testing the red cells present after centrifugation by blood grouping or fetal erythrocyte staining. Fetal serum bilirubin may give a false high value for the bilirubin concentration in the amniotic fluid. Therefore, such samples should be discarded and the procedure repeated in one to two weeks.

CONTAMINATION WITH HEMOLYZED RED BLOOD CELLS (OF FETAL OR MATERNAL ORIGIN).   Dissolved hemoglobin will result in increased O.D. peaks at 415, 540 and 575 mμ, the sum total of which may yield false high O.D. rises at 450 mμ. Immediate centrifugation of blood-tinged fluids to remove intact red cells may be sufficient to prevent hemolysis and liberation of hemoglobin. Alternately a correction factor may be applied, equivalent to 5 per cent of the deviation from linearity at 415 mμ (Liley, 1961).

EXPOSURE TO LIGHT.   The pigment concentration is reduced by exposure to light. Amniotic fluids should therefore be kept in a dark tube or box from the time of collection until the spectrophotometric examination is completed.

DILUTION DUE TO POLYHYDRAMNIOS.   Queenan et al. (1968), measuring amniotic fluid volume by a dye dilution technique, showed that falsely low spectrophotometric values may result from polyhydramnios.

TREATMENT

In 1950, Allen et al. showed that live-born erythroblastotic infants could be protected from kernicterus by exchange transfusion. Not content with this measure of success, further fetal salvage was sought by focusing on the threats to life of the unborn infant—namely, severe anemia and hydrops fetalis. Early delivery, guided by maternal history, antibody titers, and amniotic fluid findings, saved many of these infants. There still remained those infants so severely affected that intrauterine death before 30 weeks gestation was most certain. The technique of intrauterine intraperitoneal transfusion developed by Liley (1963) prolongs the life of many of these infants until they are sufficiently mature to be delivered safely, with minimal risk from the dual hazards of severe anemia and prematurity.

It is evident from this that optimal management of the sensitized mother and her infant requires a continuing antenatal and postnatal effort, with responsibility shared equally by a team consisting of obstetrician, pediatrician, and serologist. In no other area of neonatology is this concept so clearly brought out. The main points of this antenatal diagnostic and therapeutic program are summarized in Table 7–4.

Exchange Transfusion

Objectives. The chief object of the initial exchange transfusion is the removal of antibody-coated red cells, which if allowed to remain in the infant, would break down and yield large amounts of bilirubin. Approximately 85 per cent of the infant's cells may be removed by this procedure. Removal of bilirubin is accomplished less

Table 7–4 Antenatal Management of the Rh-sensitized Mother

ON THE BASIS OF:	DECIDE—ONE OF THREE COURSES OF ACTION:

1. History
   Previous blood transfusions or injections
   Previous pregnancies and outcome
 	
2. Serological tests
   Father's Rh zygosity
   Maternal antibody titer
     at approximately 16 weeks, 28 weeks, etc.
 	
3. Amniocentesis
   In first sensitized pregnancy
   (Coombs titer > 1:32), at 28–29 weeks
   If previously severely affected infant—as early as 20–23 weeks
   Trend of repeat values important
	1. Favorable: wait until 38 weeks then induce labor
	
	2. Risk of hydrops fetalis or stillbirth: early induction of labor between 34 and 38 weeks
	
	3. Risk of hydrops fetalis or stillbirth before 34 weeks: intrauterine intraperitoneal transfusion(s), and induce labor at 34–35 weeks.

efficiently, although this becomes the main object of second and later exchange transfusions. The addition of albumin has substantially improved the efficiency of removal of bilirubin (Odell et al., 1962; Waters and Porter, 1964; Comley and Wood, 1968). Also, in the severely anemic, hydropic, or prehydropic infant, heart failure may be dramatically reversed by exchange transfusion designed to rapidly reduce the elevated venous pressure.

Criteria. Precise criteria for exchange transfusion vary among different workers. Certain principles are at present common to most, and a synthesis of these is attempted here. In general, when presented with a newborn with a positive direct Coombs test on the cord blood, the question is whether exchange transfusion should be performed immediately or deferred until the subsequent course of the disease becomes evident. The information generally considered necessary to make this decision includes the history of previous offspring, maternal Rh antibody titer, clinical status at birth, and cord hemoglobin and bilirubin concentrations. In Table 7–5 are the criteria selected by McKay (1964); they enable a reasonable decision to be made on the basis of the foregoing information. However, certain

Table 7–5 Need for Exchange Transfusion in Infants with a Positive Coombs Test[*]

	OBSERVE	CONSIDER EXCHANGE	DO EXCHANGE
At Birth			
History of previous offspring	No need for exchange transfusion	Exchange transfusion necessary or kernicterus	Death or near death from erythroblastosis
Maternal Rh antibody titer	<1:64	>1:64	
Clinical situation	Apparently normal	Induced or spontaneous delivery of premature infant	Jaundice, fetal hydrops
Cord hemoglobin	>14 gm./100 ml.	12–14 gm./100 ml.	<12 gm./100 ml.
Cord bilirubin	<4 mg./100 ml.	4–5 mg./100 ml.	>5 mg./100 ml.
After Birth			
Capillary blood hemoglobin	>12 gm./100 ml.	<12 gm./100 ml.	<12 gm./100 ml. and falling in first 24 hours
Serum bilirubin	<18 mg./100 ml.	18–20 mg./100 ml.	20 mg./100 ml. in first 48 hours or 22 mg./100 ml. on two successive determinations at 6–8 hr. intervals after 48 hrs. Clinical signs suggesting kernicterus at any time or any bilirubin level

[*]From McKay, R. J.: Pediatrics, 33:763, 1964.

reservations must be kept in mind. A history of the need for exchange transfusion in a previous sibling does not necessarily reflect severity of disease in that infant since the exchange may have been performed unnecessarily or for jaundice due in part to nonhemolytic factors such as immaturity or infection. Also, succeeding infants are not always as severely affected as previous siblings. The predictive value of the maternal antibody titer in individual cases is sufficiently imperfect that it is of little help in guiding one to a decision of the need for exchange transfusion. Limiting the criteria for early exchange to the presence of either clinical evidence of disease or a cord hemoglobin below 13.5 grams per 100 ml. *and* a cord bilirubin level above 3.5 mg. per 100 ml., Dunn (1966) found that over half of the infants born to sensitized mothers could safely get along without exchange transfusion.

Following birth, serum indirect bilirubin values are best evaluated by plotting individual determinations on a graph against the infant's age in order to estimate the rate of rise toward an anticipated peak (Fig. 7–4). The need for *repeat* exchange transfusions may be determined by reference to such a graph, the aim being to keep serum indirect bilirubin levels under 20 mg./100 ml.

In borderline cases, the use of one of the tests of bilirubin binding capacity (or reserve albumin binding capacity), as discussed earlier, may aid further in deciding on the need for exchange transfusion. In the hands of Odell et al. (1970) and Johnson and Boggs (1970), such tests correlate better with the risk of late neurologic toxicity than does the serum bilirubin level. Although these tests are less easy to perform in the routine clinical laboratory than is the serum bilirubin, their improved predictive value points to the importance of including a test of bilirubin binding in the laboratory evaluation of the jaundiced newborn. Their ultimate value awaits experience derived from their use under the usual circumstances and personnel of the average clinical laboratory.

Technique. The simplest and most widely used technique is that outlined by Allen and Diamond (1957), the details of which are given in their monograph. Minor improvements in equipment and procedure have been introduced since then and have been reviewed by Odell et al. (1962) and Bowman and Friesen (1970). One of the most important factors in the smooth performance of exchange transfusion is the experience and skill of the operator. Unfortunately, with increasing use of phototherapy and the anti-D gamma globulin, the immediate benefits of reduced need for exchange transfusion will be attended by the long term consequence of a reduction in the number of pediatricians with sufficient experience to perform this procedure with confidence. It is important that pediatricians responsible for newborn care take cognizance of this fact now and insure that exchange transfusions continue to be performed by or under the close supervision of experienced personnel. In the absence of such personnel, newborns for possible exchange are best referred to centers where experience and expertise in this procedure are concentrated.

When the decision for exchange has been made, it is wise to substitute glucose water for the infant's formula. Immediately before exchange, the gastric contents should be aspirated. Suction apparatus should be on hand during the exchange in case excessive mucus or regurgitation develops.

Except for the severely anemic newborn who requires packed red blood cells, whole blood is used, in a volume of 160 to 180 ml./ kg. body weight. The chief advantage of whole blood lies in the presence of unbound albumin in the plasma and its ability to bind a maximal quantity of free bilirubin. Generally, the blood should be less than three days old. In the very sick or hydropic infant, improved oxygen delivery to the tissues may be obtained by using very fresh blood less than 24 hours old (Delivoria-Papadopoulos et al., 1971a).

Although heparinized blood is preferable because it eliminates the metabolic hazards of acid-citrate-dextrose (ACD) anticoagulant, the need for such blood to be fresh (less than 24 hours old) is a difficult one to satisfy in most blood banks; therefore, ACD blood (less than three to four days old) is generally used. The blood should be group O, Rh-negative, and cross-matched by an indirect Coombs test *against the mother's serum prior to delivery.* In centers where a large proportion of the donor population is Negro, a sickle cell preparation on the donor blood should be considered part of the cross-match procedure. Exchange transfusion with sickle cell trait blood has produced fatal intravascular sickling (Veiga and Vaithianathan, 1963). Prior to use the blood should be warmed to room temperature (see p. 218).

Albumin should be given when the need for more than one exchange is anticipated. The simplest procedure is to replace 50 ml. of supernatant plasma (of whole blood) with 50 ml. of 25 per cent salt-poor human albumin (Waters and Porter, 1964). Albumin is contraindicated in severely anemic or hydropic infants for fear of increasing plasma volume and aggravating congestive heart failure.

The equipment for exchange transfusion is now available commercially as the Pharmaseal Sterile Exchange Transfusion Tray.* This equipment functions well and offers many advantages over standard equipment. A recent modification simplifying the three-way stopcock has been of great value.

Placement of the tip of the umbilical venous catheter is critical. Optimally, it should be passed through the ductus venosus into the inferior vena cava (Fig. 7–12) in order to avoid the complications

---

*Pharmaseal Laboratories, Glendale, California.

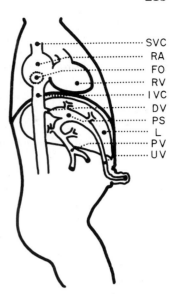

Figure 7–12 Umbilical venous system in the newborn. SVC, superior vena cava; RA, right atrium; FO, foramen ovale; RV, right ventricle; IVC, inferior vena cava; DV, ductus venosus; PS, portal sinus; L, liver; PV, portal vein; UV, umbilical vein. (From Kitterman et al., Pediat. Clin. N. Amer. 17:895, 1970.)

that may arise with a catheter tip in the portal vein or one of its branches (Kitterman et al., 1970). The location of the catheter should be verified by x-ray.

The need for an alert, competent assistant who is familiar with resuscitative techniques cannot be too strongly emphasized.

Syringe volumes exchanged are generally 20 ml. for term infants and 10 ml. for smaller prematures. The entire exchange should be accomplished in about one hour.

In the infant (usually a premature) with *hydrops fetalis*, a number of disturbances exist which require special consideration in treatment. The main problem is the severe anemia resulting in congestive heart failure with edema, ascites, and pleural effusions. Hypoxia and acidosis (mixed metabolic and respiratory) may be associated with peripheral and probable pulmonary vasoconstriction which is responsible for the elevated venous pressure in the face of a normal blood volume (Phibbs and Toohey, 1968). Hepatic insufficiency associated with severe hemolysis may contribute to hypoalbuminemia, hypoglycemia, and coagulation defects. A rational plan of management of the hydropic infant should, therefore, include the following measures:

1. Prompt establishment of respirations and administration of oxygen by positive pressure, through tracheal intubation if necessary. If ascites is severe, sufficient fluid should be removed to ease respirations.

2. Rapid correction of acidosis.

3. Keep baby warm and use prewarmed donor blood (p. 218).

4. Blood for exchange transfusion should consist of fresh (under 24 hours) packed cells, preferably anticoagulated with heparin to avoid the acidosis associated with ACD (acid–citrate–dextrose) blood. If only ACD blood is available, this should be first buffered with tris (hydroxymethyl) aminomethane (THAM) (see p. 216). Acidosis may also be averted by using blood anticoagulated with citrate–phosphate–dextrose (CPD). Elevated venous pressure should be reduced by first removing approximately 20 ml. of blood for each 10 ml. infused until the venous pressure is normalized (a deficit of 40 to 80 ml. may be necessary by the end of the exchange). The total volume of this first critical exchange should be 1 to 1½ times the infant's estimated blood volume, rather than the usual two-volume exchange. Albumin is contraindicated in the first exchange.

5. After the exchange, it is wise to maintain the infant with an infusion of 10 per cent glucose in water (65 ml. per kg. per day) by scalp vein. Depending on the clinical condition, frequent monitoring of blood gases, pH, and glucose may be necessary, with the addition of sodium bicarbonate or extra glucose as required.

6. Serum indirect bilirubin levels must be watched frequently (at intervals of 4 to 8 hours) in the first few days after birth to determine the need for repeat exchange transfusion. Decisions regarding exchange should take into consideration factors that may compromise serum binding of bilirubin such as hypoalbuminemia, acidosis, hypoxia, and the presence of visible heme pigments in the plasma. Once the infant's cardiorespiratory status has been stabilized, albumin may be added to the whole blood used for exchange transfusion, as described earlier.

7. If bleeding should develop in association with severe thrombocytopenia or coagulation defects, the possibility of disseminated intravascular coagulation should be considered (Chessels and Wigglesworth, 1971). If confirmed, this could be treated by exchange transfusion with heparinized blood, followed by transfusion of fresh platelet-rich plasma.

8. Measures of questionable value in such infants include digitalis, diuretics, and peritoneal dialysis (Nathan, 1968; Parkin and Walker, 1968).

Although the chance of survival of hydropic infants is generally very poor, the report of salvage of 6 out of 19 such infants by Bowman and his group in Winnipeg (1969) suggests that aggressive management may at times be rewarding. Additional measures used by these workers included instillation of digoxin in the fetal peritoneal cavity at the time of intrauterine transfusion along with administration of digoxin and diuretics to the mother. Further studies are necessary to evaluate the relative importance of these measures and to explore other measures.

Prophylactic antibiotics after exchange should not be necessary with good aseptic technique. Although positive blood cultures are frequent in postexchange blood obtained not only from the umbilical vein catheter but also from peripheral veins (Lipsitz and Cornet, 1960; Nelson et al., 1965), this probably represents a transient bacteremia due to contamination of the catheter with bacteria in the umbilical stump. Because clinical signs of septicemia are rare among such patients, it seems wise to observe them closely and institute antibiotic therapy only if suspicious signs develop. In the infants followed by Nelson (1965), treated with and without antibiotics, there was no difference in the incidence of infection.

Biochemical Changes. The occurrence of sudden unexpected death during exchange transfusion suggests that biochemical disturbances may be at fault. Those that have been observed include:

1. *Hyperkalemia* resulting from aged blood may cause cardiac arrest. However, the use of blood under four days of age has almost eliminated this complication.

2. *Hypocalcemia* may occur secondary to the removal of calcium by binding with the citrate of the ACD blood. This has given rise to the common practice of infusing approximately 1 ml. of 10 per cent calcium gluconate after every 100 to 150 ml. of blood exchanged. Cardiac monitoring is critical. Recent studies in which *ionized* calcium has been measured in addition to total calcium indicate that reduced calcium ion concentrations are common during exchange (especially in the premature), are rarely associated with symptoms, and are only transiently raised by the infusion of calcium gluconate (Maisels et al., 1971; Radde et al., 1971). Further studies are necessary, however, before it can be recommended that the practice of adding calcium be modified or abandoned.

3. *Hypomagnesemia* has also been observed (Bajpai et al., 1967). As yet, there is no evidence that this is of sufficient significance to warrant the routine infusion of magnesium during exchange transfusion.

4. *Increased blood citrate*, along with increased blood pyruvate, has been demonstrated by Anderson et al. (1963). However, they did not observe tetany or other complications associated with this.

5. *Acidosis* during exchange with ACD blood has been observed by several workers (Povey, 1964; Barrie, 1964; Calladine and Gairdner, 1964). When ACD solution is added to freshly drawn blood, there is an initial pH drop from 7.4 to about 7.0, with a further decrease to about 6.4 during storage for three weeks. In three of six infants studied by Povey, the pH fell during exchange to dangerously low levels — 7.06, 7.04, and 6.95. Similar pH values were observed by Barrie (1964) but in only two of 20 exchange transfusions. He attributed this lower incidence to variations in technique, including removal of 80

per cent of the supernatant plasma and a slower rate of exchange. In a more recent study, Barrie (1965) showed that acidosis could largely be prevented by the administration of sodium bicarbonate, either as a separate injection of 1 mEq. after every 100 ml. of blood, or mixed with the donor blood in similar amounts. Because sodium bicarbonate may cause hypernatremia and elevation of the pCO_2, it has been recommended that THAM be used instead (Pierson et al., 1968). These workers advise that when ACD blood is used for exchange transfusion, even for low-risk infants, it should be buffered to physiologic pH by the addition of 8 ml. of hypertonic (1.2M) THAM,* added immediately before transfusion. Alternatively, we have found that blood anticoagulated with CPD is well tolerated without drop in blood pH by small prematures and has the advantage of not requiring addition of alkli.

Calladine and Gairdner (1964) observed a rise in pH due to metabolism of citrate to bicarbonate. This resulted in a pronounced alkalosis developing within half an hour after completion of an exchange transfusion and lasting several days. In Barrie's study (1965), the alkalosis was also observed but it was milder, pH values not rising over 7.5. Use of sodium bicarbonate or THAM does not augment this alkalosis.

6. *Hypoglycemia* may be present before exchange transfusion and may be aggravated afterward when ACD blood has been used (see p. 195).

In spite of the large amount of information gathered on the biochemical changes occurring with exchange transfusion, a definite relation to sudden death during the procedure has not yet been proven. Although it might seem that heparinized blood has an advantage because it avoids some of these changes, the possibility that it may aggravate hypoglycemia and raise the level of free fatty acids (which compete with bilirubin for binding to albumin), and the difficulty in assuring its ready availability in most blood banks make it difficult to recommend for general use. In a study by Schiff et al. (1971), the metabolic effects of heparinized and ACD blood have been compared.

Electrocardiographic Changes. Robinson and Barrie (1963) used the electrocardiograph to monitor 30 exchange transfusions and found frequent elevation of the P wave and slight tachycardia. Serious alterations, such as bradycardia, abnormal QRS complexes, and ST segment changes, were occasionally observed and were regarded as danger signs of ventricular embarrassment. They recommended use of electrocardiographic monitoring for the early detection of such changes.

---

*THAM-E (tromethamine with electrolytes), Abbott Laboratories, North Chicago, Illinois. To prepare a 1.2 M solution add 250 ml. of 10 per cent dextrose in water to the bottle containing 36 grams of powder. Discard after use.

Table 7-6 Potential Hazards of Exchange Transfusion*

TYPE OF HAZARD	PROBLEMS ENCOUNTERED
Vascular	Embolization with air or clots Thrombosis Hemorrhagic infarction of the colon
Cardiac	Arrhythmias Volume overload Arrest
Metabolic	Hyperkalemia Hypernatremia Hypocalcemia Hypomagnesemia Acidosis Hypoglycemia
Clotting	Overheparinization Thrombocytopenia
Infections	Bacteremia Serum hepatitis Malaria (Czapek et al., 1968)
Miscellaneous	Mechanical injury to donor cells Perforation Hypothermia

*Modified from Odell, G. B., et al.: Pediat. Clin. N. Amer., 9:605, 1962.

Potential Hazards. These are listed in Table 7-6.

Thrombosis, when it occurs, usually develops in the portal vein in association with difficult or traumatic insertion of the catheter, prolonged retention of the catheter after exchange, or infection. Portal hypertension with splenomegaly and esophageal varices may develop, becoming manifest within the first year or two of life (Oski et al., 1963). In uncomplicated exchange transfusions, this sequela is rare (Thompson and Sherlock, 1964).

Another vascular complication that has been reported recently is hemorrhagic infarction of the colon (Corkery et al., 1968; Friedman et al., 1970). This probably results from the presence of a catheter in the portal system producing retrograde microembolism or obstructive hemodynamic changes, leading to hemorrhagic infarction of the colon with perforation. Clinical manifestations include abdominal distention, passage of blood by rectum, and symptoms of sepsis. Free air in the peritoneal cavity has been demonstrated on flat x-ray films of the abdomen in about half of the reported cases. This complication adds weight to recommendations that the catheter location for exchange transfusion be verified by x-ray (or fluoroscope).

Hypothermia, both general and cardiac, may result from infusion of unwarmed blood. The possibility that the latter may be a factor in the unexplained cardiac arrhythmias and circulatory collapse occasionally observed during exchange transfusion points to the need for preventive measures. Hey and co-workers recommend the following:

1. Ambient temperature should be approximately 28 to 30°C. (80 to 86°F.) in a draft-free room. 2. Donor blood should be removed from the refrigerator and left at room temperature for 3 to 5 hours before the exchange. (More rapid warming can be obtained by placing the donor bag in a 37°C. water bath with gentle mixing by inversion every 30 minutes for 1 to 2 hours). To prevent recooling of donor blood during its passage from the bag down the infusion tubing, the latter should be either enclosed in a thermally regulated water jacket or connected to at least a six foot long section of coiled tubing immersed in a 37°C. water bath.

Mortality. The mortality rate of the exchange transfusion procedure itself has been defined by Boggs and Westphal (1960) as the number of infants who died during or within six hours after an exchange transfusion. This may be expressed in relation either to the total number of infants exchanged or to the total number of exchanges. Most workers exclude from this figure infants who are hydropic, kernicteric, or otherwise moribund at the time of exchange. By this definition, it is generally agreed that the mortality rate of exchange transfusion should be less than 1 per cent. The most important factor in maintaining this low figure is the experience and skill of the persons performing the exchange. Prevention of acidosis, hypothermia and hypoglycemia may further diminish the morbidity and mortality risks of the procedure.

Anemia After Exchange Transfusion. A moderate degree of anemia is common after exchange transfusion. This probably results from a combination of factors that include degree of anemia at birth, dilution of infant's blood by whole blood of lower hematocrit used for the exchange, and persistence of Rh antibody, causing not only hemolysis of remaining Rh-positive erythrocytes but also destruction of newly formed reticulocytes from the bone marrow. Destruction of reticulocytes probably accounts for the observation of low reticulocyte counts in peripheral blood in the presence of increased erythroid activity in the bone marrow.

Simple transfusion is rarely necessary for this type of anemia. In the immediate postexchange period, if the hemoglobin concentration falls below 10 gm./100 ml., a small transfusion of Rh-negative packed red cells may be given, sufficient to raise the hemoglobin to 12 to 13 gm./100 ml. Following discharge from hospital, a further decrease in hemoglobin to levels as low as 5 to 6 gm./100 ml. by six to eight weeks of life may occur. This is tolerated surprisingly well and is almost always corrected spontaneously, heralded by an increase in reticulocyte count at about this time. Only if the infant is lethargic, feeding poorly, and not thriving in the presence of persistent reticulocytopenia should blood transfusion be considered. Again, only Rh-negative blood should be given. Hematinics, such as iron, folic acid, and vitamin B_{12}, are of no value in this type of anemia.

Selective Induction of Labor—Early Delivery

The purpose of early delivery is to prevent stillbirth from severe anemia. Allen et al. (1954) showed that 10 per cent of babies who were still alive in utero at 37 weeks of gestation were subsequently stillborn. Presumably, most of these infants could be saved by delivery at 37 weeks.

Which infants are at risk and potentially salvageable? In the past, attempts to answer this question have been based mainly on information regarding the history of previous stillbirths, maternal antibody titers, and zygosity of the father. Chown and Bowman (1958) state that the risk of stillbirth in the next Rh-positive infant of a woman with one previous stillbirth is 75 per cent, and this rises to 90 per cent following two previous stillbirths. In addition, hydrops fetalis is frequent among the remaining newborn infants. Similar figures are given by Allen et al. (1954), who in addition showed the predictive value of maternal antibody titers. The value of early delivery of infants judged to be at risk (on the basis of previous pregnancy outcome) has been well shown in a large retrospective study by Boggs (1964). But must we wait for the knowledge derived by sacrificing one infant by stillbirth in order to save subsequent infants by early delivery? Recent experience with amniotic fluid examination has shown that this need not be so. It has been shown that the findings on amniocentesis give the best correlation with the severity of anemia in the infant, and are therefore of greater value in determining the risk of stillbirth at any stage of gestation. Knowing which infants are at risk and delivering them sufficiently early to avert severe anemia should theoretically prevent stillbirth and hydrops fetalis. However, the risks of prematurity—in particular hyaline membrane disease and pulmonary immaturity—are large enough to render delivery before 34 weeks unrewarding. In infants of this age or older, however, with good obstetrical and pediatric management, the outlook should be good.

In Rh-sensitized mothers not requiring early delivery, Allen and Diamond recommend "pre-term" induction at about 38 weeks of gestation. This practice not only spares some infants the risk of further intrauterine exposure to antibody, but also enables mother and infant to reap the benefits of an alert, well-prepared "first" team of obstetrician, pediatrician, and nursing and technical staff, rather than suffer the uncertainties surrounding a middle-of-the-night spontaneous delivery.

Intrauterine Intraperitoneal Transfusion

What can be done for those infants so severely affected that they would die in utero before 34 weeks of gestation? Liley (1963) reasoned that because the main threat to survival of these infants was severe anemia, efforts to prolong intrauterine life should concentrate on blood transfusion for amelioration of the anemia. With this in mind, the technique of intrauterine intraperitoneal transfusion was developed. In essence, this represents a form of partial exchange transfusion because the addition of Rh-negative donor cells is balanced by the removal of antibody-coated Rh-positive fetal cells by hemolysis. Erythrocytes introduced into the peritoneal cavity of the infant are absorbed intact into the fetal circulation. *This procedure should be reserved for the small group of infants who from the findings on amniocentesis are almost certain to die before 34 weeks of gestation.*

Indications and Technique

The technique of intrauterine intraperitoneal transfusion is not one to be undertaken by any but an experienced obstetrical and pediatric team. The details, first reported by Liley in 1963, have been brought up to date more recently (Liley, 1965, 1968; Queenan, 1967). The ideal candidate is a fetus between 28 and 33 weeks of gestation whose trend of optical density values obtained from two amniocenteses one week apart is high (upper zone 2 or zone 3 of Liley's graph and either flat or rising [see Fig. 7–9]). In the fetus under 28 weeks of gestation, transfusion is technically difficult because of the small size and mobility of the fetus. The two-needle technique of Liggins (1966), whereby the fetus is transfixed with one needle while blood is injected through the other needle, has helped to overcome this problem, enabling successful transfusion of fetuses as young as 20 weeks. As with amniocentesis, accurate localization of the placenta is important. A 16 gauge 18 cm. Tuohy needle is inserted into the abdominal wall under local anesthesia and is introduced into the amniotic cavity; radiopaque dye is then injected. This serves to outline more accurately the placental site, to detect signs of fetal hydrops, and to demonstrate the fetal gastrointestinal tract (and peritoneal cavity). When the latter is localized, the needle is advanced cautiously through the anterior abdominal wall of the fetus into the peritoneal cavity and after replacement of the needle by a 50 cm. nylon epidural catheter, blood is then injected. This should be fresh group O Rh-negative packed red blood cells, anticoagulated with ACD and cross matched against maternal serum. The volume required has been reduced somewhat from the initial figures of 80 to 120 ml. to volumes more in keeping with recent estimates of peritoneal blood volume. Depending on the stage of gestation, the volume required varies from 20 ml. at 20 to 22 weeks to 75 ml. at 33 weeks (Queenan, 1967). Improved survival of fetuses receiving smaller volumes suggests that some of the earlier fetal deaths after intrauterine transfusion may have been due to an excessive volume of infused blood leading to abdominal distention, elevation of the diaphragm and cardiothoracic embarrassment. Antibiotics are administered to the fetal peritoneum, the amniotic cavity, and the mother. Depending on the severity of fetal affliction and the interval before planned delivery, repeat transfusions may be necessary. These transfusions are usually performed at intervals of 1½ to 3 weeks. When the infant is finally delivered at about 34 to 35 weeks of gestation, the cord blood should be analyzed for the proportion of nonfetal donor erythrocytes by estimating the concentration of Hb F chemically or by the red cell staining technique of Kleihauer et al. (1957). Instead of the usual proportion of adult hemoglobin of 15 to 40 per cent, much higher values are found, of the order of 55 to 95 per cent in most reported cases.

Results. The early results of intrauterine transfusion by Liley (1965) showed survival rates of approximately 50 per cent among infants in whom death in utero or postnatally with hydrops fetalis was felt to be otherwise inevitable. The initial enthusiasm, however, has been tempered somewhat by further experience over the years. With the knowledge that predictions based on *single* amniotic fluid examinations are less reliable than those based on the *slope of two or more* plotted values, we have learned how better to select infants truly at risk and to avoid unnecessary transfusion of infants likely to survive beyond 34 weeks of gestation. With the knowledge that hydropic infants subjected to this procedure have a very low salvage rate, of the order of 10 to 15 per cent (Lucey, 1966), most workers have in the past regarded this as a contraindication to intrauterine transfusion. Accumulated experience has, in addition to improved selection of infants for the procedure, led to improved technical skill in performing it and also better management of the prematurely born infant.

In Table 7–7 are listed the results of intrauterine transfusion compiled from the experience of 11 university hospital groups during 1964 and 1965 (Lucey, 1966). Of 238 fetuses receiving intrauterine transfusions, the survival rate for non-hydropic fetuses was 45.3 per cent and for hydropic fetuses, it was only 13.6 per cent. Subsequent results of other groups have been summarized by Walker and Ellis

Table 7–7   Cooperative Report on Intrauterine Transfusions
in Erythroblastosis Fetalis*

	Total Number of Fetuses Receiving I.U.T.'s 238		
Hydrops Fetalis 110		Nonhydropic 128	
Deaths 81	Survivors 29	Survivors 77	Deaths 51
$\frac{14}{95}$	14 Neonatal Deaths 19 33		$\frac{19}{70}$
	15 Neonatal Survivors 58 73		
	Final percent of Infants Salvaged		
13.6%	30.7%		45.3%

*From Lucey, J. F., in Intrauterine Transfusion and Erythroblastosis Fetalis, Report of the Fifty-third Ross Conference on Pediatric Research, Lucey J. F., and Butterfield, L. J., eds., Columbus. Ross Laboratories, 1966, p. 14.

(1970). As discussed earlier, increasing experience resulting in better patient selection and improved technical skill has increased survival rates in some centers to as high as 62 per cent (Bowman et al., 1969). Even among hydropic infants, Bowman and co-workers, by a combination of aggressive measures as outlined on p. 213, have succeeded in salvaging 6 out of 19 such infants. Results such as this, if confirmed in other centers, suggest the value of not abandoning the infant found to be hydropic at the time of an initial intrauterine transfusion.

Risks.   Fetal risks are mainly a result of needle injury to the soft tissues and viscera and are now of the order of 5 per cent per procedure. Misplaced injection of radiopaque dye prior to transfusion has resulted in localized areas of necrosis of kidney, spleen, and liver (Craig and Fellers, 1970). These authors also described two surviving infants with renal insufficiency attributable to this complication. The hazard of infection after intrauterine transfusion appears to be small and not influenced by the use of prophylactic antibiotics (Lucey, 1966).

The presence of viable lymphocytes in normal donor blood transfused to young fetuses whose immunologic competence is perhaps incompletely developed has raised the question of the risk of a graft versus host reaction after intrauterine transfusion (Hathaway et al., 1965). Among the many hundreds of infants who have received intrauterine transfusions, only two possible examples of such a complication have been reported (Marini et al., 1967; Naiman et al., 1969). Admittedly rare, this complication nevertheless justifies in our opinion reasonable efforts to remove immunocompetent lymphocytes from donor blood intended for transfusion to the very young fetus.

Premature onset of labor has been a serious consequence of intrauterine transfusion in the experience of Boggs (1970), and has been a great deterrent in selection of cases for this procedure.

Maternal complications are infrequent, occurring in only 9 of 238 mothers in the cooperative study summarized by Lucey (1966): infections and bleeding accounted for most of these complications.

The Infant Born After Intrauterine Transfusion. Such infants are usually the more generally severely affected and show high levels of bilirubin (especially the conjugated fraction) in cord blood. This reflects the severity of hemolysis and its effects on the liver. Anemia, usually proportional to the hyperbilirubinemia, may be masked to a great degree by the intrauterine transfusion. In some infants, the cord blood hemoglobin level may be almost normal, with negative direct Coombs test and predominantly non-fetal red cells, indicating almost complete replacement by donor blood. Although in rare instances an infant such as this does not require exchange transfusion, the vast majority do and multiple exchange transfusions are usually necessary.

Late complications among the survivors of intrauterine transfusion are surprisingly few in proportion to the number and seriousness of the risk factors (prematurity, hypoxia, hypoglycemia, cardiorespiratory distress, and severe hyperbilirubinemia). Studies of growth, development, and neurologic status have yielded normal findings in the vast majority of such infants (Gregg and Hutchinson, 1969; Phibbs et al., 1971). The importance of vigorous management of the above risk factors was emphasized by Phibbs and his associates. Persistent anemia in the first few months is to be anticipated in these infants and in some cases may require transfusion of Rh-negative packed cells. In a fascinating case studied by Cohen et al. (1970), the development of Rh reactivity of the infant's red cells was delayed for over five months; they attributed this phenomenon to suppression of Rh antigen by maternal Rh antibody. An increased incidence of inguinal hernias has also been noted, presumably a consequence of abdominal distention due to intraperitoneal blood.

PREVENTION OF Rh HEMOLYTIC DISEASE

The many theoretic approaches to the prevention of Rh hemolytic disease have been reviewed by Allen (1963). Of these the one showing greatest promise concerns the initial phase of pathogenesis of the disease—namely, maternal sensitization by Rh-positive fetal erythrocytes.

The basis for this approach lies in the observation that ABO incompatibility offers protection against the development of Rh sensitization, probably by allowing destruction of the fetal red cells in the mother before they can stimulate Rh antibody formation. Finn et al. (1961), in Liverpool, were the first to suggest that Rh sensitization might be prevented by destroying the fetal red cells as rapidly as possible after they entered the maternal circulation. Because most, but not all, transfer of fetal cells occurs at delivery, efforts to destroy such cells might best be undertaken soon after delivery. Injections of Rh antibody-containing plasma were proposed initially. In preliminary experiments in Rh-negative adult males, Finn and co-workers showed that chromium-51 labeled Rh-positive red cells could be rapidly eliminated if potent anti-D serum were injected shortly afterward. Later experiments by this group showed also that subsequent antibody production could be diminished greatly by this method (Clarke et al., 1963). The mechanism of suppression of development of Rh antibodies appears now to be more complex than originally supposed. The theory that antibody production is prevented by destruction of cells containing antigen is weakened by the observation of Brody et al. (1967), who showed that when *two* antigenic determinants on a single molecule are injected, together with antibody against only one of them, antibody formation against this one determinant only is suppressed, and the animal forms antibody against the second antigen. This suggested an alternate explanation, that passively administered antibody binds antigen (probably after it has been "processed" by macrophages) and prevents it from combining with receptors of the same specificity on particular antibody-forming cells (Mollison, 1968). This subject has been well reviewed by Clarke (1968).

Subsequent work by Freda et al. (1964), in New York, led to the development of a gamma globulin concentrate of anti-D*. This preparation has several advantages: the possibility of serum hepatitis is eliminated, sterility is assured and a small intramuscular injection could be given instead of a large intravenous injection of whole plasma. Successful prevention of isoimmunization following injection of this preparation in Rh-negative mothers soon after delivery was first demonstrated by Clarke and Sheppard (1965) and Freda et al. (1966). Since then, large scale studies throughout the world have confirmed the excellent degree of protection offered by this anti-D gamma globulin. In general, 1 ml. (equivalent to 300 micrograms of anti-D antibody) is injected intramuscularly to the unsensitized *mother* within 72 hours of delivery of an Rh-positive infant. The most

---

*Rhogam, Rh_o (D) Immune globulin (Human), Ortho Diagnostics, Raritan, New Jersey.

Table 7–8   Prevention of Rh Sensitization by Anti-D
Gamma Globulin*

GROUP	AFTER FIRST PREGNANCY			AFTER NEXT RH-POSITIVE PREGNANCY		
		Antibodies			Antibodies**	
	Total	No.	%	Total	No.	%
Treated	15,114	47	0.31	1,265	15	1.2
Control	6,701	354	5.3	712	81	11.4

*Pooled results of world-wide trial and Combined Study (1971).
**Cumulative incidence.

recent results of such a program have been pooled from various centers (Combined Study, 1971) and are shown in Table 7–8. Although there is some heterogeneity in patient material and study design among trials from different countries, there is general agreement about the high success rate. The protection rate (ratio of immunized patients in treated group versus control group) is of the order of 90 per cent. The effectiveness of the anti-D gamma globulin has been amply sustained through subsequent pregnancies. Of importance in interpreting the results of such trials is the fact, demonstrated earlier by Woodrow and Donohue (1968) and Ascari et al. (1969), that the true incidence of sensitization by an Rh-negative pregnancy can only be assessed by the incidence of antibodies at the end of the next Rh-positive pregnancy. Thus, although most treated mothers who did not show antibodies when tested six months after their first pregnancy were also free of antibodies after the next Rh-positive pregnancy, a small number emerged with what appeared to be de novo antibody formation. In all likelihood, these were women sensitized during their first pregnancy but since they did not show antibodies at the time of delivery by the usual methods of detection, they were assumed to be unsensitized and were given the anti-D gamma globulin. The failure of protection in this situation is readily understood. Most workers are of the opinion that such sensitization results from trans-placental hemorrhage occurring *during* the first pregnancy; this raises the question of the need for antenatal as well as postpartum administration of the anti-D gamma globulin. The safety of antenatal administration has been well shown in the studies of Zipursky and Israels (1967) and Buchanan et al. (1969). Its optimal timing and effectiveness in further reducing the already low failure rate of the current prophylactic program is presently under study and will presumably require a rather large number of patients to demonstrate a significant difference.

Another factor of possible importance in failure of protection by the anti-D gamma globulin is the occurrence at delivery of a transplacental hemorrhage too large to be neutralized by the standard 300 microgram dose of anti-D. Such hemorrhages are probably quite rare (of the order of 0.3 per cent) and would generally be detected only if maternal blood films were routinely scrutinized for fetal erythrocytes by the acid-elution technique. The larger of such hemorrhages might be recognized more easily if the infant were anemic or if the mother's blood showed a conversion in Rh type from negative to weakly positive (caused by a large number of Rh-positive fetal cells in the maternal circulation). It has been estimated that 1 ml. of anti-D gamma globulin (300 micrograms) is sufficient to inactivate up to 10 ml. of fetal cells (Pollack et al., 1969). The average volume of fetomaternal bleeding during labor is approximately 1 ml.; volumes in excess of this would require proportionately more anti-D gamma globulin (Woodrow et al., 1968).

Erroneous administration of this preparation to the infant has been reported on several occasions (Niederhoff et al., 1969; Sansone and Veneziano, 1970; Marsh et al., 1970). Although no serious consequences resulted, such accidents are inexcusable.

Because of the small but significant incidence of transplacental hemorrhage during abortions, both spontaneous and therapeutic, it is generally recommended that all Rh-negative women aborting after eight weeks of gestation receive anti-D gamma globulin, 300 micrograms, within three days of the procedure.

The current status of prevention of Rh isoimmunization is well summarized in a recent invitational symposium edited by Schumacher and Schneider (1971).

In spite of all that we now know about the prevention of Rh erythroblastosis, our efforts will amount to little unless we ensure that all physicians responsible for antenatal and obstetrical delivery care are aware of the value of anti-D gamma globulin and offer it to all Rh-negative mothers at risk. This discrepancy between knowledge and practice was strikingly documented in the Winnipeg region, where among women from the rural area only 27 per cent received Rh prophylaxis compared to 87 per cent among women in the urban area around the Rh Laboratory (Bowman, 1969). Clearly, the eradication of Rh erythroblastosis is within our grasp within the next decade.

HEMOLYTIC DISEASE OF THE NEWBORN DUE TO ABO INCOMPATIBILITY

In comparison with Rh hemolytic disease, knowledge concerning ABO incompatibility has advanced little since the condition was first recognized by Halbrecht in 1944. Several excellent reviews of the subject have appeared since then (Zuelzer and Cohen, 1957; Mollison and Cutbush, 1959). Hemolytic disease due to ABO incompatibility is more common than that due to Rh incompatibility, but generally it is much milder.

Pathogenesis

Hemolytic disease results from the action of maternal anti-A or anti-B antibodies upon fetal erythrocytes of the corresponding blood group. Several combinations of mother-infant blood groups may be involved (Table 7–9). Statistically about 20 per cent of all pregnancies involve ABO incompatibility, and of these, half consist of group O mothers and infants who have group A or B blood. However, only in about 10 per cent of ABO incompatible pregnancies does hemolytic disease manifest itself, and such cases are virtually limited to the A or B infants of group O mothers. This peculiar characteristic of group O sera resides in the nature and molecular size of the antibodies present. Abelson and Rawson (1961) demonstrated that the anti-A activity and anti-B activity of O sera were predominantly in the 7S (IgG) gamma globulin fraction, whereas those in sera from group A or B persons were predominantly in the 19S (IgM) macroglobulin fraction. Because 7S antibodies cross the placenta and 19S antibodies generally do not, the capacity of such antibodies to cause hemolytic disease in the newborn is readily apparent. Furthermore, the presence of 7S antibodies in the serum of women who have not been sensitized by previous pregnancy explains why ABO hemolytic disease frequently occurs in first-born infants. In contrast, Rh hemolytic disease is rare in first-born infants.

In addition to molecular size, the anti-A and anti-B antibodies possess distinct serologic properties, which have led to their classification as "natural" or "immune." The natural antibodies (19S) agglutinate best in saline, do not produce hemolysis in vitro, and are neutralized by A and B blood group substances. The immune antibodies (7S) agglutinate better in protein media, frequently produce hemolysis in vitro, and resist neutralization by A and B substances. Hemolysis is not complement-dependent (Wang and Desforges, 1971). Sera of group O mothers whose infants have ABO hemolytic disease frequently show one or more of the properties of such immune sera.

Table 7–9 Possible Combinations Resulting in ABO Incompatibility

MOTHER	INFANT
O	A, B
A	B, AB
B	A, AB

Clinical Manifestations

The chief manifestation of ABO hemolytic disease is jaundice. This occurs in only about 10 to 20 per cent of ABO incompatible pregnancies. It usually appears within the first 24 hours of life and is generally much milder than that seen in Rh hemolytic disease. Rarely, it may be sufficiently severe to cause kernicterus and death.

Because anemia is usually mild or absent, pallor is uncommon. Hydrops fetalis and stillbirth are, therefore, exceedingly rare; one such case was reported by Miller and Petrie (1963) in an infant still-born at 40 weeks of gestation.

Hepatosplenomegaly may occur, but it is generally less than that seen in Rh hemolytic disease. Boineau and Hallock reported two infants with severe disease associated with marked hepatospleno-megaly. Interestingly, both were of blood group B; the increased severity of hemolysis in such infants compared to group A infants has been noted by others (Mollison, 1967; Clifford et al., 1968).

First-born infants are affected in about 40 to 50 per cent of cases. Subsequent infants may or may not be affected. In an analysis of several hundred families who have had ABO incompatible infants subsequent to an infant with ABO hemolytic disease, the severity of hemolysis was greater in about one third of the cases, about the same in one third, and less (or absent) in the remaining third (Molthan, 1971).

Laboratory Findings

Hematologic Findings.   Anemia is uncommon. The hemoglobin concentration is usually normal, but rarely it may be as low as 8 gm. per 100 ml. (Boineau and Hallock, 1971). Evidence of a mild compensated hemolytic state consists of polychromasia, reticulocytosis (10 to 30 per cent), and increased numbers of nucleated red cells.

Microspherocytosis is usually present in ABO hemolytic disease and stands out against the background of normal macrocytic cells of the newborn (Fig. 7–13). The number of spherocytes often requires careful scrutiny of a well prepared blood smear. Mann and Graven (1965) attempted to quantitate this by measuring mean erythrocyte diameters on peripheral blood smear. Among infants with ABO hemolytic disease, they found a significant decrease compared to normal newborns and infants with Rh hemolytic disease.

Accompanying the spherocytosis, increased osmotic fragility may be found, thus introducing possible confusion with hereditary spherocytosis. Increased autohemolysis may be found in both conditions, but in ABO hemolytic disease it is *not* corrected by glucose whereas in hereditary spherocytosis, autohemolysis returns to normal with

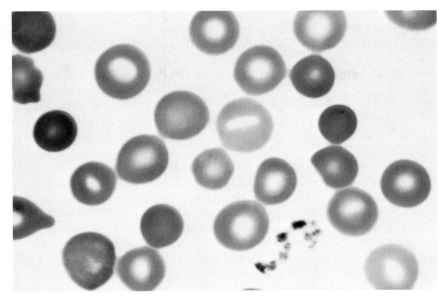

Figure 7-13   Spherocytes in ABO hemolytic disease.

the addition of glucose (Kostinas et al., 1967). Demonstration of the carrier state in the parents and persistence of hemolytic anemia in the infant will usually resolve any doubts (see Chapter Five, p. 120).

Elevated Serum Bilirubin Levels. These are often the only indication that a hemolytic process is taking place. As in Rh hemolytic disease, this involves mainly the indirect fraction. Occasionally, when jaundice is severe and prolonged, elevation of the direct fraction may also develop.

Serologic Findings. DEMONSTRATION OF INCOMPATIBLE BLOOD GROUPS. The usual situation consists of a group O mother and an infant who is group A or B. Rarely, other combinations may occur, as shown in Table 7-9.

DIRECT COOMBS TEST ON INFANT'S RED CELLS. Depending on slight variations in method, this test gives results varying from negative to moderately positive; in general, the test is weakly positive. In contrast, the infant's serum may readily show free antibody (by the indirect Coombs test) against *adult* erythrocytes possessing the corresponding A or B antigen; likewise, eluates of the infant's coated erythrocytes readily react with antigens on adult erythrocytes (Haberman et al., 1960). A possible explanation for this disparity may be found in the later studies of Voak and Williams (1971). Using ferritin-conjugated IgG anti-A and anti-B, they were able to show by electron microscopy that the A and B antigen sites on infant cells were farther apart than on adult cells, resulting in a weaker antiglobulin reaction. Enhanced pinocytosis of antibody by infant cells (Haberman et al., 1967) was felt to be insignificant. Although modifications of the Coombs test have been introduced in order to improve its sensitivity (Haberman et al., 1960; Chan et al., 1961; Cohen and Nelken, 1964), the fact that a positive direct Coombs test may frequently occur in the absence of hemolysis renders it of limited diagnostic value in such infants. With the more sensitive tests, however, a *negative* test may be of value in excluding ABO incompatibility as a cause of jaundice.

DEMONSTRATION OF ANTIBODY IN INFANT'S SERUM. Normally, group A infants of group O mothers possess anti-B but not anti-A, and group B infants of group O mothers possess anti-A but not anti-B in their serum. However, when free anti-A is present in a group A infant or anti-B in a group B infant, ABO hemolytic disease may be presumed. Gunson (1957) demonstrated such antibody by both an indirect Coombs test and Löw's papain test. In jaundiced ABO-incompatible infants, the indirect Coombs test was positive in 39 of 42 infants under 24 hours of age, with a decreasing incidence of positive reactions after this. The papain test was positive in 17 of 17 infants under 24 hours of age, 18 of 20 infants between 24 to 48 hours of age, and in none of three beyond this age. ABO incompatible infants without jaundice gave negative results with these tests. Similar results have been obtained by Zuelzer (1956) using the indirect Coombs test.

DEMONSTRATION OF ANTIBODIES IN MATERNAL SERUM. When the infant has signs of a hemolytic process, the mother's serum acquires "immune" characteristics, as evidenced by the presence of agglutinins persisting after neutralization with A and B substance, and hemolysins. These tests do not usually become positive until the postpartum period, reaching their peak by about seven to 10 days. However, only one of three infants born of mothers with such antibodies shows hemolytic disease. The main value of these tests appears to be that, when they are negative, ABO incompatibility in the infant can be virtually excluded. To be valid in this regard, early tests must be supplemented by repeat tests later to avoid missing peak titers.

Because only the 7S (IgG) anti-A or anti-B in maternal serum is significant in relation to disease in the infant, the ideal test of maternal serum should estimate only this fracton. Kochwa et al. (1961) used column chromatography, followed by partial neutralization with AB substance for this purpose, and they showed in a small number of cases good correlation with the occurrence of hemolytic disease in the infant. The procedure is difficult and requires two days to perform, thereby rendering it practical only for prenatal diagnosis. Polley et al. (1965) devised a rapid simple modification of this test that was positive (titer of 1000 or more) in 13 of 18 infants requiring exchange transfusion, in four of 15 who did not require exchange transfusion, and in only one of 16 healthy incompatible infants. A simple modification of this test employs 2-mercaptoethanol to inhibit reactivity due to 19S (IgM) natural anti-A or anti-B (Moores et al., 1970). In their experience, hemolytic disease due to ABO incompatibility was virtually confined to the infants of mothers whose sera contained non-inhibitable anti-A or anti-B. However, among such mothers only about 25 per cent of the infants showed evidence of hemolytic disease. Like the direct Coombs test on infant's erythrocytes, this test is of only negative diagnostic value.

VALUE OF SEROLOGIC TESTS. Because only a small proportion of sensitized infants develop sufficient jaundice to require exchange transfusion and severe anemia is not usually a problem, the value of such serologic tests in the diagnosis and treatment of ABO hemolytic disease may be questioned. Their main value seems to be in deciding to what extent other causes of neonatal jaundice should be pursued in an otherwise well newborn.

Erythrocyte Acetylcholinesterase Activity. Kaplan et al. (1964) have demonstrated reduced activity of this stromal enzyme in 10 of 12 infants with proven ABO hemolytic disease, and normal activity in 19 of 20 infants with Rh hemolytic disease. Stocker et al. (1969) confirmed these observations and showed further that the reduction in enzyme activity correlated well with the need for exchange transfusion. The practical value of this test depends on its adaptability to the circumstances of the routine clinical laboratory. Interestingly, reduced acetylcholinesterase activity has also been found in certain types of acquired autoimmune hemolytic anemia (Sirchia et al., 1970).

Amniocentesis. There is no need for this procedure in the antenatal management of ABO hemolytic disease.

Treatment

Management of the infant with ABO hemolytic disease is directed toward control of hyperbilirubinemia by frequent determinations of serum indirect bilirubin levels (and bilirubin binding capacity) with a view to the need for exchange transfusion. The principles and methods are the same as those described for Rh hemolytic disease. Group O blood of the same Rh type as that of the infant should be used. Whole blood is preferable in order to allow maximum bilirubin removal by albumin. Where the disease appears of sufficient severity to anticipate the need for multiple exchange transfusions, 25 per cent human albumin may be added to the donor blood (see p. 212). If the titer of anti-A and anti-B in the group O blood is low, it is not necessary to add group A and B substance. Replacement of the donor plasma with AB plasma offers no additional advantage (Goldfarb et al., 1964).

In selected infants whose serum indirect bilirubin levels appear likely to rise to levels over 20 mg. per 100 ml., a trial of phototherapy seems worthwhile (Kaplan et al., 1971; Sisson et al., 1971). This should only be used early in the course of the disease, and not at a time when definite indications for exchange transfusion already exist. Should the serum indirect bilirubin continue to rise in spite of phototherapy, there should be no delay in carrying out exchange transfusion when the usual indications are present (Patel et al., 1970).

There is no need to consider early delivery in mothers who have had previous infants with jaundice due to ABO hemolytic disease.

Summary

The main differences between hemolytic disease of the newborn due to Rh and ABO incompatibility are summarized in Table 7–10.

Table 7–10   Comparison of Rh and ABO Incompatibility

	RH	ABO
Blood Group Set-up		
Mother	Negative	O
Infant	Positive	A or B
Type of Antibody	Incomplete (7S)	Immune (7S)
Clinical Aspects		
Occurrence in first-born	5%	40–50%
Predictable severity in subsequent pregnancies	Usually	No
Stillbirth and/or hydrops	Frequent	Rare
Severe anemia	Frequent	Rare
Degree of jaundice	+++	+
Hepatosplenomegaly	+++	+
Laboratory Findings		
Direct Coombs test (infant)	+	(+) or O
Maternal antibodies	Always present	Not clear-cut
Spherocytes	O	+
Treatment		
Need for antenatal measures	Yes	No
Exchange transfusion		
Frequency	Approx. $^2/_3$	Approx. $^1/_{10}$
Donor blood type	Rh-negative Group-specific, when possible	Rh — same as infant Group O *only*
Incidence of late anemia	Common	Rare

HEMOLYTIC DISEASE OF THE NEWBORN DUE TO OTHER ANTIBODIES

Approximately 2 per cent of cases of erythroblastosis fetalis involve antibodies other than those of the Rh(D) or ABO systems. The most important of these are anti-c, anti-Kell, and anti-E.

Because routine antenatal blood typing generally includes only ABO and D factors, these less frequent incompatibilities are not likely to be detected until after the birth of an erythroblastotic infant. The finding of a positive direct Coombs test in an infant born of an Rh(D)-positive mother should direct suspicion to one of these incompatibilities. A specific diagnosis can be made by further typing of red cells from the mother and *father*, and by testing mother's serum with a panel of standard test cells and also father's cells. In the event of a rare "private" antigen incompatibility, antibody reactions may be demonstrable only with red cells of the father. Father's cells are preferable in this regard because the antibody coating the infant's red cells will confuse the interpretation of positive reactions.

The occurrence of hemolytic disease of the newborn due to anti-c indicates the need to consider this antigen when administering Rh-negative blood to an Rh-positive female recipient. In this situation the recipient's red cells should be tested with anti-c serum, and if the reaction is negative, such blood should not be given.

ADJUNCTS IN THE MANAGEMENT OF HYPERBILIRUBINEMIA

The mainstay in the treatment of hyperbilirubinemia due to erythroblastosis fetalis is exchange transfusion to remove sensitized erythrocytes destined for destruction and, to a lesser extent, bilirubin. The risks of exchange transfusion are small but significant (especially in the premature infant) and have stimulated the search for alternate methods of reducing serum bilirubin levels to prevent brain damage. Phototherapy and phenobarbital have received the greatest attention and their initial success in the prevention of hyperbilirubinemia among prematures has led to their trial in infants with hemolysis due to isoimmunization and other disorders. Therefore, a brief review of these therapeutic adjuncts seems appropriate here.

Phenobarbital

Phenobarbital increases hepatic clearance of bilirubin mainly by inducing synthesis of glucuronyl transferase; an effect on hepatic uptake and excretion of bilirubin has also been suggested. The activity of other hepatic enzymes which influence the metabolism of drugs and endogenous steroid hormones is also increased by phenobarbital (Wilson, 1969).

The observation by Trolle (1968a) that infants born of mothers receiving barbiturates for various reasons during late pregnancy showed a reduced incidence of jaundice led a number of workers to explore the use of this drug in the prevention of neonatal hyperbilirubinemia. The results have shown, in general, that when the drug is administered to mothers in doses ranging from 30 to 180 mg. a day for two weeks or more before delivery, there is a significant reduction in serum bilirubin levels among the newborn offspring (Trolle, 1968b; Maurer et al. 1968; Ramboer et al., 1969). Postnatal administration of the drug to the newborn has been less effective. Yeung and Field (1969) used a larger dose of phenobarbital in Chinese newborns with jaundice due to a variety of causes including ABO incompatibility and glucose-6-phosphate dehydrogenase deficiency; this produced a significant reduction in serum bilirubin levels and a decrease in the need for exchange transfusion compared to a group of control infants. Subsequently, McMullin and co-workers (1970), in a controlled trial with an even larger dose of phenobarbital in infants with Rh erythroblastosis, showed a reduced need for late exchange transfusions among the treated infants. The statistical soundness of both these studies has since been challenged by Behrman and Fisher (1970) and Walker (1970), respectively. Although phenobarbital may eventually prove to be of use in lowering serum bilirubin levels among milder cases of erythroblastosis and perhaps reducing the need for repeat exchange transfusion, the present data are insufficient to recommend it for general use. In addition, the potential adverse effects, both immediate and late, constitute a further deterrent to its use in the developing newborn (see p. 50).

Phototherapy

Serum bilirubin concentrations of newborn infants can be lowered by exposure to sunlight or artificial blue light (Cremer et al., 1958). Both in vitro and in vivo, there is evidence that bilirubin undergoes gradual decomposition to a series of derivatives that exhibit progressively less yellow color and diazo reactivity but increased water solubility. These degradation products do not bind albumin, are rapidly excreted from the body (in bile and urine), and as far as is known from experimental and clinical studies, they are non-toxic. This subject has been well reviewed by Behrman and Hsia (1969) and Lucey (1970). Specific guidelines for phototherapy are given in the review by Behrman and Hsia, and should be consulted by all physicians concerned with its use.

The effect of light on serum bilirubin is relatively slow and therefore its main clinical usefulness is in conditions associated with a relatively slow accumulation of bilirubin, such as hyperbilirubinemia of prematurity (Lucey et al., 1968). In the face of severe hemolytic disease of the newborn, it has been found to be relatively ineffective (Obes-Polleri and Hill, 1964; Kaplan et al., 1971). From present experience with phototherapy in Rh and ABO hemolytic disease, we would reserve its use for those mild cases in which the rate of rise in serum bilirubin is relatively slow, and following exchange transfusion in the hope of reducing the need for repeat exchange. When exchange transfusion is definitely indicated in an infant, it should not be delayed for a trial of phototherapy. Infants with Rh hemolytic disease in whom exchange transfusion has been avoided as a result of phototherapy should be followed closely for the development of delayed severe anemia, since the hemolytic process itself has not been influenced by such therapy.

Chapter Eight

BLOOD COAGULATION
AND ITS DISORDERS
IN THE NEWBORN

Disorders of the coagulation mechanism with their attendant complications — hemorrhage and thrombosis — may be observed in as many as 1 per cent of all admissions to a newborn nursery (Hathaway, 1970). Hemorrhage and thrombosis may result from a variety of pathological processes; thus prompt and orderly attempts at diagnosis are essential for most effective treatment.

Bleeding in the newborn period can be broadly classified into six major categories. Bleeding may result from:

1. Accentuation of the transitory deficiencies of the coagulation mechanism that are characteristic of the newborn period.

2. Transitory disturbances of the coagulation mechanism that are a result of associated disease processes (disseminated intravascular coagulation — D.I.C.).

3. Inherited, permanent abnormalities of the coagulation mechanism.

4. Quantitative or qualitative abnormalities of the platelets.

5. Vascular abnormalities.

6. Trauma alone or in association with any of the other factors.

The problem of platelet abnormalities is extensive and therefore is discussed separately in Chapter Nine.

NORMAL BLOOD CLOTTING MECHANISMS

As blood flows from an injured vessel, it tends to form a gelatinous coagulum of fibrin that plugs the defect and stops further bleeding.

236

Table 8-1   The Blood Clotting Factors*

FACTOR NUMBER	SYNONYMS	DEFINITION
I	Fibrinogen	A protein that, when modified by thrombin, forms the clot (fibrin).
II	Prothrombin	An alpha globulin that, when acted on by thromboplastin accelerators and calcium, is converted to thrombin.
III	Thromboplastin	An unidentified substance or substances present in tissues that promote pro-thrombin conversion to thrombin. In plasma it is formed only by interaction of several factors and is quickly destroyed.
IV	Calcium	Necessary in the first and second stages of coagulation.
V	Proaccelerin, labile factor, Ac globulin	A plasma factor that participates in the first and second stages of coagulation.
VI	Accelerin, serum Ac globulin	Active form of factor V. Terms no longer employed.
VII	Proconvertin, stable factor, SPCA, auto-prothrombin I	A plasma factor required for the conversion of prothrombin to thrombin. Increases $2\frac{1}{2}$ times in the process of clotting.
VIII	Antihemophiliac factor (AHF), antihemo-philiac globulin (AHG)	A thromboplastic precursor the deficiency of which is responsible for classic hemophilia. It is found in the beta globulin fraction.
IX	Plasma thromboplastin component (PTC), Christmas factor, autopro-thrombin II	A factor that participates in thromboplastin formation. An alpha globulin.
X	Stuart-Prower factor, Stuart factor, Prower-Stuart factor	Participates in thromboplastin formation and prothrombin conversion.
XI	Plasma thromboplastin antecedent (PTA)	Reacts with activated Hageman factor and forms thromboplastic substance.
XII	Hageman factor, contact factor	A factor concerned with initiation of clotting in vitro. Becomes activated by contact with rough surface. Deficiency unaccompanied by clinical manifestations.
XIII	Fibrin-stabilizing factor	A serum factor responsible for the stabilization of the fibrin clot.

*Modified from Aballi, A. J., and DeLamerens, S.: Pediat. Clin. N. Amer., 9:785, 1962.

If the initial defect is small, platelet clumping alone is sufficient to seal the wound. The flow of blood is also controlled by the constriction of afferent vessels in the wound area, as well as by the pressure of extravascular tissues.

Although our knowledge of the normal coagulation mechanism and the process of clot lysis is still incomplete, sufficient facts are available to construct schemas of coagulation and fibrinolysis that enable the clinician to understand the hemorrhagic phenomena in his patients.

The use of a standard nomenclature for the coagulation factors has greatly facilitated the learning process for the non-hematologist. Table 8–1 lists the coagulation factors with their Roman numerals, common synonyms, abbreviations, and a brief definition of their mode of action.

According to current concepts, two major pathways exist to activate the coagulation system. In Figure 8–1, a simplified version of the entire sequence of clotting is depicted, based on the formulation of Stormorken and Owren (1971).

An intrinsic pathway, occurring within the vascular lumen, and not requiring the presence of tissue juices, is triggered off by the activation of Factor XII (Hageman Factor) and Factor XI (PTA) through surface contact, collagen, or other negatively charged substances. This complex, in the presence of calcium, then activates Factor IX

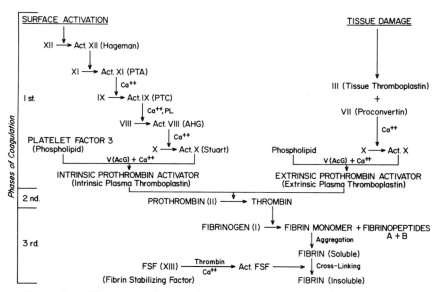

Figure 8–1   The steps in the coagulation process. The intrinsic pathway is initiated by surface activation and the extrinsic pathway is initiated by tissue damage.

(PTC). Activated Factor IX, in turn, interacts with Factor VIII (AHG), platelet phospholipid, and calcium to form a complex which activates Factor X (Stuart–Prower factor).

In the extrinsic system, tissue thromboplastin, along with Factor VII (proconvertin) and calcium, forms a complex which also activates Factor X. From this point on, both the intrinsic and extrinsic systems proceed in a similar fashion.

In the next major phase of coagulation, Factor II (prothrombin) is activated to thrombin by a complex which includes activated Factor X, Factor V (proaccelerin), platelet phospholipid, and calcium.

Thrombin, in turn, cleaves fibrinogen into fibrinopeptides and fibrin monomers, which then polymerize and are stabilized as insoluble fibrin by means of activated Factor XIII (fibrin stabilizing factor) and calcium.

Although precise details remain to be experimentally defined, there appear to be plasma inhibitors for each activated stage in the coagulation mechanism. The best studied of these naturally occurring inhibitors is a group of antithrombins.

THE FIBRINOLYTIC SYSTEM

Under normal circumstances, when fibrin is deposited upon vessel walls or in tissues, it is slowly broken down into soluble fibrin split products (FSP) by plasmin (Figure 8–2). Plasmin is a proteolytic enzyme which splits arginine and lysine bonds. Although plasmin has a high affinity for insoluble fibrin, it can also attack fibrinogen and Factors V and VIII. Plasminogen is the inactive precursor of plasmin that is normally present in plasma. It is activated to plasmin by a variety of factors present in plasma, urine, and tissue. Like the coagulation system, the fibrinolytic system is also normally held in check by a series of inhibitors. Normal blood contains inhibitors of plasminogen activators and of plasmin. Thus, both the coagulation mechanism and the fibrinolytic system are held in a state of dynamic equilibrium. This precarious state can be upset by a wide variety of stimuli.

THE LABORATORY TESTS OF BLOOD COAGULATION

The clinican should familiarize himself with the tests available in the study of the bleeding infant, recognize their usefulness as well as their limitations, and thus be in a position to select only those most likely to provide interpretable information in light of the clinical situation.

Bleeding from a coagulation disturbance can manifest itself at

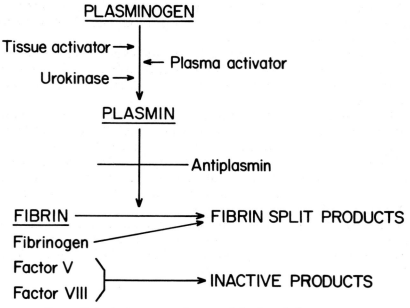

Figure 8–2   Activation mechanism of the thrombolytic system.

any time after birth. When bleeding from the gastrointestinal tract occurs in the first few hours after delivery, it is necessary to determine if the blood has originated from the mother (having been swallowed by the infant) or is coming from the neonate and represents actual hemorrhage. This distinction should be made before proceeding with other laboratory studies. Vomitus, gastric aspirate, or stool containing red blood may be used for this purpose employing the alkali denaturation test popularized by Apt and Downey (1955).

Technique.   To lyse the erythrocytes and to prepare the hemoglobin solution, a small amount of stool or vomitus is mixed with water. Generally, one part of stool or vomitus is mixed with five to ten parts of water. The test tube is centrifuged for several minutes at approximately 2000 rpm to separate the debris. The supernatant solution, which must be pink, is then decanted or filtered. About 1 ml. of 0.25 N (1 per cent) sodium hydroxide is then mixed with 5 ml. of the hemoglobin solution.

The color change is read in two minutes. Blood containing adult hemoglobin (Hb A) changes from pink to brown-yellow, while blood containing predominantly Hb F remains pink. It is helpful to run a control tube containing the peripheral blood of the infant being studied.

Screening Tests

The Platelet Count

In all bleeding infants, one of the initial steps in the laboratory investigation should be the preparation and inspection of a well prepared cover slip smear of the peripheral blood for an estimation of platelet numbers. The presence of platelets in clumps or the presence of multiple platelets in a single oil immersion field indicates that thrombocytopenia is not a factor in the bleeding disorder. One should examine both sides of the cover slip preparation before concluding that platelets are inadequate because of the occasional tendency for platelets to adhere to only one surface of the cover slip pair. The facilities for the preparation and inspection of a blood film are generally available, and every physician caring for newborns should be capable of preparing a blood film and evaluating platelet numbers. If the findings of a blood film inspection should prove equivocal, a direct platelet count should be performed.

The Whole Blood Coagulation Time

This test determines the time taken by whole blood to clot in a glass tube or siliconized or plastic tube under standard conditions of obtaining the sample and conducting the test. The clotting time may be prolonged in severe hemophilia, afibrinogenemia, Stuart-Prower factor deficiency, thrombocytopenia, and in hemorrhagic disease of the newborn. *It is often normal in these disorders, even when the defect is moderately severe.* The test is nonspecific, requires careful techniques of blood drawing and laboratory methodology, and consumes relatively large quantities of blood; it therefore cannot be recommended as a useful part of the initial diagnostic evaluation of a bleeding infant.

The Bleeding Time

This test measures the length of time required for a wound of standardized size to stop bleeding. The individual's capacity to seal off small wounds is a measure of his platelet numbers and platelet function. The bleeding time generally is prolonged in thrombocytopenia, thrombasthenias, von Willebrand's disease, and in disseminated intravascular coagulation. This test is always normal in patients with hemophilia or patients with congenital deficiencies of factors mediating the second or third stages of coagulation unless aspirin has been recently administered.

In the Ivy method of determining the bleeding time, the standard cut is made on the dorsal surface of the forearm, while in the Duke method the puncture is made in the earlobe. Earlobe punctures should never be done in infants and children because of the difficulty in applying pressure to the wound in case bleeding should persist. The bleeding time test should not be performed in patients with, or suspected of having, thrombocytopenia.

TESTS OF THE FIRST PHASE OF COAGULATION

The tests of the first phase of coagulation are primarily designed to differentiate the three types of hemophilia—hemophilia due to deficiencies of Factor VIII (antihemophiliac factor), Factor IX (plasma thromboplastin component), or Factor XI (plasma thromboplastin antecedent). In this category are the thromboplastin generation test, the prothrombin consumption test, and the partial thromboplastin time. Modifications of the thromboplastin generation test and the partial thromboplastin time may be used for the assay of Factor VIII and Factor IX activity.

The Thromboplastin Generation Test. This test introduced by Biggs and Douglas (1953) is considered to be the most sensitive test of the first phase of coagulation. It estimates the thromboplastin (intrinsic prothrombin activator) generated from a prothrombin-free incubation mixture. A generating mixture comprised of all factors necessary for Phase 1 is incubated at 37° C., and at intervals aliquots of this generating mixture are added to recalcified normal plasma and the clotting time is noted. In principle, the thromboplastin generation test is similar to the prothrombin time. Both utilize the property of thromboplastin to shorten the clotting time of normal plasma. In the prothrombin time, plasma is tested with known active thromboplastin, while the plasma in the thromboplastin generation test is obtained from a normal subject and the thromboplastic activity of the generation mixture is unknown.

Three reagents are used to supply generating mixtures with the factors necessary for the first phase of coagulation—the patient's adsorbed plasma, the patient's serum, and the patient's platelets or a platelet substitute such as cephalin.

In Table 8–2, the factors normally present in each of the reagents employed are listed. If abnormalities of thromboplastin generation are detected, normal adsorbed plasma or serum can be substituted for the patient's plasma or serum in order to determine which factor or factors are deficient. Serum or adsorbed plasma from patients with known deficiencies can also be employed in this test, so that by substitution or mutual correction studies the precise defect can be demonstrated.

Table 8–2 Constituents of Reagents Prepared from Normal
Whole Blood and Their Effect on the Correction of
Abnormalities of the Thromboplastin Generation Test

	EFFECT OF ADDED REAGENT IN THE THROMBOPLASTIN GENERATION TEST		
	---	---	---
REAGENT	Factor VIII (AHG) Deficiency	Factor IX (PTC) Deficiency	Factor XI (PTA) Deficiency
Whole plasma (Contains Factors VIII, IX , X, and XI)	Corrects	Corrects	Corrects
Adsorbed plasma (Contains Factors VIII and XI)	Corrects	No correction	Corrects
Serum (Contains Factors IX, X, and XI)	No correction	Corrects	Corrects

The thromboplastin generation test is particularly useful for the
demonstration of mild deficiencies that cannot be detected by other
methods.

The Prothrombin Consumption Test. During normal coagulation, thrombin production continues after the blood has clotted, so
that after one hour of incubation at 37° C. approximately 75 per cent
of the prothrombin originally present is converted to thrombin. A
prothrombin time performed with this incubated serum will then
demonstrate a prothrombin concentration of less than 25 per cent of
normal. Patients with moderate or severe defects in the first phase of
coagulation do not convert prothrombin to thrombin at a normal rate as
a result of their impaired thromboplastin generation, and thus their
serum, after standing for one hours, contains more than 25 per cent
of its original plasma prothrombin concentration. When this serum
is used to measure prothrombin time, a rapid result is obtained.

Thrombocytopenia or qualitative defects of platelet function may
also result in an abnormal prothrombin consumption, as do Factor
V or Factor VII deficiencies. These two deficiencies are not detected
in the serum prothrombin time unless the missing second phase
factors are added to the final test system.

The prothrombin consumption test is relatively simple to perform
but is not as sensitive as the thromboplastin generation test. The test
is of little value in detecting deficiencies in the first phase of coagulation during the neonatal period because of the initially low levels
of plasma prothrombin present (McElfresh, 1961). When the prothrombin is low to start with, misleading results are obtained when

one attempts to interpret the residual prothrombin content after one hour of incubation.

The Partial Thromboplastin Time. In this test, the effect of adding a weak or partial thromboplastin to the clotting time of plasma is estimated. The effect of such an addition to normal plasma is much greater than that observed in cases associated with a defect in the first phase of coagulation in which thromboplastin generation is impaired. The differences between normals and first phase deficients are, of course, obliterated when full strength thromboplastin is employed. This deceptively simple test is moderately sensitive and of great value as a screening test for the presence of first phase defects, provided that well standardized partial thromboplastin is employed. Mild defects in the first phase of coagulation may be missed by this test.

Assay for Factor VIII in Plasma. The assay is performed by comparing the effects of dilutions of unknown and standard adsorbed plasma in serial thromboplastin generation tests. Patients with severe Factor VIII deficiency have less than 1 per cent of normal activity, while patients with moderately severe hemophilia assay between 1 and 5 per cent and those with mild hemophilia assay above 5 per cent.

Tests of the Second Phase of Coagulation

Tests of the second phase of coagulation measure the conversion of prothrombin to thrombin. In addition to prothrombin, Factor V (proaccelerin), Factor VII (proconvertin), and Factor X (Stuart-Prower) must be present in sufficient concentration for this reaction to proceed at a maximal rate.

The One-stage Prothrombin Time (Quick's Method). This test is performed by adding thromboplastin and calcium to citrated or oxalated plasma and noting the time of appearance of the first fibrin strand. Obviously, abnormalities in the first phase of clotting are not reflected by a prolonged prothrombin time because the addition of thromboplastin by-passes the contribution of the first phase.

This test does not measure a specific clotting factor but measures the overall activity of both the second and third phases of coagulation. The third phase of coagulation is introduced into this test because the end point requires fibrin formation. A severe fibrinogen deficiency thus results in a prolonged prothrombin time as do any deficiencies of prothrombin, Factor V, Factor VII, or Factor X.

Differential tests can be performed in conjunction with the one-stage prothrombin time in order to discern specific abnormalities in the second phase. These substitution and mutual correction tests are similar in principle to those employed in the detection of first phase defects and are summarized in Table 8–3.

Table 8–3 Constituents of Reagents Prepared from Normal
Whole Blood and Their Effect on the Correction
of the Second Phase of Coagulation
(Prolonged Prothrombin Time)

| | EFFECT OF ADDED REAGENT IN CORRECTING THE PROLONGED PROTHROMBIN TIME | | |
REAGENT	Prothrombin Deficiency	Factor V (proaccelerin) Deficiency	Factor VII (proconvertin) Deficiency
Whole plasma (Contains prothrombin and Factors V, VII, and X)	Corrects	Corrects	Corrects
Adsorbed plasma (Contains Factor V)	No correction	Corrects	No correction
Serum (Contains Factors VII and X)	No correction	No correction	Corrects

TESTS OF THE THIRD PHASE OF COAGULATION

In the third phase of coagulation, fibrinogen is converted to fibrin in the presence of thrombin.

The Thrombin Clotting Time. This test determines the time plasma takes to clot after the addition of thrombin. Prolongation of the thrombin time occurs in the presence of a fibrinogen deficiency or in the presence of certain inhibitors of coagulation such as heparin or fibrin split products.

Fibrinogen itself can be measured by several methods.

A summary of the factors involved in the three stages of coagulation and the preferred tests for their detection appear in Table 8–4. For details regarding the performance of these tests, as well as the assay of specific factors, the reader is advised to consult standard texts of blood coagulation such as that of Biggs and Macfarlane (1966).

TESTS OF THE FIBRINOLYTIC SYSTEM

When a bleeding infant is suspected of hemorrhaging as a result of pathological activation of either the coagulation system or the fibrinolytic mechanism, additional laboratory tests may be necessary to establish the diagnosis. These may include the measurement of fibrin degradation products and the euglobulin lysis time.

Fibrin Degradation Products. When the fibrin formed intravascularly, as a result of the coagulation process, is broken down by

Table 8–4   Factors Involved in Coagulation and Their
Laboratory Evaluation*

	FIRST PHASE	SECOND PHASE	THIRD PHASE
Purpose	Generation of thromboplastin	Conversion of pro-thrombin to thrombin	Conversion of fibrinogen to fibrin clot
Factors Involved	Platelet thrombo-plastic factor Factor XII (Hageman) Factor XI (PTA) Factor X (Stuart-Prower) Factor IX (PTC) Factor VIII (AHG) Factor V (proaccelerin) Calcium	Prothrombin Factor V (proaccelerin) Factor VII (proconvertin) Factor X (Stuart-Prower) Calcium Thromboplastin†	Thrombin† Fibrinogen
Preferred Test	Thromboplastin generation test	One-stage prothrombin time	Fibrinogen determination
Other Methods	Prothrombin consumption Partial thromboplastin time Assay of factors	Two-stage prothrombin time Assay of factors	Thrombin time

*Modified from Aballi, A. J., and DeLamerens, S.: Pediat. Clin. N. Amer., 9:785, 1962.
†Not normally present in blood.

Table 8–5   Coagulation Factor and Test Values in Normal
Pregnant Women and Newborn Infants*

CATEGORY	FIBRINOGEN (MG./100 ML.)	FACTORS								
		II (%)	V (%)	VII (%)	VIII (%)	IX (%)	X (%)	XI (%)	XII (%)	XIII (Titer)
Normal adult or child	190–420	100	100	100	100	100	100	100	100	1/16
Term pregnancy	483	92	108	170	196	130	130	69	–	1/16
Premature (1500–2500 gm.) cord blood	233	25	67	37	80	Dec.***	29	–	–	1/8
Term infant cord blood	216	41	92	56	100	27	55	36	–	1/8
Term infant, 48 hours	210	46	105	20	100	Dec.	45	39	25	–

*From Hathaway, 1970 (Pediat Clin. N.A. 17:929, 1970)
Note: All levels expressed as means or ranges.
**Kaolin PTT
***Dec. = decreased

plasmin, degradation products appear in the blood. The presence of increased quantities of degradation products in serum indicates that fibrinolysis is occurring. This most commonly occurs secondary to disseminated intravascular coagulation. The presence of increased quantities of degradation products rarely indicates acute primary fibrinolysis. Many techniques have been developed for the measurement of these degradation products. The most sensitive of these methods appears to be the tanned red cell hemagglutination inhibition technique (Mersky et al., 1969).

Euglobulin Lysis Time. The euglobulin lysis time is an indicator of the amount of plasminogen activator present in the blood. If the level of activator is increased, the euglobulin lysis time becomes shorter than normal. When free plasmin is present in the blood it becomes very short. The euglobulin lysis time is usually normal in the presence of disseminated intravascular coagulation, but is significantly shortened when primary pathological fibrinolysis is present. Unfortunately, a shortened euglobulin lysis time is not in itself diagnostic of primary fibrinolysis.

BLOOD COAGULATION IN THE NEWBORN

Even at the moment of birth, significant alterations in the normal coagulation mechanism may be present. During the first few days of

Table 8–5   Coagulation Factor and Test Values in Normal Pregnant Women and Newborn Infants (*Continued*)

Category	Platelet Count (Cu. mm.)	Euglobulin Lysis Time (Min.)	Partial Thrombo-plastin Time°° (Sec.)	Prothrombin Time (Sec.)	Thrombin Time (Sec.)
Normal adult or child	200,000–450,000	90–300	37–50	12–14	8–10
Term pregnancy	290,000	278	44	13	8.0
Premature (1500–2500 gm.) cord blood	220,000	214	90	17(12–21)	14(11–17)
Term infant cord blood	190,000	84	71	16(13–20)	12(10–16)
Term infant, 48 hours	200,000	105	65	17.5(12–21)	13(10–16)

life, these alterations, specifically the decreases of the vitamin K dependent factors, may become profound. When the changes that normally occur become exaggerated, hemorrhage may result.

Table 8–5 summarizes the results of coagulation studies performed on the cord blood of term and premature infants and compares them with values observed in term infants at 48 hours of life, in pregnant women at term, and with normal values for older children and adults. Note that the platelet count and the levels of Factor V, Factor VIII, and fibrinogen are all in the normal adult range in term infants. The vitamin K dependent factors — that is, prothrombin, Factor VII, Factor IX, and Factor X — may already be lower than that observed in the adult, as is Factor XI.

The Hageman factor (Factor XII) shows a wide range of variability (Kurkcouglu and McElfresh, 1960) and may be depressed in the newborn. The whole blood clotting time is normal (Fresh et al., 1956), as is the capillary bleeding time (Aballi and De Lamerens, 1962).

Bleyer et al. (1971) have traced the development of hemostasis in the human fetus. Their work should be consulted for details of changes in coagulation and coagulation factors that accompany intrauterine development.

The First Phase of Coagulation

The generation of thromboplastin is usually abnormal at birth and may become progressively more abnormal during the first two or three days of life (Van Creveld et al., 1954). The deficient generation of thromboplastic activity is a result of deficiencies of Factor IX and Factor X, the serum factors involved in the first phase of coagulation. Factor XI deficiency may also play a role. A coexisting deficiency of Hageman factor, if present, accentuates this abnormal thromboplastin generation.

Infants who receive vitamin K demonstrate improved thromboplastin generation, but complete normality may not be reached for as long as three to six months (the response of these factors is illustrated in Fig. 8–3). The premature infant does not show as marked a response to vitamin K as does the term infant.

The Second Phase of Coagulation

Brinkhous et al. (1937) were the first to demonstrate a decrease in true prothrombin *content* in the newborn period. The concentration of prothrombin is low in the cord blood and becomes progressively lower during the first three days of life. The prothrombin *time*, which measures the activity of Factors V, VII, and X as well as prothrombin, may be normal or prolonged at birth and becomes progressively longer during the first few days of life. This prolongation of the prothrombin time is a result of increasing deficiencies of Factors VII and X. Loeliger and Koller (1952) found that cord blood contained an average of only 24 per cent of the normal adult content of Factor VII. Dyggve (1958) also observed that cord blood contained only 23 per cent of the Factor VII activity observed in normal adult blood and that this value fell to approximately 15 per cent by the third day of life.

Administration of vitamin K to the newborn will increase the levels of prothrombin, Factor VII, Factor IX, and Factor X, but it will not raise them to normal adult levels. The response to vitamin K in premature infants is generally much less than that observed in the term infant (Van Creveld et al., 1954).

In the normal infant, the level of Factor V is similar to or often higher than that observed in the adult, and plays no role in the prolongation of the prothrombin time that characterizes the newborn period.

The Third Phase of Coagulation

Fibrinogen levels are in the normal adult range or just slightly below adult values throughout the newborn period. Therefore, this factor cannot be implicated in the bleeding disturbances that accompany this period of life, except in the rare instances of congenital afibrinogenemia.

Despite the normal levels of fibrinogen, the thrombin time is generally abnormal in the neonate (Roberts and associates, 1966). Since this test measures the conversion of fibrinogen to fibrin, it can be influenced by a decrease in the quantity of fibrinogen, an abnormality of the fibrinogen, an increase in antithrombins, or the presence of fibrin degradation products. The reason, or reasons, for the prolongation of the thrombin time in the newborn is unclear. Aballi and De Lamerens (1962) have gathered evidence to indicate that this delayed thrombin time is a result of increased heparin activity during this period. These authors found no correlation between the prolonged thrombin time and any coagulation defect, and they concluded that it was devoid of clinical significance. Salazar de Sousa (1954) was also able to demonstrate increased heparin-like activity as well as increased antithrombin activity in the blood of neonates. Witt and associates (1969) have presented evidence for the existence of a "fetal fibrinogen" that they believe is responsible for the prolongation of the thrombin time. Others (von Felten and Straub, 1969; Gmür et al., 1970) demonstrated, instead, that the abnormality of the thrombin time was caused by the presence of increased quantities of fibrin degradation products.

Most investigators (Hathaway, 1970; Chessells and Pitney, 1970; Ecklund et al., 1970; and Karpatkin, 1970), however, have failed to demonstrate the presence of increased quantities of fibrin degradation products in the serum of healthy term infants at the time of birth.

The blood of the newborn infant possesses increased fibrinolytic activity and decreased plasminogen levels (Markerian et al., 1967; Ecklund et al., 1970). The fibrinolytic activity decreased rapidly during the first hours of life (Engström and Kager, 1964).

In summary, defects in all three phases of coagulation can be demonstrated during the newborn period. The defects in the first and second phases of coagulation appear to be primarily the result of deficiencies in the vitamin K dependent factors. Despite the decreased levels of clotting factors, the whole blood of most newborn infants is hypercoagulable, as measured by the Lee–White clotting time and thromboelastograph (Koch, 1962).

THE ROLE OF VITAMIN K

Vitamin K is required for the hepatic synthesis of prothrombin, Factor VII (proconvertin), Factor IX (plasma thromboplastin component), and Factor X (Stuart-Prower). Table 8–6 describes the characteristics of the natural and synthetic compounds with vitamin K activity.

It is now generally agreed that administration of vitamin K to the healthy term infant prevents the decrease in prothrombin activity and the prolongation of the prothrombin time that are normally observed during the first few days of life (Aballi and De Lamerens, 1962; Dam et al., 1952).

Response to vitamin K is not limited to its effect on the one-stage prothrombin time. It has been observed that administration of vitamin K also prevents a decrease in the activity of the Factor VII and X complex (Van Creveld et al., 1954; Douglas and Davis, 1955; Haupt, 1960), of prothrombin, and of Factor IX (Aballi et al., 1957). Treatment with vitamin K can therefore be expected to result in normal or near normal values for both the prothrombin time and the thromboplastin generation test in the healthy term infant, although normal adult values for the specific factors (prothrombin, VII, IX, and X) may not be reached for many weeks (Van Creveld et al., 1954; Fresh et al., 1957; Dyggve, 1958). This is understandable when one appreciates that values for both the prothrombin time and the thromboplastin generation test fall into the normal range when the concentrations of the specific factors involved in these tests range from 50 to 200 per cent of the adult standard.

In the premature infant, particularly the very small premature infant, the response to vitamin K is less predictable (Lelong et al., 1955; Aballi et al., 1957). Their levels of prothrombin are often lower

Table 8–6   Characteristics and Routes of Administration
of Natural Vitamin K Compounds and Some Synthetic
Water-Soluble Analogues*

	NATURAL VITAMIN K COMPOUNDS	
	Vitamin K_1	*Vitamin K_2*
Chemical term	2-Methyl-3-phytyl-1,4-naphtho-quinone	2-Methyl-3-difarnesyl-1,4 naphthoquinone
Official term (U.S.P. XVI)	Phytonadione	–
Solubility	Fat	Fat
Source	Green plants	Gastrointestinal microorganisms
Preparations	Phytonadione (U.S.P. XVI) and Mephyton are oily preparations; AquaMephyton and Konakion are clear aqueous colloidal suspensions.	None available
Routes of administration	Phytonadione and Mephyton: oral or intravenous. AquaMephyton and Konakion; oral, intramuscular, subcutaneous, intravenous.	–

	WATER-SOLUBLE ANALOGUES OF VITAMIN K		
Chemical term	2-Methyl-1,4 naphtho-quinone	2-Methyl-2-sodium bisulfite-3-dehydro-1,4-naphthoquinone	2-Methyl-1,4-naphthalendiol tetrasodium diphosphate hexahydrate
Official term (U.S.P. XVI)	Menadione	Menadione sodium bisulfite	Menadiol sodium diphosphate
Solubility	Water	Water	Water
Preparations	Menadione (U.S.P. XVI)	Hykinone and menadione sodium bisulfite (U.S.P. XVI)	Synkayvite and menadiol sodium diphosphate (U.S.P. XVI)
Routes of administration	Intravenous or intramuscular	Oral, intravenous or intramuscular	Oral, intravenous, or intramuscular

*From Report of Committee on Nutrition, American Academy of Pediatrics. Pediatrics, 28:501, 1961.

than those observed in the term infant, and their response to vitamin K may be minimal. Factor IX activity is also generally lower, and vitamin K often does not normalize the thromboplastin generation test during the first week of life (McElfresh, 1961). Van Creveld and associates (1954) observed that Factor VII levels were often below 30 per cent of adult values at eight weeks of age in prematurely born infants, despite vitamin K therapy during the newborn period. The inadequate response to vitamin K in these small infants suggests that the immature liver is incapable of optimal synthesis of many of the coagulation factors. This conclusion was reached by Pool and Robinson (1959) after demonstrating with in vitro methods that the liver of fetal and newborn rats was relatively deficient in Factor VII synthesis, despite the presence of adequate amounts of vitamin K in the incubation mixture.

Although some investigators (Hardwicke, 1944; Sells et al., 1941) have demonstrated that doses of as little as 2.5 to 5.0 μg. of vitamin K exert a beneficial effect on the coagulation mechanism during the neonatal period in the term infant, Aballi and co-workers (1962) found that 25 μg. is necessary to protect all infants from a prolonged prothrombin time. Hundred-fold doses of 2.5 mg. were no more effective.

It is well recognized that large doses of the synthetic water-soluble vitamin K analogues may result in hyperbilirubinemia and kernicterus, as discussed in Chapter Five, but small doses of the natural vitamin K compounds have not been found to be associated with any signs of toxicity.

Controversy still exists as to whether vitamin K administration to the pregnant mother exerts a beneficial effect on her offspring. Because of the uncertainties of optimum dose, timing, and duration of therapy required in the mother to prevent a decrease in the level of the vitamin K dependent factors in the newborn, the Committee on Nutrition of the American Academy of Pediatrics recommends that vitamin K be administered to the newborn. Their report states:

Commonly employed synthetic water-soluble analogues (menadione, menadione sodium bisulfite, and menadione sodium diphosphate) are all probably safe and effective when administered in proper dosage. However, the margin of safety is almost certainly greatest with vitamin K_1, and this derivative is considered the drug of choice. A single parenteral dose of 0.5 to 1 mg. or an oral dose of 1.0 to 2.0 mg. is probably adequate for prophylaxis, but it may be necessary at times to repeat this dosage for treatment, and larger doses will generally be necessary for treatment of infants whose mothers received anticoagulant therapy. Oral, intramuscular, or intravenous routes are feasible for vitamin K_1 and all synthetic analogues except menadione. This is not used orally. At the present time it is recommended that vitamin K be given to the infant at birth, rather than administering it to the mother prenatally.

Hemorrhage due to vitamin K deficiency in the newborn can be safely and easily prevented. Deaths as a result of hemorrhage still occur and should be prevented by uniform adoption of the Committee's recommendations.

HEMORRHAGIC DISEASE OF THE NEWBORN

In 1894, Townsend introduced the term "haemorrhagic disease of the newborn" to distinguish a form of generalized bleeding that was observed during the newborn period that was self-limited in nature and thus could be distinguished from hemophilia with its lifelong complications. Townsend analyzed his experience with 50 cases of which 31 had proven fatal. The majority of infants initially manifested bleeding on the second or third day of life, although in two infants bleeding was noted on the first day and in one infant it occurred for the first time on the fourteenth day. Bleeding from the gastrointestinal tract was the most common manifestation of the disease, but bleeding from the umbilicus and nose, and into the skin and internal organs was also recorded.

Townsend, although admitting that the hemorrhages may have had a variety of etiologies, chose to lump them under a single descriptive term. Included in his series were infants born after difficult deliveries, febrile infants, and infants with congenital syphilis. Although much credit must be given to Townsend for calling attention to this syndrome, much of the confusion in later years concerning etiology and proper therapy stems from his broad classification of neonatal bleeding.

Hemorrhage in the newborn may occur with thrombocytopenia, vitamin K deficiency, transient inability of the liver to synthesize the necessary coagulation factors, disseminated intravascular coagulation in association with infections, acidosis, or hypoxia, or as a result of an inherited abnormality of the coagulation mechanism. To include all but the congenital disorders under the term hemorrhagic disease of the newborn can only lead to confusion.

The Committee on Nutrition of the American Academy of Pediatrics (1961) has chosen to define the disease in the following way: "Hemorrhagic disease of the newborn is a hemorrhagic disorder of the first days of life caused by a deficiency of vitamin K and characterized by deficiency of prothrombin, proconvertin, and probably other factors."

Within the limits of this definition, it is difficult to define the true incidence of this disease. Many of the older studies in the literature did not attempt to separate bleeding caused by vitamin K deficiency from bleeding that may have been caused by other factors. Also, it has not always been recognized that, if early artificial feedings are instituted, withholding of vitamin K may not necessarily result in laboratory evidence of a severe deficiency state. Therefore, comparison of groups to determine incidence of bleeding merely on the basis of whether or not they received vitamin K can result in erroneous conclusions.

The diet of the infant exerts a great effect on the coagulation process. In 1932, Sanford and associates observed that the incidence of hemorrhage could be reduced by starting supplemental feedings at four hours of age. Gellis and Lyon (1941) also demonstrated the beneficial effect of early feedings on the prothrombin time. In Table 8–7 are recorded the results of a study by Aballi (1965) on the effects of early introduction of milk feedings on the prothrombin time. In infants fed at eight hours of age, only 2 per cent had prothrombin values of less than 20 per cent at three days of age, while in the group not fed until 36 hours of age 11 per cent fell below this value.

Dam et al. (1942) reported that cow's milk contains approximately 6 μg. of vitamin K per 100 ml., while breast milk contains only 1.5 μg. Aballi has demonstrated that the administration of as little as 25 μg. of vitamin K can prevent the lengthening of the prothrombin time of normal term infants so that ingestion of eight to ten ounces of milk during the first 48 hours of life can have a profound effect on the coagulation status. Sutherland and associates (1967) observed that bleeding associated with hypoprothrombinemia was confined to breast-fed infants who had not received vitamin K. These authors found that

Table 8–7   Influence of Time of Onset of Feedings on the Prothrombin Time During the First Three Days of Life[*]

MILK FEEDINGS STARTED 8 HOURS AFTER BIRTH (50 INFANTS)			
Prothrombin Time (%)	*Per Cent of Infants with This Value*		
	Initially	*2nd Day*	*3rd Day*
Over 50	68	54	72
20–49	25	37	26
Less than 20	7	9	2
Mean activity	61	52	68

MILK FEEDINGS STARTED 18 HOURS AFTER BIRTH (30 INFANTS)			
Prothrombin Time (%)	*Per Cent of Infants with This Value*		
	Initially	*2nd Day*	*3rd Day*
Over 50	65	35	76
20–49	29	59	20
Less than 20	6	6	4
Mean activity	58	47	63

MILK FEEDINGS STARTED 36 HOURS AFTER BIRTH (80 INFANTS)			
Prothrombin Time (%)	*Per Cent of Infants with This Value*		
	Initially	*2nd Day*	*3rd Day*
Over 50	76	41	40
20–49	24	46	40
Less than 20	0	13	11
Mean activity	59	43	48

[*]From Aballi, A. J.: South. Med. J. 58:52, 1965.

there were twice as many bleeding episodes among the breast-fed infants who received no vitamin K as among infants who received vitamin K or a cow's milk formula, or both. Similarly, Keenan and associates (1971) demonstrated that the prothrombin activity of infants 24 hours after the first feeding of a cow's milk formula did not differ significantly from that of infants given vitamin K at birth. This effect of early feeding must be taken into account when one evaluates reports of lack of deleterious effects from the withholding of vitamin K.

After Townsend's original description of hemorrhagic disease of the newborn, Schwartz and Ottenburg (1910) reported a prolonged coagulation time in newborn infants with this entity. In 1912, based on his autopsy study of two infants who had died with melena, Whipple postulated that the defect was due to a lack of prothrombin. Gelston (1921) found a lowered prothrombin level in an infant with an umbilical hemorrhage, and later Kugelmass et al. (1930) demonstrated a decrease in prothrombin concentration as a cause of newborn bleeding. Brinkhous and associates (1937) were the first to demonstrate that the true prothrombin level was low in normal newborns as well. Soon afterward, several groups of investigators (Hellman and Shettles, 1939; Nygaard, 1939; Dam et al., 1939) showed that administration of vitamin K could prevent and cure the hypoprothrombinemia of both normal newborns and those with hemorrhagic disease.

The estimates of the incidence of hemorrhagic disease of the newborn in infants not receiving vitamin K reveal tremendous variability and range, from 0.84 per cent (Salomonsen, 1940) to none in approximately 6000 (Potter, 1945). Sutherland and co-workers (1967) reported that 1.7 per cent of infants not receiving vitamin K had moderate or severe bleeding while approximately 0.4 per cent of those who were vitamin K sufficient demonstrated similar bleeding phenomena. Serious bleeding involving the central nervous system or the adrenal, or sufficient to produce anemia was observed only in vitamin K-deficient infants and occurred with a frequency of 0.7 per cent. Most estimates of the incidence of the disease are in the range of one in 200 to one in 400 (Smith, 1960).

Bleeding may occur on the first day of life but is more commonly observed on the second or third day of life. Bleeding from the gastrointestinal tract, umbilical cord, circumcision site and nose, and into the scalp, as well as generalized ecchymosis, is the most frequent external manifestation of the disease. Prolonged oozing from the deep puncture wounds inflicted for capillary bilirubin determinations may be the earliest sign of the disease. Internal hemorrhage may also occur.

The laboratory features of the disease are summarized in Table 8–8 and are contrasted with the findings in neonates with disseminated intravascular coagulation. Vitamin K deficiency is characterized

Table 8–8   Differential Features of Hemorrhagic
Disease of the Newborn

FEATURES	VITAMIN K DEFICIENCY	DISSEMINATED INTRAVASCULAR COAGULATION
Uniformity of clotting defect	Constant	Variable
Capillary fragility	Normal	Usually abnormal
Bleeding time	Normal	Often prolonged
Clotting time	Prolonged	Variable
One-stage prothrombin	Very prolonged (5% or less)	Moderately prolonged
Partial thromboplastin time	Prolonged	Prolonged
Thrombin time	Normal for age	Usually prolonged
Fibrin degradation products	Not present	Present
Factor V	Normal	Decreased
Fibrinogen	Normal	Often decreased
Platelets	Normal	Often decreased
Red cell fragmentation	Not present	Usually present
Response to vitamin K	Spectacular	Diminished or absent
Associated disease	Usually trivial (trauma may be precipitating factor)	Severe. May include sepsis, hypoxia, acidosis, or obstetric accident
Previous history	No vitamin K given or mother receiving barbiturates or anticonvulsants	Above illnesses. Vitamin K given

by a prolonged clotting time and a very prolonged prothrombin time, with decreases in Factors II, VII, IX, and X. Vitamin K deficiency should be suspected as the cause of hemorrhage in any apparently newborn infant who has not received this vitamin at birth.

Treatment consists in the intravenous or intramuscular administration of 1 to 2 mg. of vitamin K_1 (Table 8–6). The intravenous route is preferred for treatment if a superficial vessel is easily available because intramuscular injections may result in a large hematoma. The intravenous route is also advisable, because one can not always be certain at the time of treatment that the hemorrhage is due to vitamin K deficiency and intramuscular injections are always to be avoided in the event that a defect of the coagulation mechanism is the cause of the bleeding.

If vitamin K deficiency is responsible for the coagulation disturbance, the response to treatment is striking (Fig. 8–3). The rise in clotting factors can be demonstrated in two to four hours. Within 24 hours almost complete correction of the coagulation abnormalities can be expected.

As detailed in the final section of this chapter, blood, preferably fresh, should also be administered if the hemorrhage has been severe.

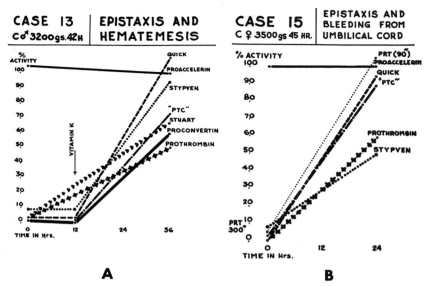

Figure 8–3 Response of the coagulation factors to vitamin K administration in hemorrhagic disease of the newborn. (From Aballi, A. J., and De Lamerens, S.: *Pediatric Clinics of North America,* 9:785, 1962.)

DISSEMINATED INTRAVASCULAR COAGULATION

In 1962, Aballi and De Lamerens introduced the useful term "secondary hemorrhagic disease of the newborn" to emphasize that not all bleeding in the neonate was a result of vitamin K deficiency. They indicated that this form of hemorrhage occurred commonly in premature infants of low birth weight, but was also seen in any infant who was anoxic, acidotic, or septic. Hemorrhage into the lungs and central nervous system was more frequent than that seen with the bleeding associated with vitamin K deficiency. Coagulation defects included alterations in capillary fragility, thrombocytopenia, depression of the vitamin K dependent factors, and decreased levels of Factor V and fibrinogen.

What Aballi and De Lamerens called "secondary hemorrhagic disease of the newborn" now is recognized, in most instances, as being similar to, or the same as, the entity termed disseminated intravascular coagulation. Disseminated intravascular coagulation is an acquired pathophysiologic process characterized by the intravascular consumption of platelets and plasma clotting factors (Factors II, V, VIII, XIII, and fibrinogen). This widespread coagulation within the vasculature results in the deposition of fibrin thrombi and the production of a hemorrhagic state when the rapid utilization of platelets and clotting factors results in levels that are inadequate to maintain hemostasis. The accumulation of fibrin in the microcirculation produces mechanical injury to the red cells, leading to erythrocyte fragmentation and the microangiopathic anemia described in Chapter Three. Disseminated intravascular coagulation is now being diagnosed with increasing frequency in the neonatal period and has been the subject of several excellent reviews (Abildgaard, 1969; Karpatkin, 1971; Lascari and Wallace, 1971).

Etiology. Disseminated intravascular coagulation is not in itself a primary disease process but a response to certain stimuli. The process can be initiated by endotoxin, endothelial damage, the introduction of thromboplastic substances into the circulation, proteolytic enzymes, foreign particulate matter, and platelet aggregation. Disseminated intravascular coagulation has now been described in association with a myriad of conditions that occur in the neonatal period. A list of the clinical situations which may be associated with disseminated intravascular coagulation is presented in Table 8–9. Whaun and associates (1971) have found that septicemia due to gram-negative organisms is probably the single most common cause of this condition in neonates. Hypoxia and acidosis are also extremely common initiating events. Transplacental passage of thromboplastic material may occur in the eclamptic or preeclamptic mother and may also initiate the process in the newborn infant.

Clinical Manifestations. The clinical manifestations are extremely variable and, in part, are determined by the associated dis-

TABLE 8–9   Conditions Associated with Disseminated Intravascular Coagulation in the Newborn

OBSTETRIC COMPLICATIONS
    Abruptio placentae
    Preeclampsia and eclampsia
    Dead twin fetus
    Fetal distress during delivery
    Amniotic fluid embolism
    Breech delivery

NEONATAL INFECTIONS
    Bacterial, both gram-negative and gram-positive
    Disseminated herpes simplex
    Cytomegalovirus infections
    Rubella
    Toxoplasmosis
    Syphilis

MISCELLANEOUS CONDITIONS
    Respiratory distress syndrome
    Severe erythroblastosis fetalis
    Giant hemangioma
    Renal vein thrombosis
    Severe acidosis and hypoxemia
    Indwelling catheters

ease process and, in part, by the severity of the coagulation disturbance. In the typical case, oozing at puncture sites is noted in a sick infant. Closer physical examination then frequently reveals the presence of petechiae. Clinical manifestations, however, may include pulmonary, cerebral, and intraventricular hemorrhages, bleeding from the umbilical stump and body orifices, purpura, ecchymoses, and thrombosis of peripheral or central vessels with tissue necrosis and gangrene (Glaun et al., 1971).

Laboratory Diagnosis. Laboratory abnormalities include the presence of a hemolytic anemia with red cell fragmentation visible in the peripheral smear (Fig. 8–4), variable degrees of thrombocytopenia, and a prolongation of the prothrombin, partial thromboplastin, and thrombin times. The level of Factor V is generally decreased, while Factor VIII and fibrinogen levels may be decreased. The leukocytes frequently show toxic granulation and the white count may be elevated with a predominance of immature forms; such abnormalities may provide an early clue to the presence of sepsis.

The presence of elevated levels of fibrin degradation products (fibrin split products) occurs invariably in older infants, children, and adults with disseminated intravascular coagulation, but may not always be present in the neonate. Whaun and associates (1971) found the presence of anemia, thrombocytopenia, fibrin split products,

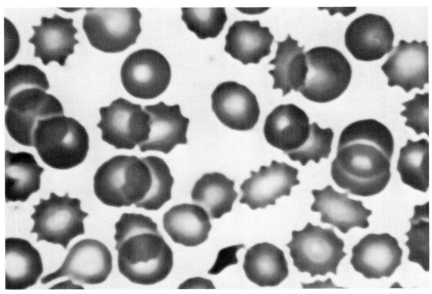

Figure 8–4   Peripheral blood smear from an infant with disseminated intravascular coagulation demonstrating the presence of irregularly contracted and fragmented erythrocytes.

a decreased Factor II (prothrombin), a decreased Factor V, a prolonged thrombin time, and the presence of red cell fragmentation to be the most useful laboratory abnormalities for the diagnosis of disseminated intravascular coagulation in newborns. The laboratory diagnosis of disseminated intravascular coagulation in the neonatal period may be difficult because of the commonly seen physiologic alterations that are also present during this period of life. Fortunately, many of the factors which are normally consumed in disseminated intravascular coagulation, such as platelets, Factor V, Factor VIII, and fibrinogen, are present in normal or near normal adult values in the neonate so that deviations from these values are of great diagnostic significance. The laboratory findings that distinguish disseminated intravascular coagulation from vitamin K deficiency are listed in Table 8–8.

Therapy. Treatment must be directed toward both the underlying disease and the coagulation abnormality. In general, success will depend on the ability to correct the condition that initiated the process of disseminated intravascular coagulation rather than on the management of the hematologic abnormalities. If the condition which underlies disseminated intravascular coagulation is brought under control, then intravascular coagulation will cease. Thus, management of the patient may include the administration of appropriate antibiotics, correction of abnormalities of pH and electrolytes, and maintenance of adequate oxygenation and blood pressure.

The decision to treat the coagulation abnormality must be based on the clinical findings in conjunction with the laboratory findings, and not on the presence of laboratory abnormalities alone. If the infant is bleeding or has evidence of definite thrombotic complications, and laboratory studies support the diagnosis of disseminated intravascular coagulation, then treatment is indicated.

Heparin, a potent anticoagulant that acts as both an antithrombin and an inhibitor of other steps of the coagulation process (the activation of Factor IX by XI, the activation of Factor VIII by IX), has been used with success to halt the process of disseminated intravascular coagulation. When the consumption of coagulation factors is stopped their levels return to normal and the bleeding caused by their depletion ceases. Heparin should be administered intravenously as an initial dose of 100 units per kilogram of body weight and then at a maintenance dose of 600 units per kilogram per day. The maintenance dose may be administered continuously or given as 100 units per kilogram at four hour intervals.

The aim of heparin therapy is to maintain the whole blood clotting time in the range of 20 to 30 minutes, or the activated partial thromboplastin time in the range of 60 to 70 seconds (Stuart and Michel, 1971), depending on each individual laboratory's own normal values.

The dose of heparin can be increased or decreased, depending on the results of these studies. The effectiveness of heparin therapy can be judged most simply by repeated platelet counts. If the consumption process has been halted the platelet count should remain stable and then, after a variable period, often two to three days, begin to rise and eventually reach supranormal levels.

Heparin therapy should be continued until the process of disseminated intravascular coagulation has been halted. This, in large part, will depend on the treatment of the underlying disease. When the process is believed to be under control, heparin is discontinued and four to five hours after the last dose, the platelet count, prothrombin, partial thromboplastin, and thrombin times are determined. If these are in the normal range, the tests should be repeated in six to eight hours. If they continue to remain normal it can be assumed that the process of consumption is over.

On occasion, it may be necessary to administer platelets and coagulation factors to replace those that have been consumed during the process of disseminated intravascular coagulation. This should not be attempted until the patient has received an adequate dose of heparin. Replacement prior to that time will merely provide more fuel for the process of disseminated intravascular coagulation and increase the deposition of fibrin. The administration of fresh frozen plasma in a dose of 10 ml. per kilogram and one unit of a platelet concentrate per 5 kilograms of body weight should be sufficient to restore them to hemostatic levels. Coagulation factors usually return to normal levels during heparin therapy; thus it is rarely necessary to replace them on more than one occasion unless hepatic function is impaired.

Exchange transfusion with relatively fresh blood (Skyberg and Jacobson, 1969; Gross and Melhorn, 1971) has also been successfully employed in the management of disseminated intravascular coagulation. This procedure serves to simultaneously anticoagulate the patient, replace coagulation factors, and clear the body of fibrin degradation products that may serve to inhibit coagulation.

More controlled experience will be necessary before the optimum form of treatment for disseminated intravascular coagulation in the newborn can be established. Infants frequently recover without anticoagulation when the primary disease is treated successfully. Similarly, the mortality rate in infants with disseminated intravascular coagulation has been found to be close to 60 per cent (Whaun et al., 1971) despite adequate heparin therapy. At the present, the best method of success remains an appreciation of the conditions associated with disseminated intravascular coagulation, their prompt recognition, and early treatment. We have found that frequent platelet counts, hemoglobin determinations, and examination of peripheral smears for signs of red cell fragmentation provide a useful surveillance system for the early detection of disseminated intravascular coagulation. It should be employed in all infants born after difficult deliveries, in those born after complicated pregnancies, in those with congenital abnormalities that may predispose to infections, and in those infants with problems of acidosis or hypoxia.

CONGENITAL DEFICIENCIES OF THE COAGULATION FACTORS

Although the majority of infants with congenital deficiencies of the coagulation factors go through the first weeks of life with no difficulty, all the congenital defects may manifest themselves by bleeding in the newborn period.

Factor VIII (antihemophiliac factor, AHF) deficiency and Factor IX (plasma thromboplastin component, PTC) deficiency account for approximately 90 per cent of all the congenital disorders of the coagulation mechanism (Didisheim and Lewis, 1958; Diamond, 1961). Factor VIII deficiency is approximately six times as frequent as Factor IX deficiency.

Schulman (1962) observed that 11 of 25 children with severe AHF or PTC deficiency had hemorrhagic symptoms during the first week of life. In contrast, only three of 22 infants with mild hemophilia (defined as hemophilia with a normal whole blood clotting time) had hemorrhagic manifestations in the neonatal period. Hartmann and Diamond (1957) observed hemorrhage in 33 of 94 infants with AHF or PTC deficiency. Of these, the majority occurred following circumcision, being seen in 30 patients, while intracranial hemorrhage was observed in two and umbilical hemorrhage in one. Massive hemorrhage into the scalp is another well recognized site of bleeding in newborns with Factor VIII deficiency (Kozinn et al., 1965).

Strauss (1965) interviewed the parents of 65 patients with AHF deficiency in order to determine the frequency of neonatal bleeding. Of this group, 36 patients had a circumcision performed during the first 10 days of life. Of the 16 patients with mild or moderate hemophilia (Factor VIII levels in excess of 1 per cent of normal), only two had mild bleeding. In 20 infants with severe hemophilia, 10 had mild bleeding and four had severe prolonged bleeding from the circumcision site.

Baehner and Strauss (1966) reviewed the neonatal records of 192 patients with either Factor VIII or Factor IX deficiency. Only nine of these patients experienced bleeding unrelated to circumcision during the first week of life. Even after circumcision, only 26 of 61 infants with severe hemophilia and five of 46 infants with less severe disease had serious bleeding complications. When circumcision was delayed beyond the neonatal period in seven instances, moderate or severe bleeding occurred in each patient.

The reason that all hemophiliacs do not bleed in the newborn period is not clear. Didisheim and Lewis (1958), Strauss (1965) and Baehner and Strauss (1966) have recorded the virtual absence of Factor VIII in the cord blood of infants with hemophilia. It may be concluded from these observations, as well as from those of Cade and associates (1969), that no significant transplacental passage of Factor VIII or any of the other coagulation factors takes place. Thus, the old theory that maternal antihemophiliac factor crossed the placenta to protect the newborn hemophiliac is no longer tenable. Bleeding following circumcision may be prevented owing to the liberation of tissue thromboplastin caused by the pressure of the circumcision clamp.

In addition to AHF and PTC deficiency, von Willebrand's disease (pseudohemophilia), Factor V (proaccelerin) deficiency, Factor VII (proconvertin) deficiency, Factor X (Stuart-Prower) deficiency, Factor XI (plasma thromboplastin antecedent) deficiency, Factor XIII (fibrin stabilizing factor) deficiency, and afibrinogenemia (Manios et al., 1968) may all present themselves in the newborn period. Factor XIII deficiency is the most recently recognized addition to the list of inherited coagulation disturbances that may cause protracted hemorrhage during the early weeks of life (Duckert et al., 1960; Barry and Delâge, 1965; Fischer et al., 1966; Britten, 1967). This latter deficiency state commonly manifests itself by a continuous ooze from the umbilical stump.

It must be remembered that these congenital deficiencies are comparatively rare and should only be considered after excluding the more common causes of bleeding in the newborn. Githens and Ferrier (1959) reviewed their experience with significant external hemorrhage during a five year period at the nurseries of the Colorado General Hospital, where vitamin K had been administered to all infants. Four babies out of a total of 5192 full-term infants had manifested marked external bleeding. Of these four infants, one was found to have a Factor IX (PTC) deficiency, two had thrombocytopenia, and one was bleeding from a rectal fissure.

Hartmann et al. (1955) reviewed their experience with 34 patients referred for study because of abnormal bleeding during the first week of life. Nineteen of these 34 suffered from congenital disorders. Of these, 14 patients had Factor VIII (AHF) deficiency, two had Factor IX (PTC) deficiency, one had Factor VII (proconvertin) deficiency, and two patients had congenital afibrinogenemia. Of the remaining 15 patients, six had thrombocytopenic purpura, four had vitamin K deficiency, one suffered from acquired hypofibrinogenemia, and four were infants with severe erythroblastosis (three of whom had thrombocytopenia and low levels of prothrombin, Factor V, and Factor VII, while one infant also had low levels of fibrinogen).

THE BLEEDING INFANT: DIAGNOSIS AND MANAGEMENT

The diagnosis and rational treatment of the bleeding infant require a thoughtful synthesis of facts obtained from family history, maternal history, physical examination, and a few carefully chosen laboratory tests.

A method of approach to this problem is outlined in Figure 8–5

If hemorrhage occurs from the gastrointestinal tract during the first day of life, it must be established whether the blood is of infant or maternal origin. This procedure (the Apt test) is described on page 240. One should appreciate that melena may occur as late as 30 hours after swallowing as little as 30 ml. of whole blood (Apt and Downey, 1955).

The sex of the newborn should be noted and correlated with available information concerning the inheritance of the coagulation defects (Table 8–10). Although cases of Factor VIII (AHF) deficiency (Choremis, 1956; Mellman et al., 1961; Whissell et al., 1965; Lusher, 1969) and Factor IX (PTC) deficiency (Strauss and Olson, 1969) have been reported in females, the chances of abnormal bleeding in a female being due to Factor VIII (AHF) or Factor IX (PTC) deficiency are extremely remote.

Family History.   In approximately 50 to 75 per cent of patients with Factor VIII or Factor IX deficiency, a positive family history

Table 8–10   Mode of Transmission of the Hereditary
Coagulation Disorders

Sex-Linked Recessive (disorders primarily of males)
   Factor VIII (AHF) deficiency
   Factor IX (PTC) deficiency

Autosomal Dominant (disorders of both sexes; one parent affected)
   Factor XI (PTA) deficiency
   Von Willebrand's disease

Autosomal Recessive (disorders of both sexes; parents appear normal)
   Prothrombin deficiency
   Factor V (proaccelerin) deficiency
   Factor VII (proconvertin) deficiency
   Factor X (Stuart-Prower) deficiency
   Factor XII (Hageman) deficiency—No bleeding associated with this disorder
   Factor XIII (fibrin stabilizing factor) deficiency
   Afibrinogenemia, congenital

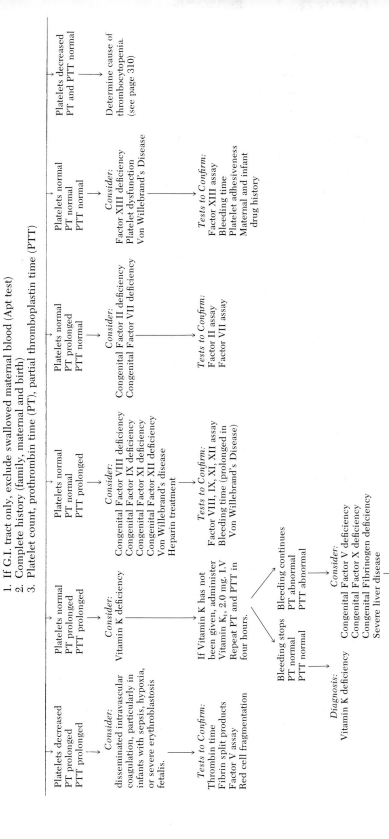

Figure 8–5 A Diagnostic Approach to the Bleeding Newborn

265

of other male members with bleeding manifestations can be obtained (Schulman, 1962; Biggs and Macfarlane, 1962).

Maternal History.   A careful inquiry should be made into drug ingestion by the mother. Maternal ingestion of coumarin anticoagulants, barbiturates, and certain anticonvulsants (Mountain et al., 1970) has been implicated as causes of neonatal hemorrhage (see Chapter Two). Many drugs also may produce thrombocytopenia in the newborn (Chapter Nine) or impair platelet function (Bleyer and Breckenridge, 1970). The most common of the drugs leading to platelet dysfunction is aspirin. The mother should also be questioned as to the recent or past history of thrombocytopenia, rubella during the first trimester, syphilis, or a history suggestive of preeclampsia.

Infant History.   In reviewing the patient's record, information concerning vitamin K administration, birth trauma, prolonged anoxia, degree of prematurity, and sites of bleeding should be noted.

Physical Examination.   Particular attention should be paid to the type and sites of bleeding. In infants with hemophilia, the skin lesions are generally cutaneous and subcutaneous hematomas (Schaffer, 1960) rather than flat petechiae or ecchymoses. Muscle and joint hemorrhages and cephalhematomas (Kozinn et al., 1965) may also be observed in newborn hemophiliacs, although this is uncommon. Oozing from puncture sites should be looked for.

Signs of sepsis, jaundice, or hepatosplenomegaly should also be noted, for their presence suggests that the bleeding is part of a generalized disturbance resulting either in thrombocytopenia or impaired hepatic synthesis of the coagulation factors—for example, cytomegalic inclusion disease, toxoplasmosis, herpes simplex, and syphilis. Jaundice may be solely the result of a large enclosed hemorrhage (Rausen and Diamond, 1961).

Syndactylism has been observed in association with congenital deficiency of Factor V (de Vries et al., 1951).

Cephalhematomas have been observed in infants with congenital disturbances of the coagulation mechanism, and in vitamin K deficiency. Oozing of blood from the umbilical stump or from the circumcision site is characteristic of the bleeding that occurs with vitamin K deficiency and Factor XIII deficiency.

Hemorrhage in more than one area suggests a generalized disturbance as the cause rather than a local problem such as a bleeding vessel in a circumcision.

Laboratory Studies.   The first step in the laboratory evaluation should be a determination of platelet adequacy, either by examination of a well prepared cover slip smear of the peripheral blood or by a direct platelet count, and the determination of the prothrombin time and partial thromboplastin time. If the infant has not received vitamin

K it should be given in a dose of one to two milligrams, intravenously, while the results of the laboratory tests are awaited.

If the platelet count alone is abnormal, then the causes of isolated thrombocytopenia, as described in Chapter Nine, should be investigated.

If the platelet count is decreased and is associated with a prolongation of the prothrombin time and partial thromboplastin time, it is strongly suggestive of the presence of disseminated intravascular coagulation. As previously discussed on page 258, this diagnosis should be strongly suspected in the presence of sepsis, hypoxia, or acidosis in a critically ill infant. The diagnosis can be firmly established by the demonstration of a prolonged thrombin time, a decrease in the level of Factor V, VIII, or fibrinogen, the presence of fibrin split products in the serum, and the finding of red cell fragmentation.

If the platelet count is found to be normal, while the prothrombin time and partial thromboplastin time are prolonged, a diagnosis of vitamin K deficiency may be considered as a cause of the bleeding (Fig. 8–4). Generally, bleeding cannot be attributed to vitamin K deficiency unless the prothrombin time is markedly prolonged (at least greater than 25 to 30 seconds). If the prothrombin and partial thromboplastin times are prolonged, the tests should be repeated four to eight hours after the administration of vitamin K. A significant decrease in the prothrombin and partial thromboplastin times confirms the diagnosis and cessation of bleeding can be expected shortly thereafter.

When the prothrombin time and partial thromboplastin time remain prolonged after the administration of vitamin K, and the platelet count is normal, then congenital deficiencies of Factor V, X, or fibrinogen must be considered diagnostic possibilities. Caution must always be exercised in the diagnosis of a congenital defect in the vitamin K-dependent factors or Factor V until it can be established that vitamin K therapy has been adequate and hepatic dysfunction is not present. In general, deficiencies of the vitamin K-dependent factors tend to parallel each other in their degree of severity if the deficiency is caused by a lack of vitamin K or is a result of liver immaturity or impairment. If three of the vitamin K-dependent factors are normal while one is persistently abnormal, this is evidence of a congenital deficiency of this factor.

When a prolonged prothrombin time is the only laboratory abnormality present in the bleeding infant, a congenital deficiency of either Factor II (prothrombin) or Factor VII should be considered. Similarly, when a prolonged partial thromboplastin time is the only laboratory abnormality, congenital deficiencies of Factors VIII, IX, XI, or XII should be considered along with Von Willebrand's disease. Inadvertent administration of an overdose of heparin to the infant may also produce a similar isolated laboratory abnormality (Galant, 1967).

Mutual correction studies (Table 8–3) or specific factor assays can be employed to determine the presence of a specific defect in coagulation.

When a congenital defect is suggested by the laboratory findings, family studies should be undertaken in an attempt to further substantiate the diagnosis. Often the genetic pattern may provide a clue to the type of defect that can be anticipated (Table 8–10). If the diagnosis remains in doubt, studies on the infant can always be repeated at a later age when the needs for prompt treatment are not as pressing.

In Table 8–11 are listed the usual laboratory findings in the congenital coagulation defects. These studies must be carefully interpreted against the background of the physiologic variations seen in the neonatal period.

On occasion, neonatal bleeding may be present in the absence of any abnormalities in the platelet count, prothrombin time, or partial thromboplastin time. In these situations a congenital deficiency of Factor XIII (fibrin stabilizing factor) or a defect in platelet function should be suspected. Transient neonatal platelet dysfunction produced by maternal aspirin ingestion has been associated with gastrointestinal bleeding, cephalohematoma, and periorbital purpura (Bleyer and Breckenridge, 1970). It is anticipated that the frequency and severity of this phenomenon will be better appreciated in the near future.

Table 8–11 The Differentiation of Congenital Deficiencies of the Coagulation Factors

DEFICIENCY	COAGULATION TIME	THROMBOPLASTIN GENERATION TEST	PROTHROMBIN TIME	DEFECT CORRECTED BY PLASMA	
				Fresh	*Stored*
Fibrinogen	Prolonged	Normal	Prolonged	Yes	Yes
Factor V	Variable	Prolonged	Prolonged	Yes	No
Factor VII	Normal	Normal	Prolonged	Yes	Yes
Factor VIII (AHF)	Variable	Prolonged	Normal	Yes	No
Factor IX (PTC)	Variable	Prolonged	Normal	Yes	Yes
Factor X	Prolonged	Prolonged	Prolonged	Yes	Yes
Factor XI (PTA)	Variable	Prolonged	Normal	Yes	Yes
Factor XII (Hageman)	Prolonged	Prolonged	Normal	Yes	Yes

Management of the Bleeding Infant

In many instances, hemorrhage may be of such a profound nature that transfusion therapy must be instituted before a precise diagnosis has been made. In all instances in which hemorrhage has occurred in the absence of prior vitamin K therapy, this vitamin should be administered before the start of the transfusion. Fresh whole blood or plasma can only temporarily correct the defects caused by vitamin K deficiency, while therapy with the vitamin permanently corrects the defects, provided that liver function is normal.

When it is apparent that vitamin K deficiency plays no etiologic role in the coagulation disturbance, a prompt judgment must be made as to whether the patient has disseminated intravascular coagulation or an as yet undiagnosed, but specific, congenital deficiency of a coagulation factor.

The management of disseminated intravascular coagulation with either heparin or exchange transfusion has been described on pages 260 and 261. When preliminary studies suggest the presence of a congenital coagulation disturbance, but a specific diagnosis has not yet been established, administration of fresh frozen plasma or fresh whole blood can be relied on to correct the disturbance. Fresh frozen plasma in a dosage of 5 ml. per pound administered every 12 hours generally supplies the necessary amounts of the deficient factor to stem bleeding of nonsurgical origin. If anemia is profound and red cells must also be administered, they may be given in the form of packed red cells alone during the intervals between plasma therapy. In this way, the plasma may be administered rapidly to minimize deterioration of labile factors such as Factor VIII (AHF). If whole blood is used, it should be fresh (less than 24 hours old) and given in amounts adequate to supply approximately 5 ml. of plasma per pound every 12 hours.

When the exact nature of the congenital deficiency has been established, stored plasma cryoprecipitate, commercial Factor VIII concentrates, or fibrinogen may be substituted for fresh frozen plasma when appropriate (see Table 8–10). Despite the fact that Factor IX is relatively stable in stored plasma, many centers prefer to use fresh frozen plasma when treating Factor IX (PTC) deficiency, because of the higher plasma levels obtained and the better therapeutic responses observed. A Factor IX concentrate (Konyne, Cutter Laboratories) is also available for the treatment of patients with Factor IX deficiency. Its use should be reserved for those situations where high levels of Factor IX need to be maintained for prolonged periods of time such as in life-threatening hemorrhages or in the preparation of and postoperative control of bleeding in patients requiring surgical procedures.

The relative potency of available sources of Factor VIII for replacement therapy are compared in Table 8–12. Pertinent details of these products and their uses are described in a comprehensive article dealing with the management of bleeding in hemophilia by Abildgaard (1969). One unit of Factor VIII activity is defined as the Factor VIII activity present in one milliliter of average normal human plasma. Transfusion of one unit of Factor VIII activity per kilogram of body weight will usually produce a 2 per cent rise in the circulating Factor VIII level. The estimated biologic half-life of Factor VIII following infusion is approximately 14 hours.

To achieve hemostasis it is desirable to raise the Factor VIII level to a minimum value of 20 per cent. This is achieved by providing the patient with 10 units of Factor VIII per kilogram of body weight, either in the form of fresh plasma, cryoprecipitate, or Factor VIII concentrate. The advantage of cryoprecipitate and Factor VIII concentrates lies in their ability to achieve levels of Factor VIII activity with small volumes of infusate, thus decreasing the risks of circulatory overload due either to hypervolemia or hyperproteinemia.

In the infant with a minor bleeding problem, such as a prolonged ooze from a circumcision site, therapy designed to achieve a Factor VIII level of 20 per cent, with maintenance of this level for 24 to 48 hours, is satisfactory. This can be achieved by the administration of 10 units per kilogram every 12 hours, or by a single infusion of 40 units per kilogram.

For more serious bleeding, such as is observed with large cephalohematomas or gastrointestinal or umbilical bleeding, therapy should be designed to achieve a Factor VIII level of 40 to 50 per cent, maintained for a period of 48 hours.

For life-threatening hemorrhages, such as intracranial bleeding or intra-abdominal hemorrhaging associated with organ injury, and for the provision of hemostasis during and after a surgical procedure, replacement therapy should be designed to achieve and maintain Factor VIII levels in the range of 80 to 100 per cent.

Similar guidelines may be applied to the treatment of infants with Factor IX (PTC) deficiency, although in the treatment of this congenital deficiency it appears that the infusion of one unit of Factor IX produces only a 1 per cent rise in the circulating level of Factor IX. Daily infusions of fresh frozen plasma in a dose of 10 ml. per kilogram of body weight appear to be adequate in the maintenance of hemostasis in patients with Factor XI (PTA) deficiency.

Topical therapy to bleeding wounds such as circumcisions is best achieved by the use of thrombin or an absorbable gauze such as Gelfoam or Oxycel. Nonabsorbable materials should be avoided because their removal may precipitate another bleeding episode. Circumcisions and other superficial wounds that are bleeding in a hemo-

Table 8–12   Sources of Factor VIII for Replacement Therapy

MATERIAL	APPROXIMATE FACTOR VIII ACTIVITY (Units/Ml.)	AVERAGE PROTEIN CONCENTRATION FACTOR VIII ACTIVITY (Gm./100 Units)	VOLUME OF USUAL DOSAGE FORM (Ml./Bottle or Bag)	AVERAGE TOTAL FACTOR VIII ACTIVITY (Units/Bottle or Bag)
Plasma*	1 (variable)†	7.0	250	200
Cryoprecipitate	7 (variable)†	0.42	15	100
Concentrates				
Antihemophilic factor (human)–Hyland	7	0.35	30	200
Antihemophilic factor (human) method four–Hyland‡	30–45	0.1	10;30	250;500;1,000
Antihemophilic factor (human)–Courtland	8	?	25	200
Fibro–AHF-rich fibrinogen)–Merck, Sharpe and Dohme	1	1.0	100 (1 Gm.) 200 (2 Gm.)	100 200

*Fresh, fresh frozen, or lyophilized antihemophilic plasma.
†Depends on starting potency (normal Factor VIII varies from 50 to 200 per cent) and variable loss during preparation.
‡This product is available in three dosage forms: 10 ml. = 250 units; 10 ml. = 500 units; 30 ml. = 1000 units.
(From Abildgaard, C.: Advances in Pediatrics, *16*:370, 1969)

philiac should not be sutured or cauterized because this results in further tissue trauma and thus more bleeding.

In the treatment of afibrinogenemia, bleeding can generally be controlled by raising the plasma level of fibrinogen to 80 to 100 mg./100 ml. This level can be achieved by the administration of 100 mg./kg. of fibrinogen.

ROUTINE COAGULATION STUDIES PRIOR TO CIRCUMCISION

Routine bleeding times and whole blood coagulation times are of little value in predicting which child may safely undergo circumcision. If the time spent in these procedures was instead employed in the careful questioning of the mother regarding a personal or family history of bleeding and in the examination of a peripheral blood film for the determination of platelet adequacy, more infants would escape the hemorrhagic hazards of circumcision and less time of the technician would be wasted.

Chapter Nine

THROMBOCYTOPENIA
IN THE NEWBORN

Effective hemostasis in the newborn infant is dependent on three interrelated factors: the coagulation proteins of the plasma and serum, the blood vessels, and the platelets.

Hemorrhage due to defects of the first two has been discussed in Chapter Seven. A deficiency in the numbers of platelets and qualitative impairment of platelet function are the remaining important causes of neonatal hemorrhage. This type of hemorrhage should be suspected when bleeding in the newborn is characterized by cutaneous petechiae and purpuric spots (Fig. 9–1). These lesions are usually generalized and may recur in crops over the first few days of life, in contrast to the petechiae commonly seen in normal newborns, which are localized to the head and upper chest and do not recur (Poley and Stickler, 1961).

Certain peculiarities of platelets of the newborn, such as their slightly lower numbers (especially in prematures), their susceptibility to maternal influences, and their participation in congenital disorders manifesting at birth, place them in a unique position deserving special consideration. Before beginning to discuss these quantitative aspects, it seems appropriate to review briefly the current status of our knowledge of platelet function and its disturbances in the newborn.

Normal Platelet Function

When a small blood vessel is injured there is an immediate response consisting of a series of reactions between the vessel wall

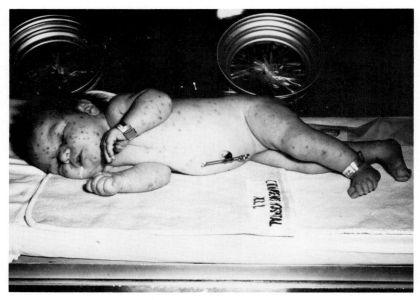

Figure 9–1   Extensive purpura in a thrombocytopenic newborn.

and the circulating platelets and terminating in the formation of a temporary hemostatic plug (Marcus, 1969). Initially, platelets adhere to the collagen exposed beneath the vessel intima. Adenosine diphosphate (ADP) released from such platelets leads to further aggregation of platelets, with the formation of a mass which seals the leak in the vessel wall. Breakdown of platelets then releases lipid thromboplastin, which activates the intrinsic clotting system of the plasma to form the fibrin component of the hemostatic plug. Based on the above reactions the major tests of platelet function include:

1. Bleeding time – an overall test of primary hemostasis.
2. Platelet adhesiveness (to a foreign surface such as glass beads).
3. Platelet aggregation (to each other).
4. Thromboplastic activity (platelet factor 3).
5. Clot retraction (dependent on 3, above).

Platelet Function in the Newborn. Clinical observations of abnormal "capillary fragility" of normal and ill newborns (especially prematures) have prompted a number of studies of platelet function in this age group (Hrodek, 1966; Hilgartner, 1968; and Mull and Hathaway, 1970). Abnormalities common to most of these studies included impaired platelet aggregation in response to collagen and exogenous ADP, impaired clot retraction, and decreased platelet factor 3 activity. Bleeding time was generally normal. The clinical significance of such abnormalities remains unclear, however, in view of the absence of bleeding tendency (Mull and Hathaway, 1970).

At least one of the above functional abnormalities can now be attributed to drugs received by the mother. Both acetylsalicylic acid (ASA) and chlorpromazine interfere with release of ADP and may therefore impair platelet aggregation (Weiss et al., 1968; Mills et al., 1968). Two groups of workers studying paired samples of maternal and cord blood discovered that impaired platelet aggregation was found only in the infants of mothers who had received ASA during the one to two week period before delivery; infants of mothers who had not received drugs showed normal platelet aggregation (Corby and Schulman, 1971), Bleyer and Breckenridge, 1970). The effect of ASA on maternal platelets was milder and of shorter duration. In addition to ASA, Corby and Schulman observed a similar impairment of platelet aggregation among infants of mothers who had received promethazine, alphaprodine and meperidine. The effect of promethazine was also demonstrated in vitro.

Aspirin is frequently taken by mothers during pregnancy without knowledge of the physician. Among 67 pregnant women who kept drug diaries, Bleyer et al. (1970) noted that 69 per cent had received ASA during the last trimester. The occurrence of three incidents of bleeding (cephalhematoma, melena and periorbital purpura) among 14 infants whose mothers received ASA suggested that ASA-induced platelet dysfunction may be of clinical significance in the newborn. Until this question is resolved, it would seem wise to discourage the use of ASA by mothers during the last month of pregnancy.

Disturbances of Platelet Function

A number of inherited defects of platelet function have been delineated by application of the above tests in the study of patients with bleeding disorders associated with a normal platelet count but an increased bleeding time. From the pediatric point of view, the type known as Glanzmann's thrombasthenia seems the most important of these. This is a rare disorder characterized by prolonged bleeding time, defective clot retraction and inability of platelets to aggregate in response to ADP. Bleeding in the newborn period has been described (Bowie et al., 1965; Zaizov et al., 1968).

Impaired platelet function may result from peculiarities of the neonatal blood environment. The role of drugs administered via the mother during labor certainly cannot be overlooked, as illustrated above. In addition, the effects of bilirubin, so commonly increased in the blood of newborns, deserve special consideration. Suvansri et al. (1969) demonstrated that bilirubin concentrations exceeding 15 to 20 mg. per 100 ml. were associated with morphologic abnormalities of platelets, along with impaired platelet thromboplastic activity and clot retraction. Maurer et al. (1970) showed that the impairment of platelet aggregation induced by unconjugated bilirubin occurred only with the free fraction and not with albumin-bound bilirubin.

Platelet Counts in the Normal Newborn Infant

Accurate enumeration of platelets depends on several technical factors, the most important of which is the use of the phase microscope to facilitate the distinction of platelets from other particulate matter. Counts by this method are therefore generally slightly lower and in a narrower range than those obtained by conventional microscopy. In the older child and adult, normal platelet counts range from 150,000 to 450,000/cu. mm., with a mean value of 250,000/cu. mm. (Brecher et al., 1953). Only recently have data on platelet counts in normal newborns been obtained by this method. The values for full-term and premature infants have been found to differ.

Full-term Newborns. Ablin et al. (1961) studied 105 full-term white and Negro newborns during the first four days of life. Platelet counts ranged from 84,000 to 478,000/cu. mm. The mean value was 200,000/cu. mm. ± two standard deviations, extending the range from 100,000 to 300,000/cu. mm. These values are only slightly lower than those of older children and adults. Similar results were obtained by Aballi et al. (1968) in a study of 88 term infants during the first 48 hours of life. The mean platelet count in this group was 251,000/cu. mm. and the range was 117,000 to 450,000/cu. mm.

Premature Infants. A number of studies have suggested that platelet counts under 100,000/cu. mm. are sufficiently common in premature infants to be considered physiologic. In Medoff's study of 26 premature infants in Philadelphia (1964), platelet counts at birth ranged from 31,000 to 197,000/cu. mm., fell to less than 50,000/cu. mm. by the tenth to twentieth day of age (especially among the smaller infants), and rose to normal by one month of age. Similar observations were made in Baltimore by Kaplan and Klein (1962) and in Boston by Desforges (1964). However, in the Baltimore study, the low platelet counts were confined to one nursery among serveral in that city, and suggested an unrecognized chemical or infectious agent in the environment. More recent studies have not confirmed the above observations of a "physiologic" thrombocytopenia of prematurity. Fogel et al. (1968) obtained serial counts in 73 random prematures in Miami and found only four with platelet counts less than 100,000/cu. mm., all among infants weighing under 1700 gm. at birth. The thrombocytopenia did not develop in these infants until between the tenth and twentieth days of life, and it disappeared by one month of age. In a larger study by Aballi et al. (1968) of 273 thriving premature infants in Memphis, the incidence of platelet counts less than 100,000 at varying times from birth to one month of age was only 1.5 to 3.6

per cent. The mean platelet counts at birth and in the second week of life were 220,000 and 260,000/cu. mm., respectively. No significant differences were found between infants with birth weights above and below 1500 gm.

The above data suggest that the thrombocytopenia observed in the earlier studies may well have been the result of an unrecognized infectious or other toxic agent in the nursery at that time. Premature infants whose platelet counts fall below 100,000/cu. mm. deserve investigation for some of the etiologic factors discussed later in this chapter.

Pathogenesis of Thrombocytopenia

The level of platelets in the blood reflects a balance between their production and their destruction. Platelets are produced in the bone marrow by the megakaryocytes, possibly under the regulatory influence of a plasma humoral substance (Schulman et al., 1960). Once they are released into the circulation, they survive under normal circumstances for approximately eight days, at the end of which time they are removed by the reticuloendothelial cells of the liver and spleen (Aster and Jandl, 1964).

Thrombocytopenia, therefore, may result from a decreased production of platelets, increased destruction of platelets, or a combination of the two. Included in this category of increased destruction are those disorders leading to disseminated intravascular coagulation, in which there is excessive consumption of platelets along with clotting factors (see p. 257). Platelet production is evaluated chiefly by inspection of the number and appearance of the megakaryocytes in a carefully collected sample of bone marrow. In this respect, it is essential that clotting of the marrow sample be avoided; otherwise megakaryocyte breakdown may occur and give the false impression of a decrease in number. Platelet destruction may be evaluated by determination of the platelet survival, using platelets labeled with isotopes such as chromium-51. The technical problems of obtaining adequate blood samples make this technique impractical in the newborn, and therefore for most clinical purposes the pathogenesis of the thrombocytopenia is inferred from the appearance of the bone marrow. Alternatively, measurement of the plasma concentration of a substance ordinarily contained in platelets, such as the enzyme acid phosphatase, may confirm the presence of increased platelet destruction (Oski et al., 1963).

An additional clue to the mechanism of thrombocytopenia may be obtained from an evaluation of platelet size (Garg, et al., 1971). Generally, young platelets are larger than old platelets, just as young reticulocytes are larger than mature erythrocytes. A predominance of

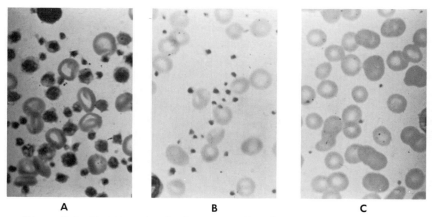

A   **B**   **C**

Figure 9–2 Variations in platelet size in thrombocytopenia. *A*, Large platelets in acquired "destructive" thrombocytopenia. *B*, Normal platelets. *C*, Small platelets in the Wiskott-Aldrich syndrome.

large platelets on peripheral blood smear (preferably from venous samples collected in ethylenediamine tetra-acetate [EDTA] therefore suggests that the thrombocytopenia is a result of peripheral platelet destruction with compensatory marrow release of young platelets. Conversely (with the exception of certain hereditary thrombocytopenic defects), normal or small platelets in a thrombocytopenic infant suggest a marrow disorder resulting in impaired production of platelets. Examples of such changes are shown in Figure 9–2.

The infant's response to a transfusion of normal platelets may also be of value in differentiating peripheral destruction from decreased production in the newborn (Gill and Schwartz, 1970). This will be discussed further on p. 311.

The pathogenesis of thrombocytopenia due to specific causes is discussed further under the appropriate sections.

ETIOLOGIC CLASSIFICATION OF NEONATAL THROMBOCYTOPENIA

The causes of thrombocytopenia in the newborn are numerous (Table 9–1). In many, maternal influences operate, such as immune platelet disorders, infections, and drugs, and therefore the thrombocytopenia presents at birth and is usually confined to the neonatal period. In others, such as the congenital or hereditary disorders, thrombocytopenia may not present clinically for several months after birth, but it remains a problem throughout the life of the child. This subject has been well reviewed by O'Gorman Hughes (1967) and Pochedly (1971).

Table 9–1 Etiologic Classification of Neonatal
Thrombocytopenia

Immune Disorders
    Passive (acquired from mother) — ITP, drug-induced thrombo-
    cytopenia, systemic lupus erythematosus.
    Active
        Isoimmune — platelet group incompatibility.
        Associated with erythroblastosis fetalis — due to the
        disease or to exchange transfusion.

Infections (? mediated in part by intravascular coagulation)
    Bacterial — generalized sepsis, congenital syphilis.
    Viral — cytomegalic inclusion disease, disseminated herpes
    simplex, rubella syndrome.
    Protozoal — congenital toxoplasmosis.

Drugs (administered to mother) — non-immune mechanism; e.g.,
    thiazide diuretics, tolbutamide.

Congenital Megakaryocytic Hypoplasia
    Isolated — congenital hypoplastic thrombocytopenia.
    Associated with: absent radii; microcephaly; rubella syn-
        drome; pancytopenia and congenital anomalies (Fanconi's
        anemia).
    Associated with pancytopenia but no congenital anomalies.
    Associated with trisomy syndromes — D_1 (13), E (18).

Bone Marrow Disease
    Congenital leukemia.

Disseminated Intravascular Coagulation (DIC) (See p. 258)
    Sepsis.
    Obstetrical complications — abruptio placentae, eclampsia,
        amniotic fluid embolism, dead twin fetus.
    Anoxia.
    Stasis — giant hemangioma (including placental chorangioma),
        renal vein thrombosis, polycythemia.

Inherited (Chronic) Thrombocytopenia
    Sex-linked:
        Pure.
        Aldrich's syndrome.
    Autosomal:
        Pure — dominant or recessive.
        May-Hegglin anomaly — dominant.

Miscellaneous
    Thrombotic thrombocytopenic purpura.
    Inherited metabolic disorders — glycinemia,
        methylmalonic acidemia, isovaleric acidemia
    Congenital thyrotoxicosis.

IMMUNE THROMBOCYTOPENIA

A variety of conditions are associated with the passage of antibody from the mother across the placenta to the infant, resulting in immunologic destruction of the infant's platelets, thrombocytopenia, and bleeding (Table 9–1). Although firm evidence that such an antiplatelet factor is really antibody in nature exists mainly for the drug-induced and isoimmune types of thrombocytopenia, clinical association leaves little doubt that a similar mechanism operates in the others (maternal idiopathic thrombocytopenic purpura, and others).

Etiology.   Depending on whether the antibody is formed against an antigen on the platelets of the mother (autoimmune) or those of the infant (isoimmune), these disorders may be classified as either passive or active. In the former, the infant is an innocent bystander to a disease in the mother causing thrombocytopenia. In the latter, the infant is the "troublemaker" and suffers the consequences of antibody formation that his platelets have stimulated in the otherwise well mother.

Passive Type.   The maternal disorders in which thrombocytopenia may occur in both mother and infant include idiopathic thrombocytopenic purpura, drug-induced thrombocytopenia, and systemic lupus erythematosus.

Active Type.   Thrombocytopenia in this situation is confined to the infant and occurs either alone or in conjunction with erythroblastosis fetalis. In the former, the infant possesses a platelet antigen lacking in his mother, his platelets cross the placenta to the maternal circulation, and they result in formation of antibodies by the mother against the foreign platelet antigen. When these antibodies cross the placenta to the fetal circulation, they react with the infant's platelets, resulting in the condition known as *isoimmune neonatal thrombocytopenic purpura* (Pearson et al., 1964). The immunologic mechanism is analogous to that of red cell sensitization occurring in erythroblastosis fetalis.

Thrombocytopenia in erythroblastosis fetalis, however, has not yet been shown to be on an immune basis. It usually occurs only in the more severe cases or following exchange transfusion.

NEONATAL THROMBOCYTOPENIA ASSOCIATED WITH MATERNAL IDIOPATHIC THROMBOCYTOPENIC PURPURA (ITP)

The newborn infants of women with ITP frequently manifest thrombocytopenia with varying degrees of hemorrhagic phenomena at birth. Although the thrombocytopenia is usually transient, disappearing within a few weeks to four months, fatalities have been reported. This association of thrombocytopenia in mother and infant and the demonstration of platelet agglutinins in both (Harrington et al., 1953) led to the formulation of the immune theory of etiology of this disease. The technical status and significance of the finding of platelet agglutinins have since been questioned (Corn and Upshaw, 1962; Jackson et al., 1963). However, there is little argument that the disease is in fact due to antibodies directed against the platelets. The subject of ITP in pregnancy has been well reviewed by Goodhue and Evans (1963), Schenker and Polishuk (1968), and Heys (1968).

There have now been four reports describing five infants born of women with ITP associated with autoimmune hemolytic anemia— Evans' syndrome (Silverstein et al., 1966; Letts and Kredenster, 1968 and 1969; Longpré et al., 1970). Thrombocytopenia was present in one of the four liveborn infants. Two infants showed evidence of a Coombs-positive hemolytic anemia.

Risk to the Newborn.   The most important single factor determining whether or not the offspring of mothers with ITP will be affected is the stage of activity of the maternal disease at the time of delivery. In 21 cases reviewed by Goodhue and Evans (1963) where the mother's platelet count at term was noted, the newborn infant was unaffected in each of five mothers with a normal platelet count, and was affected (purpura and/or low platelet count) in eight of 16 mothers with a low platelet count. In this limited series, the risk to the newborn seems confined to those born of mothers with thrombocytopenia at term, being approximately 50 per cent. A similar percentage of thrombocytopenic infants was found in a review of 21 such pregnancies by Heys (1968). In a report of cases of neonatal thrombocytopenia by Anthony and Krivit (1962), eight of nine pregnancies of mothers with ITP and low platelet counts at term resulted in infants with thrombocytopenia. The apparent higher risk to the newborn suggested by this series probably reflects that these pregnancies were selected on the basis of one or more infants presenting with thrombocytopenic purpura, thereby excluding women with ITP whose pregnancies yielded normal infants. Although it is often stated that affected infants may be born of mothers who have been cured of their disease or in clinical remission, documentation of this by platelet counts performed at term is generally lacking, rendering acceptance of such cases difficult. However, it is quite possible that, during periods when the mother's platelet count is normal, platelet antibody may still be present and cause thrombocytopenia in the newborn (Andre et al., 1965). In such cases, unless there is a definite history of maternal purpura, it is important to exclude the more likely possibility of an isoimmune type of thrombocytopenia resulting from active immunization of the mother by antigenically incompatible platelets of the fetus.

Clinical Manifestations.   Affected infants of mothers with ITP show maximal signs of bleeding at or shortly after delivery, because of the mechanical pressures of the birth process. In mild cases, however, there may be minimal, delayed, or no bleeding at all. Where there is no bleeding, slight depression of the platelet count may be the only evidence that the infant has been affected by the maternal disease. The commonest type of bleeding consists of petechiae and purpuric spots. These are usually generalized, and new lesions continue to occur. In contrast, the non-thrombocytopenic petechiae often seen in normal newborns are usually confined to the head and upper chest, do not recur, and are a consequence of a temporary increase in venous pressure during delivery. Bleeding from other sites may follow, such as epistaxis, melena, hematuria, and oozing from the umbilical cord or from needle punctures. Rarely, intracranial hemorrhage may develop, manifesting with episodes of twitching, apnea, cyanosis, and frequently terminating fatally. Aside from the aforementioned signs of bleeding, other physical findings are normal. The absence of hepatosplenomegaly in particular is important in excluding underlying disease that may cause thrombocytopenia, such as certain infections and congenital leukemia.

Jaundice, although usually absent, may occur in a newborn with thrombocytopenia from any cause. As an isolated finding in an infant with extensive purpura, jaundice may be explained by absorption of bilirubin from sites of enclosed hemorrhage, either in the subcutaneous tissue or internally (Rausen and Diamond, 1961). In this situation, it usually does not become prominent until after 24 hours of age. Early-appearing jaundice, on the other hand, in the presence of hepatosplenomegaly should alert the physician to the possibility of underlying infection or coincidental blood group incompatibility.

Laboratory Findings.   The platelet count is decreased, often as low as 5000 to 10,000/cu. mm. In mildly affected or asymptomatic infants, the platelet count may be only slightly lower than normal. The simplest means of demonstrating thrombocytopenia as the cause of bleeding or purpura is by careful inspection of a well prepared coverslip smear of heel-prick blood. When thrombocytopenia is the cause of the bleeding, the platelets are usually markedly reduced in number, sparse, and single. The presence of larger numbers of platelets, in particular clumps of platelets, excludes thrombocytopenia as a causative factor. All physicians caring for newborns should become adept at this simple technique as part of the effective diagnostic study of the bleeding newborn (see Chapter Eight).

Hemoglobin concentration is usually normal except where sufficient blood loss has occurred to result in anemia. In such a case, the blood smear may reveal signs of bone marrow stimulation, such as polychromasia and increased numbers of nucleated red blood cells; the reticulocyte count is accordingly elevated.

If enclosed hemorrhage should result in jaundice, the serum bilirubin is elevated; this involves the indirect fraction. In the case reported by Rausen and Diamond (1961) and one observed personally by us, jaundice was not evident until after the first 24 hours of life. This delayed onset, supported by a negative Coombs test and appropriate blood group studies, usually excludes coincidental blood group incompatibility as a factor in the jaundice.

Bone marrow examination, carefully performed to avoid clotting in the sample, usually reveals increased numbers of megakaryocytes with morphologic appearances of immaturity, as found in typical ITP in older children and adults. Decreased numbers of megakaryocytes have occasionally been observed (Hugh-Jones et al., 1960; Pearson et al., 1964).

Serologic tests for platelet antibodies in the passive form of neonatal thrombocytopenia are difficult to perform and equally difficult to interpret. Tests for platelet agglutinins are as frequently positive as they are negative in such cases. Similar criticism applies to the use of other techniques of demonstrating platelet antibodies, such as the antiglobulin consumption test and fluorescent antibody tests. The most sensitive of such tests, the complement-fixing antibody technique of Shulman et al., which is positive in about 50 per cent of patients with the isoimmune form of neonatal thrombocytopenia, has been consistently negative not only in patients with ITP but also in thrombocytopenic infants born of mothers with ITP (Shulman et al., 1964). Reasons postulated for this failure to detect antibody in this apparent immunologic situation are: the insensitivity of the method to the small amounts of antibody necessary to cause thrombocytopenia, and the possibility that such antibody may be of the incomplete or blocking variety, requiring for its demonstration a complement-fixing antibody of the same specificity that has yet to be identified (Shulman et al., 1964).

Treatment. Because this is a transient, usually mild and self-limited disorder, most cases do not require special treatment. The main justification for active therapeutic measures is to prevent or treat serious life-threatening hemorrhage, most commonly intracranial. Measures available in such a situation include exchange transfusion, transfusion of blood and platelet concentrates, corticosteroid administration, and splenectomy.

Exchange transfusion in an attempt to remove platelet antibody from the infant was attempted in two infants reported by Killander (1960) and Bridges and Carré (1961). In neither of these infants was the subsequent course of the platelet levels improved by the procedure, although in the first the purpuric manifestations subsided after the exchange transfusion. It seems that this procedure should be given further trial, but only in infants who exhibit severe bleeding or signs of impending intracranial hemorrhage. The use of *fresh* whole blood is recommended to take advantage of the additional number of viable platelets.

Transfusion of freshly prepared platelet concentrates are of definite value in treating the acutely bleeding thrombocytopenic infant. The usual precautions in obtaining and rapidly processing such concentrates apply. If the platelets cannot be used promptly, they may be stored (at room temperature, 20 to 22°C., rather than in the cold) for up to 24 hours. It has recently been suggested that such blood should be anticoagulated with a special ACD solution of pH 6.5, rather than the usual ACD solution of pH 6.8 to 7.0 or EDTA solution, to minimize clumping and thereby improve the recovery and yield of infused platelets (Aster and Jandl, 1964). The amount of platelet concentrate to be given to the average newborn should be that amount derived from two 500 cc. units of whole blood. If bleeding persists, the infusion should be repeated in six to eight hours. Should anemia develop, packed red cell transfusions may also be given.

There is no evidence as yet that corticosteroids appreciably influence the course of bleeding or thrombocytopenia in these infants. Until such evidence is available, steroid therapy does not seem to be indicated in the average infant manifesting only petechiae and thrombocytopenia (Anthony and Krivit, 1962).

Similarly, splenectomy has not been shown to be of definite value. Furthermore, in view of the self-limited nature of this disorder and the risk of fulminating infection after splenectomy in young infants, this procedure seems to be contraindicated.

In summary, the wisest course of management for most of these infants is one of watchful waiting and masterful restraint. For infants with severe bleeding or signs of intracranial hemorrhage, platelet transfusions are of help and exchange transfusion is worthy of trial.

Prognosis. Although earlier reviews (Robson and Walker, 1951; Epstein et al., 1950) state that mortalities among infants with the passive form of ITP may be as high as 30 per cent, more recent studies indicate much lower figures. Among 49 cases collected from the literature by Anthony and Krivit (1962), only five infants died. To these cases, Anthony and Krivit added 14 consecutive cases of their own with no serious morbidity and no mortalities. Three of the 11 affected infants reported by Schenkes (1968) died of their thrombocytopenia. The combined mortality from these 74 cases was approximately 10 per cent. With increasing availability of platelet transfusions, it is reasonable to expect lower mortality figures.

It is apparent that the large majority of infants suffer only mild bleeding in the form of cutaneous petechiae and purpura, and almost all recover without sequelae. The duration of thrombocytopenia varies from one week to four months. Although the thrombocytopenia may persist as long as four months, risk of active or recurrent bleeding seems to diminish greatly after the first few days of life.

NEONATAL THROMBOCYTOPENIA ASSOCIATED WITH DRUG-INDUCED THROMBOCYTOPENIA IN THE MOTHER

A variety of drugs cause thrombocytopenia in certain individuals. In most cases, thrombocytopenia occurs only in a minority of persons receiving the drug and is not dose-related, suggesting idiosyncrasy rather than toxic effect. The list of such drugs is long, but among the major offenders are sulfonamides, Sedormid, quinidine, and quinine. Quinine is of special importance with regard to the newborn because it has been used frequently in the past to induce labor.

The mechanism of thrombocytopenia induced in the mother by these drugs is generally felt to be an immune reaction in which antibody is formed against a drug-haptene complex. Such antibody attacks the mother's platelets and simultaneously crosses the placenta to destroy the infant's platelets. Early techniques used to demonstrate this antibody relied on the demonstration of platelet agglutination in a mixture of platelets, drug, and test serum. Mauer et al. (1956) reported a case of quinine-induced thrombocytopenia in a mother and infant, in both of whom platelet agglutinins were demonstrated. Although the thrombocytopenia disappeared after a few days, the antibody persisted for several months. Shulman (1958), using a complement-fixing technique, confirmed the presence of platelet antibodies in patients with quinidine-induced thrombocytopenia.

Neonatal thrombocytopenia associated with administration of thiazide diuretics to the mother is distinguished from the immune variety just described by the finding of normal platelet counts in the mother and negative tests for antibody. This is discussed on page 296.

NEONATAL THROMBOCYTOPENIA ASSOCIATED WITH SYSTEMIC LUPUS ERYTHEMATOSUS IN THE MOTHER

Although placental transmission of lupus erythematosus (L.E.) factor has been frequently documented, most infants born of mothers with systemic lupus erythematosus (S.L.E.) do not show clinical evidence of disease.

Two infants with transient thrombocytopenia have been reported. In the case described by Nathan and Snapper (1958), the mother showed signs of active S.L.E. at 34 weeks of gestation when she delivered a three pound, three ounce infant. The child showed no petechiae or other signs of illness. The L.E. phenomenon was demonstrable, lasting one week. Blood counts at 24 hours of age revealed a hemoglobin of 14.5 gm./100 ml., a white cell count of 8400/cu. mm., and a platelet count of 30,000/cu. mm. Platelet agglutinins were demonstrated in both mother and infant. The infant remained well, and the platelet count rose to normal by three weeks of age. Seip (1960) described an infant who appeared pale at birth but was not studied hematologically until two months of age, when his general health had deteriorated. At this time, pancytopenia was revealed by the following: hemoglobin, 3.3 gm./100 ml.; white-cell count, 1800/cu. mm.; and platelet count, 114,000/cu. mm. A reticulocyte count of 22.8 per cent indicated hemolysis as the basis for the anemia. Because of persistent anemia in spite of repeated blood transfusions, the infant was treated with prednisone and within two weeks the blood picture had become normal.

The true incidence of thrombocytopenia (and other cytopenias) in infants born of mothers with S.L.E. may prove to be higher than is evident from the reported cases if routine blood counts are done on such infants at birth. In the presence of symptoms, steroid therapy appears to be of value.

ISOIMMUNE NEONATAL THROMBOCYTOPENIA PURPURA

In a minority of cases of neonatal thrombocytopenia, the mother's platelet count is normal and there is no history of maternal bleeding or drug ingestion. Such cases led to the hypothesis of an immune etiologic mechanism involving incompatibility of fetal and maternal platelet antigens, analogous to that for red cell antigens in erythroblastosis fetalis. Passage of platelets (and leukocytes) from fetus to mother has been demonstrated by Desai et al. (1966). The subsequent search for platelet antibodies seemed rewarded by the demonstration of agglutinins in maternal sera against the platelets of the affected infants (Harrington et al., 1953; Schulman et al., 1954). In cases studied since that time, platelet agglutinins have not always been demonstrable. Work by Shulman et al. (1962) indicates that the aforementioned failures were probably due to the technical problems and the inherent insensitivity of the methods employed. Using a complement-fixing technique, these workers have demonstrated antibodies in a large number of cases of so-called isoimmune neonatal thrombocytopenic purpura, most of which yielded negative results from platelet agglutination tests. With the use of antisera from these mothers, Shulman and associates have typed the platelets of a large number of people and have thereby defined several different platelet antigen systems. Furthermore, certain of these platelet antisera have also been shown to react with antigens on granulocytes and lymphocytes. Such complement-fixing platelet isoantibodies have also been detected in the sera of persons receiving multiple blood transfusions.

It has been estimated that isoimmune neonatal thrombocytopenic purpura occurs about once or twice per 10,000 births (Shulman et al., 1964). The clinical and hematologic features of this disorder are the subject of an excellent review by Pearson et al. (1964). This condition has also been documented in newborn piglets (Stormorken et al., 1963).

Clinical Manifestations

As in neonatal purpura associated with maternal ITP, there is wide variation in the severity of this disease, from infants presenting only with mild petechiae to those manifesting extensive and severe hemorrhages. In general, however, bleeding manifestations appear to be more severe in the isoimmune type of purpura. Fatalities, usually due to intracranial hemorrhage, have occurred in about 14 per cent of reported cases.

First-born infants are frequently affected. In the series studied by Shulman et al. (1964), 40 to 50 per cent of the infants with isoimmune purpura were born of primiparas in whom no previous sensitizing stimuli, such as blood transfusions, had been received. Platelet isoimmunization therefore differs strikingly from erythrocyte isoimmunization due to Rh incompatibility, in which it is unusual for firstborn infants to be affected.

A generalized petechial rash is usually evident within minutes of delivery to a few hours later. Purpura and ecchymoses often follow, with large cephalhematomas occurring not infrequently. The early onset and the frequent concentration of bruising over the presenting part reflect the importance of the mechanical pressure of the birth process in the genesis of ensuing hemorrhage. In occasional severe cases, bleeding may be more widespread, resulting in hematemesis, melena, hematuria, and oozing from the umbilical cord or skin punctures. Twitching, apnea, or cyanosis should alert the physician to the possibility of an intracranial hemorrhage.

Jaundice is common, occurring in seven of the nine infants reported by Pearson et al. (1964) and in 12 of 55 cases they reviewed from the literature. Jaundice usually appeared by 24 to 48 hours of age and resulted in peak serum bilirubin levels of 15 to 20 mg./100 ml. within the next few days. Blood group incompatibility and sepsis were excluded as causes of the jaundice. They attributed the jaundice to absorption of bilirubin from sites of enclosed occult hemorrhage, as suggested earlier by Rausen and Diamond (1961). Supporting the presence of occult hemorrhage is their finding, in the icteric infants, of compensatory erythroid hyperactivity in the bone marrow, reticulocytosis, and increased numbers of nucleated red cells in the peripheral blood.

The liver and spleen are not enlarged. This is an important nega-

tive finding, differentiating this condition from others causing neonatal thrombocytopenia, such as severe erythroblastosis, infections,
and congenital leukemia.

Laboratory Findings

Hematologic. The platelet count at birth is decreased, usually
below 30,000/cu. mm. and occasionally as low as 1000/cu. mm. This
degree of thrombocytopenia is obvious on inspection of a well prepared cover slip smear of blood. In two of the infants reported by
Pearson (1964), the thrombocytopenia was documented in cord blood,
indicating the existence of platelet destruction in utero.

Anemia was uncommon in the reported cases, but it may develop
if sufficient hemorrhage has occurred. At times this may not be reflected by obvious external blood loss, suggesting instead significant
occult hemorrhage, either within the skin or internally. Reticulocytosis and increased numbers of nucleated red blood cells reflect this
and should alert one to the possibility that jaundice may develop.
The white cell count is normal despite the fact that many of the platelet antisera cross-react with leukocyte antigens (see below).

Bone marrow examination reveals, in addition to erythroid hyperplasia, two general patterns of megakaryocyte activity. In Pearson's
cases, (1964), normal or increased numbers of megakaryocytes were
seen in six infants, and no megakaryocytes were seen in two infants.
There was no correlation with the severity of the thrombocytopenia.
Shulman (1964) suggested that the decrease in megakaryocytes may
be the result of their possession of antigenic sites similar to those on
the platelets, rendering them equally susceptible to attack by the
isoantibody.

The serum (indirect) bilirubin may be elevated. In one of Pearson's cases, the serum bilirubin rose to 24.2 mg./100 ml. on the fourth
day of life, necessitating exchange transfusion.

Serologic. By the complement-fixation method—at present the
most reliable and sensitive technique for demonstrating platelet
isoantibodies (Shulman et al., 1964)—a variety of different platelet
antisera have been discovered, characterized, and used to define
a number of platelet antigen systems. These antisera have been found
not only among mothers sensitized during pregnancy, but also among
persons sensitized by drugs such as quinidine and by blood transfusions containing incompatible platelets. Other methods that have
been successful in detecting platelet antibodies (although to a lesser
degree) include platelet agglutination, antiglobulin consumption,
the mixed antiglobulin reaction, inhibition of clot retraction, fluorescent antibody techniques, and the tanned erythrocyte hemagglutination test. The limitations of these methods are discussed in greater

detail in the review by Shulman et al. (1964). Subsequent experience by these workers with the complement-fixation technique indicated that certain antibodies do not fix complement but interfere with or block the activity of complement-fixing antibodies having the same specificity. Such antibodies are analogous to the incomplete blocking antibodies in the Rh system of erythrocytes. Shulman and associates further postulate that the negative serologic findings in some cases of neonatal purpura may be due to the presence of blocking antibodies whose corresponding complement-fixing antibodies have not yet been found. All of the platelet isoantibodies studied by Shulman et al. were IgG gammaglobulins.

Platelet isoimmunization by pregnancy is not a rare occurrence. Klemperer and co-workers (1966), using the complement-fixation screening test of Aster, obtained positive results in 1.65 per cent of 6592 sera from pregnant women. Since this method detects only complete antibodies, the true incidence of platelet isoantibodies in pregnancy must be even higher. The previous low estimates of affected infants (one to two per 10,000 births) may be increased by the determination of platelet counts in newborn infants of such sensitized mothers.

Nomenclature for the newly discovered platelet isoantibodies and antigens varies among different laboratories. That proposed by Shulman appears to be the simplest and most widely accepted. In this system, the abbreviation Pl refers to platelet antigen. Each of the antigenic systems on the platelets is designated by a superscript capitalized letter of the alphabet, in order of discovery beginning with A. Within each of the alphabetically designated systems alleles are indicated by a number beside the letter. Thus, Pl^{A1} and Pl^{A2} refer to the two alleles of the A antigen system on platelets, and anti-Pl^{A1} and anti-Pl^{A2} refer to the corresponding isoantibodies. (This antigen system was first discovered in 1959 by van Loghem and co-workers, who named it Zw^a and Zw^b.)

When antisera to Pl^{B1} and Pl^{C1} were discovered, it was found that they cross-reacted with antigens on granulocytes and lymphocytes. The nomenclature was then extended for these to indicate this broader reactivity. Thus we have $PlGrLy^{B1}$ and $PlGrLy^{C1.}$ Thrombocytopenic infants in whom these antibodies were found did not manifest leukopenia, suggesting perhaps a larger leukocyte reserve to compensate for some degree of destruction.

Family studies indicate that these platelet antigens are inherited as autosomal dominant characters. In Table 9–2 are listed the frequency of positive reactors to three of the commoner platelet antisera, from the data of Shulman et al., (1964).

From the sera of 72 mothers whose infants had neonatal purpura, isoantibodies were detected in 37 (Shulman et al., 1964); four were of

Table 9–2   Platelet Antigen Systems[*]

| ANTIGEN | SOURCE OF ANTIBODY | | POSITIVE REACTORS | |
	Posttransfusion	Maternal	No. Tested	% Positive
Pl^{A1} (Zw^a)	4	17	452	97
Pl^{A2} (Zw^b)	1	–	435	26
PlGrLy^{B1}	5	8	888	46
PlGrLy^{C1}	1	2	252	30

[*]From Shulman, N. R., et al.: Progr. Hematol., 4:222, 1964.

the agglutinating type, 12 were complement-fixing, and 21 were blocking in type. The antigenic specificity of the last two types is indicated in Table 9–3 (agglutinating antibodies are not sufficiently strong to give clear-cut results in establishing antigen types). Although incompatibility of Pl^{A1} occurs in less than 3 per cent of pregnancies, anti-Pl^{A1} accounted for 46 per cent of detected antibodies and 29 per cent of the 72 suspected cases of isoimmune neonatal purpura. It is evident therefore that Pl^{A1} is a relatively potent antigen. Because anti-Pl^{A1} is an incomplete antibody that would not react in the usual complement-fixation system, a diagnosis of isoimmunization can best be made by showing that the mother's platelets do not react with a known anti-Pl^{A1} antiserum. Since Pl^{A1}-negativity occurs in only 3 per cent of the normal population, its occurrence in the mother of a thrombocytopenic infant may be considered evidence for an isoimmune etiology. As in erythrocyte isoimmunization, the platelets of the father should contain the antigen lacking in those of the mother. The less common types of platelet antibody are complete and therefore will be detected in the usual complement-fixation system (Table 9–3).

At this point, the situation with regard to platelet serology is comparable to that of erythrocyte serology in the Rh-sensitized women. An antibody has been detected in the mother's serum and used to demonstrate the presence of the corresponding antigen on the platelets of the infant and the father, and the lack of this antigen on the platelets of the mother. Because most of the positive-reacting fathers are heterozygous, not all infants of incompatible pregnancies would be expected to develop thrombocytopenia. The question arises whether information about the maternal titer of this antibody could be used to predict the occurrence of neonatal purpura in subsequent pregnancies. Shulman et al. (1964) studied eight mothers whose previous infants had isoimmune neonatal purpura and observed the following: four mothers did not develop antibodies during subsequent

Table 9-3   Antigenic Specificity of Maternal Isoantibodies[*]

Specificity	C¹-fixing Antibodies	Blocking Antibodies
Pl^{A1}	0	17
PlGrLy^{B1}	5	3
PlGrLy^{C1}	1	1
Pl^{E2}	1	0
Not established	5	–
Total	12	21

[*]From Shulman, N. R., et al.: Progr. Hematol., 4:222, 1964.

pregnancies and their infants were unaffected; four mothers did develop antibodies again—three of the infants were affected, and one was normal (even though his platelets were incompatible with those of his mother). The facts of the latter case, and the observation that maternal isoantibodies may occasionally persist at high titers for many years, suggest that the finding of a platelet isoantibody in a multiparous woman does not necessarily indicate the infant of this particular pregnancy will be affected. Nevertheless, as discussed under *Treatment*, it is still wise to anticipate and prepare for treating such infants.

In summary, isoimmune neonatal thrombocytopenic purpura should be suspected in purpuric (but otherwise normal) infants of mothers with normal platelet counts, and it can be confirmed by the demonstration in maternal serum of antibody that reacts with the platelets of the infant or the father but not with those of the mother.

Treatment

Isoimmune purpura in the majority of infants follows a mild course, and the infants usually recover without sequelae. However, the ever-present risk of intracranial hemorrhage and the significant mortality rate of 12 to 14 per cent indicate the need to seriously consider active therapeutic measures in certain cases. Those measures that have been tried include corticosteroid administration, platelet transfusions, and exchange transfusions.

At present, there has not been sufficient experience accumulated with these various forms of therapy to critically evaluate their relative effectiveness. This problem has been compounded by the variation in clinical severity not only among the different antigen-antibody systems, but also in cases caused by the same antibody. Pearson et al.

(1964) attempted to circumvent these problems by comparing the results of different modes of therapy in successive pregnancies of the same sensitized mother. From their observations in three such families, they recommend "that steroid therapy to the infant is better than no therapy; that antepartum steroids to the mother may be better than treatment of the infant alone, and that exchange transfusion should be used in severely affected infants in order to rapidly correct thrombocytopenia." The clinical course and platelet counts of three infants in one of these families are shown in Figure 9–3. In the last case in this family, the mother was given prednisone 60 mg./day for two days prior to induction of labor at 38 weeks of gestation. The rationale for antepartum steroid therapy is to offer the potential beneficial effect of steroids during the stressful descent through the birth canal. If prednisone is given to the infant, 10 mg. orally per day in divided doses should suffice.

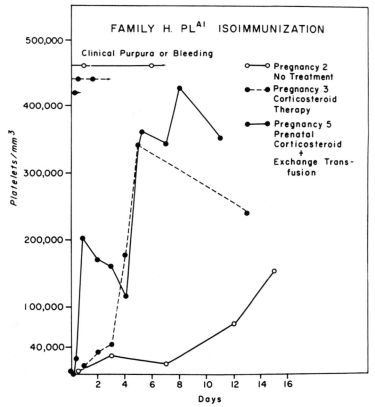

Figure 9–3 Comparison of results of three modes of therapy in successive infants with isoimmune neonatal thrombocytopenic purpura. (From Pearson, H. A., et al.: *Blood,* 23:154, 1964.)

Shulman et al. (1964) considered the following findings as indications for exchange transfusion: thrombocytopenia with a count below 30,000/cu. mm. at birth and below 10,000/cu. mm. several hours thereafter, high reticulocytosis and normoblastemia, amegakaryocytosis, early jaundice, melena or hematuria, extensive petechiae, ecchymoses, and hematomas.

The ideal transfusion regimen might be arrived at from consideration of the situation in erythroblastosis fetalis. Here one utilizes exchange transfusion with blood of a donor whose red cells lack the antigen against which antibodies have formed. This procedure not only removes antibody but also replaces sensitized red cells with cells that will survive for a normal time in the infant's circulation. In the infant with isoimmune thrombocytopenia, however, selection of compatible donor blood is difficult because the antibody is usually not known at the time of birth, and in the common type due to anti-Pl^{A1}, Pl-^{A1}-negative donors are relatively rare. Adner et al. (1969), based on their experience with an infant who received platelets from various sources, recommend a reasonable and practical compromise: exchange transfusion with fresh blood from any normal donor followed by infusion of *maternal* platelets washed with normal plasma (to remove isoantibody). In a family in which the antibody has already been identified in a previous pregnancy, one might attempt to select a compatible donor to be available at the time of delivery as a source of blood for the exchange transfusion also.

Jaundice may develop in the first few days after birth, necessitating close observation of serum bilirubin levels, with a view to the possible need for exchange transfusion to prevent kernicterus.

Prognosis

In untreated cases, there is an immediate mortality (usually from intracranial hemorrhage) of 12 to 14 per cent. Among surviving infants, the platelet count usually rises to a level above 60,000/cu. mm. by two to three weeks of age. At this platelet level, spontaneous bleeding rarely occurs. This contrasts with the passive form of neonatal thrombocytopenia associated with maternal ITP, in which platelet counts below 50,000/cu. mm. may persist for several months.

THROMBOCYTOPENIA ASSOCIATED WITH ERYTHROBLASTOSIS FETALIS OR EXCHANGE TRANSFUSION

It is not uncommon for infants born with severe Rh erythroblastosis fetalis to develop petechiae and purpura in the first few hours after birth. Most of these infants have signs of hydrops fetalis: pallor, edema, and marked hepatosplenomegaly. The occurrence of thrombocytopenia in the more severely affected infants, and a correlation with cord serum bilirubin levels (Ekert and Mathew, 1967), suggests bilirubin toxicity as a possible mechanism. Experimental evidence to support this has come from the work of Suvansri et al. (1969), who were able to induce changes in platelet morphology and function by adding solutions of bilirubin to suspensions of newborn platelets. An alternate possibility, that the thrombocytopenia may be a result of disseminated intravascular coagulation (triggered by hemolysis), was first pursued by Ekert and Mathew (1969). Unable to find a correlation between platelet counts and cord fibrinogen levels, they concluded that this mechanism was an unlikely one. A more recent study, which included a greater proportion of infants with bleeding complications and a more detailed evaluation of coagulation, led to the opposite conclusion (Chessells and Wigglesworth, 1971). An isoimmune pathogenesis remains a further possibility, for which convincing proof is lacking at present. The thrombocytopenic purpura associated with erythroblastosis fetalis is usually corrected by immediate exchange transfusion.

Another form of thrombocytopenia may occur *following* exchange transfusion and is not dependent on the severity of hemolytic disease. This occurs a few days after the procedure and is usually asymptomatic and self-limited. Although it has generally been attributed to the paucity of platelets in the stored infused blood, DeBruijne et al. (1956) found this form of thrombocytopenia even when fresh heparinized blood less than two hours old was used. They generally used two units of blood in their exchanges rather than the customary one unit, and in those cases in which one unit was used they did not observe this thrombocytopenia. They attributed the thrombocytopenia to the fact that the transfused platelets, although fresh, probably survived a shorter time than normal, so that at the end of their life span there was a short period before the infant's platelet production could compensate. Consequently, transitory thrombocytopenia resulted.

THROMBOCYTOPENIA ASSOCIATED WITH INFECTION

Thrombocytopenia, often sufficient to cause purpura and severe bleeding, frequently accompanies infections in the newborn period. Although thrombocytopenia may occur with almost any form of sepsis, it is particularly common in certain specific infections, such as cytomegalic inclusion disease, disseminated herpes simplex infection, congenital toxoplasmosis, and congenital syphilis. These are discussed in greater detail in Chapter Two.

Clinical Manifestations.   In common to most of these infections is the appearance of a sick infant with jaundice, pallor, purpura, and hepatosplenomegaly. In most cases, purpura is present at or within a few days following birth. Neurologic symptoms, such as listlessness and twitching, often accompany the microcephaly of cytomegalic inclusion disease or toxoplasmosis (hydrocephalus may also occur in the latter). In congenital syphilis, the classic signs of snuffles, rhagades, mucocutaneous lesions, and pseudoparalysis are frequently absent (Whitaker et al., 1965).

Laboratory Findings. In addition to thrombocytopenia, there is often a moderately severe hemolytic anemia evidenced by falling hemoglobin, reticulocytosis, and increased numbers of nucleated red blood cells on peripheral blood smear. The appearance of the mega-karyocytes in the bone marrow has not been well documented in most reported cases. In congenital syphilis, megakaryocytes have been reported as both increased (Whitaker et al., 1965) and decreased (Freiman and Super, 1966). In infants with cytomegalic inclusion disease in whom the bone marrow appearance was described, mega-karyocytes were virtually absent. Similar findings have been reported in the congenital rubella syndrome; the possibility that such observations represent technical artifacts was suggested by Zinkham's demonstration (1967) of normal megakaryocytes in post-mortem sections of bone marrow (see p. 301).

The specific infectious etiology may be confirmed as follows:

1. *Bacterial sepsis* — culture of organisms from blood, cerebro-spinal fluid or other sites.

2. *Congenital syphilis* — positive serology in both mother and infant, and characteristic bone changes on x-ray examination.

3. *Viral infections*

    a. *Cytomegalic inclusion disease* — demonstration of typical intranuclear inclusion-bearing cells in urinary sediment or gastric washings, isolation of virus from urine (or tissues at autopsy), presence of macroglobulin complement-fixing antibody in serum.

    b. *Disseminated herpes simplex infection* — this is usually fatal, and at autopsy intravascular and intracytoplasmic inclusions may be found in various tissues.

    c. *Congenital rubella syndrome* — isolation of rubella virus from throat washings and urine.

4. *Toxoplasmosis* — positive dye test persisting at least four months.

An additional clue to the presence of intrauterine infection is the presence of increased levels of IgM in cord serum. Because thrombocytopenia in many of the above infectious disorders may be due to disseminated intravascular coagulation, appropriate coagulation studies (see Chapter Eight, p. 259) may assist in diagnosis and management.

Pathogenesis.   The finding of decreased megakaryocytes in bone marrow aspirates from infants with these infections suggests impaired platelet production. However, the finding of normal megakaryocytes by some workers and the demonstration of coagulation defects and microthrombi in post-mortem tissues (Shershow et al., 1969; Hathaway et al., 1969, Miller et al., 1970) indicate that the thrombocytopenia may in some cases be a consequence of disseminated intravascular coagulation (see p. 257). In our experience, this is seen most frequently among newborns with sepsis due to gram-negative bacteria, such as *E. coli.*

Prognosis.   These infections are serious and often terminate fatally in the newborn. In infants who survive, particularly those with toxoplasmosis and cytomegalic inclusion disease, purpura and thrombocytopenia gradually disappear although this may take many months. In infants with congenital syphilis treated with penicillin, the thrombocytopenia usually disappears within two to three weeks as the child's general condition improves (Whitaker, 1965). Thrombocytopenia in infants with the congenital rubella syndrome usually abates by one or two months of life (see p. 301).

Treatment.   Bleeding due to thrombocytopenia in infants with these infections is generally not of sufficient severity to require specific therapy other than that for the infection. Corticosteroids have not been effective in any of these disorders. Specific antimicrobial agents should be used if available. Anemia may require blood transfusion.

THROMBOCYTOPENIA ASSOCIATED WITH ANTEPARTUM ADMINISTRATION OF DRUGS

Thiazides

This type of drug-induced neonatal thrombocytopenia differs from the immune type discussed earlier in two important respects: the maternal platelet count is normal, and platelet antibodies are absent.

Rodriguez et al. (1964) described seven thrombocytopenic newborns of mothers who had received one of the thiazides (chlorothiazide, hydrochlorothiazide, or methyclothiazide) for preeclamptic edema. In most of the cases, the drug was given for prolonged periods, up to three months, but the severity of the thrombocytopenic purpura did not correlate with the duration of therapy. Although thrombocytopenia and neutropenia have been reported previously in persons receiving these drugs, this is the first report in which the brunt of the hematologic toxicity was born by the infant while the mother remained normal.

Purpura in these infants was present at or soon after birth. It was associated with gastrointestinal and intraperitoneal bleeding in some of them. One infant died at 40 hours of age with subdural and pulmonary hemorrhages. The remainder eventually recovered, although the thrombocytopenia persisted for periods from two to 12 weeks. Platelet counts varied from 4000 to 28,000/cu. mm. Leukopenia was present in three of the seven infants. Bone marrow aspirates revealed decreased numbers of megakaryocytes in four of five infants in which this was carried out.

Corticosteroids were used in six of the seven infants with no convincing evidence of benefit.

In a recent prospective study of 84 newborn infants, there was no significant difference in the platelet counts between the infants of 37 mothers receiving thiazides and those of the remainder not receiving such drugs (Merenstein et al., 1970). This study confirms the general impression of the rarity of the above complication and suggests further that it may be due to a peculiar susceptibility of some newborn infants. The occurrence of neonatal thrombocytopenia in successive pregnancies of one mother in the report of Rodriguez et al. may support the existence of a genetic mechanism for this susceptibility.

Tolbutamide

Schiff et al. (1970) described transient thrombocytopenia in a newborn of a diabetic mother who was receiving tolbutamide. The platelet count was 26,000/cu. mm. at birth and rose to 122,000/cu. mm. by 11 days of age. The finding of elevated serum tolbutamide levels in the infant (compared to the mother) suggested marrow depression as the likely mechanism of the thrombocytopenia. Erythrocytes and leukocytes were not affected. Minor malformations of the ear and thumb were also present.

Observations such as this point to the need for a more systematic examination of the blood of newborn infants of mothers receiving drugs during pregnancy.

THROMBOCYTOPENIA DUE TO MEGAKARYOCYTIC HYPOPLASIA

As indicated in Table 9–1, a variety of syndromes are included here. They share in common a primary impairment of platelet production as the major pathogenetic mechanism of the thrombocytopenia. Bone marrow examination usually reveals decreased numbers of megakaryocytes. In some cases, however, they may appear normal in number but show decreased cytoplasmic budding, suggesting impaired release of platelets. Decreased numbers of megakaryocytes may also be seen in some of the other conditions associated with neonatal thrombocytopenia (for example, some cases of isoimmune purpura and certain infections). However, in these the megakaryocytic hypoplasia is a consequence of the primary disorder, be it immune, infectious, or other.

The conditions included in the present category may be divided into two groups, depending on whether the megakaryocytic hypoplasia occurs as an isolated phenomenon in an otherwise well child or in association with a syndrome of congenital anomalies.

Isolated Congenital Hypoplastic Thrombocytopenia

In the light of our present knowledge of causes of megakaryocytic hypoplasia in the newborn, it is now possible to reevaluate many of the cases previously reported as congenital hypoplastic thrombocytopenia and perhaps exclude some of them. The two conditions most important in this regard are the rubella syndrome and isoimmune neonatal purpura. The infant reported by Korn (1962) and the infant of Case One in the report by Hugh-Jones et al. (1960) were both born of mothers who had rubella in the first trimester of pregnancy, with the typical constellation of congenital anomalies appearing in the second infant. The rapid return to normal platelet levels in an otherwise healthy newborn of a hematologically normal mother suggests an isoimmune etiology, as in the remaining three infants of Hugh-Jones et al. (1960). True congenital hypoplastic thrombocytopenia by definition does not remit.

In most of the remaining reports of congenital hypoplastic or amegakaryocytic thrombocytopenia, the infants possessed other major congenital anomalies, the commonest of which was bilateral absence of the radii. Because this association has other characteristic hematologic features, it is discussed separately.

Congenital Hypoplastic (Amegakaryocytic) Thrombocytopenia with Associated Congenital Anomalies

This category includes thrombocytopenia occurring with bilateral absence of the radii, the rubella syndrome, and pancytopenia and multiple congenital anomalies (Fanconi's anemia).

The coincidence of megakaryocyte defect and either absent radii, congenital cardiac defect, or the other anomalies described suggest that the causative agent is an environmental factor acting at approximately six to eight weeks of gestation, the period of critical embryogenesis for these particular organs. Only in the case of the rubella virus is the nature of this causative agent known. The occurrence of more than one case in the family of some of the infants with the absent radii syndrome and Fanconi's anemia suggests the possibility of genetic factors. The recent finding by Bloom et al. (1966) of chromosome aberrations in several cases of Fanconi's anemia might further support this.

Congenital Amegakaryocytic Thrombocytopenia Associated with Bilateral Absence of the Radii. A number of cases of this syndrome have been described (Bell et al., 1956; Emery et al., 1957; Rubin, 1957; Shaw and Oliver, 1959; Nilsson and Lundholm, 1960). The subject has been well reviewed by Hall and coworkers (1969).

CLINICAL MANIFESTATIONS. Purpura is usually evident within the first few days of life, although in occasional cases the onset may be delayed for several weeks. Bilateral absence of the radii manifests as shortening of the forearms, flexion at the elbows, and radial deviation of the wrist. Occasionally, other congenital anomalies are present, such as deformities of the digits, micrognathia, dislocation of the hip, and cardiac defects. Multiple cases in a sibship have been described in a number of the reported families, suggesting an autosomal recessive inheritance; however, in none of these families was there a history of consanguinity.

LABORATORY FINDINGS. During the bleeding phase shortly after birth, platelet counts are usually in the range of 10,000 to 30,000/cu. mm. A frequent finding is an associated leukemoid blood picture, total white cell counts rising as high as 140,000/cu. mm. A marked shift to the left is seen with occasional blasts in the peripheral blood smear, often suggesting a diagnosis of congenital leukemia. Anemia may develop as a result of continued blood loss.

Bone marrow examination reveals myeloid hyperplasia and almost total absence of megakaryocytes.

Absence of the radii is evident on x-ray examination of the upper limbs. In a variant of this syndrome (Dignan et al., 1967; Hall et al., 1969), the limb deficiency included the ulna and humerus, resulting in complete (usually bilateral) phocomelia. Of interest in this regard is the absence of hematologic abnormalities in children with phocomelia resulting from maternal administration of thalidomide.

TREATMENT. Therapeutic measures in this congenital disorder are mainly supportive and include transfusion of red cells for anemia and transfusion of platelet concentrates for severe bleeding due to thrombocytopenia.

Corticosteroids and splenectomy have been tried, but without consistent benefit.

PROGNOSIS. Bleeding is usually severe, persisting for several months and often terminating in fatal intracranial hemorrhage. In some cases, gradual improvement takes place toward the end of the first year of life, and a few of these children have lived to adulthood.

Congenital Hypoplastic Thrombocytopenia with Microcephaly. Three infants have been reported with this combination (Eisenstein, 1966; Hoyeraal, 1970). The subjects of the more recent report were two brothers. The absence of other stigmata and the persistence of thrombocytopenia well past the first year of life argued against the rubella syndrome or cytomegalovirus infection as a basis for this association.

Thrombocytopenia in the Rubella Syndrome. Although cases of congenital thrombocytopenia have been described in infants whose mothers had rubella in the first trimester of pregnancy (Hugh-Jones et al., 1960; Korn, 1962), only recently has a causal relationship between the two been considered (Berge et al., 1963). In 1964, an epidemic of rubella in the United States resulted in the birth of a large number of infants with the stigmata of the intrauterine rubella infection. With accumulation of observations from several centers, the classic syndrome of congenital cardiac defects, cataracts, and deafness has been expanded to include thrombocytopenic purpura, pneumonitis, jaundice (with giant cell hepatitis), hepatosplenomegaly, and bone lesions.

INCIDENCE OF THROMBOCYTOPENIC PURPURA. In four large series, thrombocytopenia or purpura was documented in 43 to 80 per cent of newborns with the rubella syndrome. (Rudolph et al., 1965; Cooper et al., 1965; Korones et al., 1965; Plotkin et al., 1965). Since thrombocytopenia in this condition tends to abate in the weeks following birth, the lower incidence in some series may reflect a larger proportion of older infants (Zinkham et al., 1967).

CLINICAL MANIFESTATIONS. In addition to the aforementioned congenital defects, petechiae and purpura are usually present. Occasionally, the infant is asymptomatic, the thrombocytopenia being discovered only by routine platelet count in the course of study of this condition. The purpura usually appears at birth or within the first day or two of life and is not associated with severe bleeding from other sites. In most infants, the purpuric lesions fade gradually over the first week or two and do not recur. Rarely, the thrombocytopenia persists for several months.

Hepatosplenomegaly is common and of value in the clinical distinction between purpura associated with rubella or other infections and purpura due to platelet isoimmunization or maternal ITP.

In a few reports, thrombocytopenic purpura was the only finding at birth. The classical congenital anomalies were either absent (Bayer et al., 1965) or not apparent until several weeks after birth (Banatvala et al., 1965).

LABORATORY FINDINGS. Platelet counts in the purpuric infant

were usually low, ranging from 10,000 to 50,000/cu. mm. Anemia with increased reticulocytes and nucleated red blood cells has been observed and suggests a marrow response to either widespread purpura or an associated hemolytic process. The latter mechanism is supported by observations of abnormal red cell morphology (burr cells, fragmented cells, spherocytes) in the infants studied by Rausen et al. (1967) and Zinkham et al. (1967). An unusual instance of transient hypoplastic anemia developing in the first month of life was described by Lafer and Morrison (1966). White blood cell counts are usually normal, although mild leukopenia was noted in five of the 21 infants studied by Zinkham (1967).

Bone marrow examinations have generally been reported as revealing decreased numbers of megakaryocytes. Zinkham's observation of normal megakaryocytes in four post-mortem bone marrow sections suggested that the apparent reductions may be attributable to technical difficulties involved in obtaining adequate marrow samples from young infants. An impressive finding in the bone marrow of some infants studied by Zinkham was the presence of increased numbers of phagocytic histiocytes.

PATHOGENESIS. As discussed in Chapter 8 (p. 257), recent evidence suggests that the thrombocytopenia of congenital rubella syndrome (and other intrauterine infections) may be a reflection of disseminated intravascular coagulation. Such a mechanism would also explain the burr-cell hemolytic anemia described above.

TREATMENT. Because purpura in this condition is usually mild and short-lived, active treatment is usually not necessary. If severe bleeding or jaundice should develop, transfusion of blood or platelets and exchange transfusion can be performed.

PROGNOSIS. The purpura generally disappears the first week or so after birth, and platelet counts are usually normal by one or two months of age. However, in one of the infants followed by Zinkham, the thrombocytopenia persisted for six months. Late onset of thrombocytopenia at nine months of age was described in an infant followed from birth by Reiss and Pryles (1966). Recovery ensued over six weeks, followed by a brief recurrence at the age of 11 months. Deaths from hemorrhage are rare in the congenital rubella syndrome; one such case was reported by Korn (1962).

Thrombocytopenia as Part of the Syndrome of Pancytopenia with Multiple Congenital Anomalies (Fanconi's Anemia). This condition differs from the thrombocytopenia discussed in which bilateral absence of the radii is the major accompanying congenital defect. In Fanconi's anemia, all three elements of the blood are depressed and the pattern of congenital anomalies is broader, including shortness of stature, abnormal skin pigmentation, deformities of the thumbs, microcephaly, and renal anomalies.

In most of the reported cases of Fanconi's anemia, symptoms did not appear until after the first year of life.

Amegakaryocytic Thrombocytopenia with Pancytopenia but No Congenital Anomalies.   O'Gorman-Hughes and Diamond (1964) described four children, all males, who presented with amegakaryocytic thrombocytopenia in the neonatal period and later went on to develop full-blown pancytopenia. This nonfamilial form of constitutional aplastic anemia differs from the familial type first described by Estren and Dameshek (1947).

Long-term therapy with corticosteroids and testosterone resulted in improvement in two of these children.

Thrombocytopenia Associated with Trisomy Syndromes.   Mehes and Bata (1965) reported a child with D_1 (13) trisomy and congenital thrombocytopenia. Three infants with E (18) trisomy and hypoplastic thrombocytopenia have also been reported (Christodoulou and Werner, 1967; Rabinowitz et al., 1967). Absence or hypoplasia of the radii and thumbs was observed in the two infants reported by Rabinowitz.

DISEASES AFFECTING THE BONE MARROW— CONGENITAL LEUKEMIA

Because this subject is discussed in greater detail in Chapter Nine, it is mentioned here only insofar as it must be considered in the differential diagnosis when a purpuric newborn appears ill and shows hepatosplenomegaly and hyperleukocytosis (as high as 370,000/cu. mm.). Diagnosis is usually evident because of the large number of blasts on peripheral blood smear, and it is confirmed by bone marrow examination.

THROMBOCYTOPENIA ASSOCIATED WITH DISSEMINATED INTRAVASCULAR COAGULATION

A number of conditions affecting the newborn may trigger a state of disseminated intravascular coagulation, in which platelets along with certain other coagulation factors are depleted during the clotting process. These conditions are listed in Table 9–1 and are discussed in greater detail in Chapter Eight (p. 258). The syndrome of giant hemangioma and thrombocytopenia probably represents a form of localized but extensive intravascular coagulation. Since it is best known through the associated thrombocytopenia, it will be discussed in greater detail in this chapter.

THROMBOCYTOPENIA ASSOCIATED WITH GIANT HEMANGIOMA

Since this syndrome was first described by Kasabach and Merritt in 1940, there have been over 50 cases reported. These have been reviewed recently by Lelong et al. (1964).

Clinical Manifestations

The hemangioma is congenital and therefore always present at birth. In 27 of the 50 reported cases, the initial signs of bleeding occurred during the first month of life. In the remainder, it was delayed for several months, occasionally not appearing for several years.

The hemangiomas are usually large and solitary, but they may be smaller and appear in multiple sites. They may occur anywhere on the surface of the body. In five cases, they occurred within the viscera; three of these were malignant. When they occur in the neck, there is great risk of compression of the airway from local expansion; several infants have died of this.

The onset of bleeding is often heralded by a sudden increase in size or firmness of the hemangioma, with increasing purplish discoloration over the surface, suggesting acute vascular engorgement or hemorrhage. At this time, purpura and bleeding manifestations may appear anywhere in the body.

The liver and spleen are not usually enlarged.

Laboratory Findings

During the purpuric phase, the platelet count is usually below 50,000/cu. mm. Milder degrees of thrombocytopenia may be found if routine blood counts are done prior to the onset of purpura.

Bone marrow aspirates reveal increased numbers of megakaryocytes, which may appear normal or immature. The picture is identical to that of acute idiopathic thrombocytopenic purpura in older children and reflects the response to acute destruction of platelets.

Plasma fibrinogen levels are usually low, suggesting that fibrinogen (along with platelets) are "consumed" locally in the stagnated blood within the hemangioma (Rodríguez-Erdmann, 1965).

Platelet antibodies have not been found in this condition.

Pathogenesis

The acute onset of purpura, its parallel relation to the size of the tumor, and the accompanying megakaryocytic hyperplasia all suggest that the thrombocytopenia is due to increased destruction or sequestration of platelets, probably within the tumor. Evidence to support this is the finding by Gilon et al. (1959) of higher platelet counts in blood from the hemangioma compared to peripheral blood, and the observation by Kontras et al. (1963) and Brizel and Raccuglia (1965) of localization of radioactivity over the tumor following intravenous injection of chromium-51 labeled platelets. The associated hypofibrinogenemia, along with shortened survival of I^{131}-labeled fibrinogen and increased uptake of radioactivity by the hemangioma, offers further evidence for intravascular coagulation as the basis for the hemorrhagic defect (Wacksman et al., 1966; Hillman and Phillips, 1967; Thatcher et al., 1968). As expected, other consumable clotting factors (prothrombin, Factors V and VIII) may also be low in this condition. Burr-cell hemolytic anemia (resulting from traumatic injury to the red cell membrane) may also be seen (Propp and Scharf-man, 1966).

Although in the vast majority of cases this syndrome is recognized by the appearance of a large hemangioma in the infant, rarely it may result from a hemangioma on the fetal aspect of the placenta, a so-called chorangioma (Froehlich, 1971). In this situation, the thrombocytopenia is present at birth and disappears a few days afterward because of separation of the infant from the placenta.

Treatment

Like hemangiomas in general, those described above show a natural tendency to regress with time. In such cases, where surgical excision and local irradiation have not been necessary, the long-term cosmetic results have been best. Any decision to employ these forms of therapy therefore should take this into account, in addition to the potential hazards of the treatment itself. The main problems with surgery in this condition are the risks of severe bleeding during the procedure (due to thrombocytopenia and the vascular nature of the tumor) and infection after excision. With irradiation, the major risk is suppression of bone growth, which in the face or limbs may result in later asymmetry and cosmetic defect. In addition to surgery and irradiation, there has been a resurgence of interest in the use of corticosteroids, following the encouraging results reported by Fost and Esterly (1969) and Goldberg and Fonkalsrud (1969). Although hematologic abnormalities were not described in these reports, an infant with giant hemangioma and consumption coagulopathy reported by Schneider and Lascari (1968) showed a dramatic response to prednisone, consisting of a rise in platelet count from 9000 to 216,000/cu. mm. over a two week period, associated with marked shrinkage of the hemangioma. In Fost and Esterly's review of this subject, there were a number of other instances of apparent benefit from corticosteroids. However, concurrent irradiation therapy clouded interpretation of the results in many of the cases.

On the basis of the above data, we would make the following recommendations for treatment of this condition. First, all patients deserve a short trial of corticosteroids in high dosage, for example, prednisone 20 mg./day for two weeks. If a favorable response occurs, the drug should be stopped and restarted only if the hemangioma recurs. Those patients not responding or developing progressive difficulty during therapy (compression of vital structures by the hemangioma or bleeding) should receive definitive therapy to the hemangioma itself (preferably irradiation). As long as the thrombocytopenia and coagulation defect are not causing significant bleeding symptoms, heparin, in an effort to arrest clotting within the hemangioma, may be withheld. The response to irradiation varies with the dosage (Duncan and Halnan, 1964). In cases requiring rapid control of the tumor growth (within a few days), a single exposure of up to 800 rads skin dose is recommended, with careful attention to shielding vital parts. Surgery should be reserved for cases causing serious difficulty and not responsive to steroids, irradiation, or heparin. The use of heparin in this condition is directed mainly at control of the bleeding complications; it has no effect on the tumor itself. The recommended dose is 100 units/kg. intravenously every four hours, continued until bleeding ceases and the platelet count and coagulation defect show signs of improvement. Platelet concentrates and fresh frozen plasma may be necessary supplements in the management of the bleeding or in connection with surgery, along with whole blood to replace blood lost. If the anemia is largely a result of hemolysis (evidenced by the presence of burr cells and fragmented cells on smear), packed red cells will suffice.

Splenectomy has been tried in a number of cases but without convincing benefit.

Prognosis

Fatalities have occurred in a small number of cases, owing to intractable hemorrhage, infection, or airway compression. In those cases responding to irradiation, thrombocytopenia does not disappear until the size of the tumor begins to decrease. At this point, the tumor gradually decreases in size and like most infantile hemangiomas completely disappears.

Infants occasionally have shown spontaneous although slow regression of both hemangioma and thrombocytopenia (Wallerstein, 1961).

INHERITED THROMBOCYTOPENIAS

A variety of genetically distinct forms of inherited thrombocytopenia have been described. Bleeding in the newborn period has occurred rarely, and therefore only brief mention of this group of disorders is made.

Sex-linked Thrombocytopenia. In the *pure* form, a number of families have been reported (Schaar, 1963; Vestermark and Vestermark, 1964; Ata et al., 1965). One of Schaar's patients manifested purpura at birth. The presence of normal numbers of megakaryocytes in the bone marrow in most of these cases suggests that the thrombocytopenia is a result of shortened platelet survival due to an intrinsic platelet defect. This was confirmed by autologous chromium-51 survival studies in a family seen recently by us (Murphy et al., 1970).

Wiskott–Aldrich Syndrome. This consists of eczema, recurrent infections, and thrombocytopenia. Most infants are ill from the first few months of life, and eventually die in early childhood. Signs of bleeding are frequently ushered in by melena in the neonatal period, followed later by purpura. Although the thrombocytopenia was initially felt to be a result of impaired production, more recent studies using patients' (autologous) platelets have shown a shortened survival, pointing to an intrinsic platelet defect (Baldini et al., 1969). Reduced platelet size characterizes this defect and is an exception to the general observation that in "destructive" thrombocytopenias, the presence of young platelets is reflected by increased size (Murphy et al., 1970).

The possibility that some cases of apparently pure sex-linked thrombocytopenia may represent forms of the Wiskott–Aldrich syndrome is suggested by the finding of decreased levels of isohemagglutinins and increased levels of serum IgA in a family described by Canales and Maurer (1967). Neither eczema nor increased susceptibility to infections was present in the thrombocytopenic members. In the family described by Vestermark (1967) and in the one seen by us, some of the thrombocytopenic members had mild eczema. Isohemagglutinins and IgA were normal in the family seen by us.

Autosomal Thrombocytopenia. In the pure form, families with both dominant (Seip, 1963; Bithell et al., 1965; Murphy et al., 1969) and recessive (Roberts and Smith, 1950) modes of inheritance have been described. Bone marrow examination has usually revealed normal numbers of megakaryocytes. Autologous platelet survival studies in the family reported by Murphy indicated a shortened lifespan, pointing to an intrinsic platelet defect. Normal survival of autologous platelets in one of Seip's cases suggested a defect in platelet production.

May-Hegglin Anomaly. This consists of familial thrombocytopenia, giant platelets, and Döhle bodies in the cytoplasm of the granulocytes (Oski et al., 1962). Bleeding has not been described in the newborn (p. 333). Bone marrow megakaryocytes are normal and autologous platelet survival is shortened (Davis and Wilson, 1966).

MISCELLANEOUS CONDITIONS ASSOCIATED WITH NEONATAL THROMBOCYTOPENIA

Thrombotic Thrombocytopenic Purpura (TTP). This syndrome is characterized by thrombocytopenic purpura, burr-cell hemolytic

Table 9-4 Diagnostic Features of Various Types of Neonatal Thrombocytopenic Purpura

	History			Physical Findings			Associated Hematologic Abnormalities°°	Laboratory Studies			Duration of Thrombocytopenia
	Previous Infants Affected	Maternal Illness	Maternal Drugs	Jaundice°	Hepato-splenomegaly	Congenital Anomalies		Bone Marrow Megakaryocytes	Platelet Antibodies (Mother)	Maternal Thrombo-cytopenia	
Immune Disorders											
Maternal ITP	+/0	Purpura	0	0	0	0	0	↑ (or ↓)	+	+	Up to 3-4 mos.
Drug Purpura	+/0	Purpura	Quinine, quinidine Sedormid	0	0	0	0	↑ (or ↓)	+	+	Up to 1 week
Maternal S.L.E.	+/0	Rash, arthritis, renal	0	0	0	0	± Anemia, neutropenia	?	+	+	Up to 1 week
Isoimmune	+/0	0	0	+/0	0	0	0	↑ (or ↓)	+	0	Above 60,000 cu. mm. by 2-3 weeks
Infections											
Bacterial							± Coagulation defects	?	0	0	Parallels activity of infection; often months.
Viral	0	+/0	0	+	+	0	Anemia (hemolytic)		0	0	
Protozoal											
Drugs (nonimmune type)	+/0	0	Thiazides	0	0	0	± Leukopenia	→	0	0	2-12 weeks

+ Present
0 Absent
° May occur in any of types from enclosed hemorrhage.
°° Anemia in any of types if bleeding severe.

Table 9-4 Diagnostic Features of Various Types of Neonatal Thrombocytopenic Purpura (Continued)

	History			Physical Findings			Laboratory Studies				Duration of Thrombo-cytopenia
	Previous Infants Affected	Maternal Illness	Maternal Drugs	Jaundice°	Hepato-splenomegaly	Congenital Anomalies	Associated Hematologic Abnormalities°°	Bone Marrow Megakaryocytes	Platelet Antibodies (Mother)	Maternal Thrombo-cytopenia	
Congenital Megakaryo-cytic Hypoplasia											
Isolated	0	0	0	0	0	+/0	0	↓↓	0	0	Lifelong
Associated anomalies Absent radii	0	0	0	0	+/0	Cardiac, skeletal, etc.	Leukemoid reaction	↓↓ or 0	0	0	Lifelong
Rubella syndrome With pancytopenia	0	Rash in T_1	0	+/0	+/0	Eye, cardiac	± Leukopenia Later pancytopenia	↓	0	0	Up to 2 months
(no anomalies)	0		0	0	0	0		↓↓ or 0	0	0	Lifelong
Bone Marrow Disease Congenital Leukemia	0	0	0	+/0	+	0	Anemia, leukocytosis	↑ (Blasts ++)	0	0	Fatal
Giant Hemangioma (incl. chorangioma)	0	0	0	0	0	Hemangioma	Coagulation defects	↑	0	0	Disappears with hemangioma
Inherited Thrombocytopenias	+/0	Purpura only if carrier	0	0	0	0	0	Normal number	0	+/0	Lifelong, may remit with splenectomy

+ Present
0 Absent
° May occur in any of types from enclosed hemorrhage.
°° Anemia in any of types if bleeding severe.

anemia and transient focal neurologic abnormalities. Pathologically, there is widespread deposition of fibrin thrombi in the small blood vessels. As such, it has been considered by some to represent a form of disseminated intravascular coagulation, the precise etiology of which is not known. Although rare in childhood, one case of TTP was described with onset on the third day of life (Monnens and Retera, 1967). Associated with severe jaundice were purpura, hematuria, and melena. The platelet count was 4000/cu. mm. After two exchange transfusions, the infant improved but the thrombocytopenia persisted. The infant died at nine months of age, with typical lesions of TTP at post-mortem examination.

Inherited Metabolic Disorders. Thrombocytopenia (and neutropenia) are common findings in infants with methylmalonic acidemia and ketotic glycinemia (Morrow et al., 1969). Three siblings in a family with isovaleric acidemia reported by Allen et al. (1969) showed neonatal thrombocytopenia as part of a general pancytopenia with hypoplastic bone marrow. Of interest is the correction of the hematologic defect with a low-leucine diet in one surviving infant in this family. The severe acidosis common to each of the above disorders may play a role in the etiology of the hematologic complications.

Congenital Thyrotoxicosis. Zaidi and Mortimer (1965) described an interesting family in which a hyperthyroid mother gave birth to three successive newborns with thrombocytopenic purpura. Associated findings included jaundice, hepatosplenomegaly, and respiratory distress. From the reported data, it was not possible to define the mechanism of the thrombocytopenia.

DIAGNOSTIC APPROACH TO THE THROMBOCYTOPENIC NEWBORN

The important diagnostic features of the aforementioned disorders causing neonatal thrombocytopenia are summarized in Table 9-4. From this information, a rational approach to an etiologic diagnosis can be taken, as outlined in Figure 9-4.

In this scheme, it is as important to study the mother as it is the infant. Points requiring specific inquiry include: (1) a history of previous bleeding in the form of purpura, bruising, or nosebleeds that might suggest a diagnosis of maternal ITP at some time in the past; (2) ingestion of drugs that might cause thrombocytopenia in the mother and infant (for example, quinidine and quinine) or in the infant alone (thiazide diuretics, tolbutamide); (3) previous infants affected with purpura, suggesting either one of the immune or inherited thrombocytopenias; (4) skin rash or exposure to rubella in

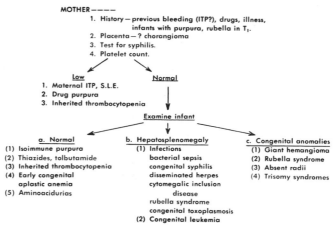

Figure 9–4   A scheme of approach to the diagnosis of the thrombocytopenic newborn.

the first eight weeks of pregnancy. The results of the routine test for syphilis should be sought and recorded, rather than left buried among the other routine laboratory results performed earlier in pregnancy. Finally, an accurate platelet count should be performed on the mother as soon as possible after delivery to separate immune neonatal thrombocytopenia due to maternal ITP from that due to platelet isoimmunization (in which case the mother's platelet count is normal).

Physical findings of importance in differential diagnosis in the affected newborn include the presence or absence of hepatosplenomegaly and congenital anomalies. Hepatosplenomegaly is often accompanied by jaundice and suggests an infectious process as the most likely cause of thrombocytopenia. In some cases, congenital leukemia may also have to be considered. Among the congenital anomalies associated with neonatal thrombocytopenia, the commonest group recognizable at birth is that occurring in the rubella syndrome (congenital heart defects, cataracts, and microcephaly). Deformity and shortening of the forearms should suggest bilateral absence of the radii with associated amegakaryocytic thrombocytopenia. A single large hemangioma or multiple smaller hemangiomas point to these tumors as the probable site of platelet trapping leading to thrombocytopenia.

Complete blood count on the infant should include hemoglobin, white cell count, platelet count, and smear. Associated anemia may be due to blood loss, concurrent hemolysis (as might occur in one of the infectious processes), or marrow infiltration due to congenital leukemia. Leukocytosis of a mild degree may accompany infection or blood loss, but when this exceeds 40,000 to 50,000/cu. mm. it should point either to congenital leukemia or to the absent radii syndrome. Bone marrow examination is essential not only for assessment of megakaryocytes, but also to exclude underlying infiltrative disorders such as leukemia. Increased numbers of megakaryocytes suggest either consumption coagulopathy or one of the immune thrombocytopenias, although megakaryocytes may be diminished in number in some infants with these disorders. A decrease in the number of megakaryocytes generally suggests one of the types of congenital megakaryocytic hypoplasia. It is important, however, to exclude the immune disorders, if possible, by serologic tests before arriving at this diagnosis because of its ominous prognosis. When in doubt, it is wise to defer such a diagnosis until follow-up observations clarify the situation. Repeat bone marrow examination may be necessary.

Serologic tests for platelet antibodies are at present difficult, time-consuming, and available only in a small number of laboratories. Should isoimmune thrombocytopenia be suspected by the finding of an otherwise normal thrombocytopenic newborn of a healthy mother with a normal platelet count, blood should be drawn from the *mother* soon after delivery and serum frozen and saved until antibody testing can be carried out. Because results of such studies are usually not available for some time, their chief value lies in the management of subsequent pregnancies, much in the manner of maternal Rh antibody tests in predicting the occurrence of erythroblastosis fetalis.

The response to platelet transfusion may be of both therapeutic *and diagnostic* aid in the thrombocytopenic newborn. Gill and Schwartz (1970) transfused several such infants with platelet concentrates derived from two units of whole blood. The subsequent platelet survival as indicated by actual platelet counts correlated well with the known pathogenetic mechanisms in several infants with thrombocytopenia associated with absent radii, cytomegalovirus infection, maternal ITP, and platelet isoimmunization. In the latter situation, maternal platelets (lacking the antigen) produced an excellent response while paternal platelets did not.

Chapter Ten

DISORDERS OF
THE LEUKOCYTES

The chief disorders of leukocytes seen in the first few days of life are neutropenia, lymphopenia, and congenital leukemia. Proper evaluation of such disorders requires a knowledge of the normal values for the total white count; the differentials for these values in the neonate differ from those observed in later infancy and childhood (see p. 18). Other aspects of white cell metabolism also show patterns characteristic of the newborn period.

NEUTROPHIL FUNCTION

General Considerations

The primary function of the neutrophil is phagocytosis. In the body's defense against bacterial invasion there is a series of steps that takes place before and after phagocytosis that eventually leads to the killing of bacteria and an immune response. This sequence is shown in Table 10–1. Until recently examination of the individual steps in this sequence has been limited by the lack of suitable methodology. Impetus for development of such methodology has arisen over the past few years from the investigation of various patients with recurrent pyogenic infections in whom commonly recognized defects such as agammaglobulinemia have been excluded. The most completely studied disorder of neutrophil function is an entity known as chronic granulomatous disease, in which there is a defect in bacterial killing (Quie et al., 1967). The neutrophils of such patients fail to show the

312

Table 10–1 Neutrophil Response to Infection

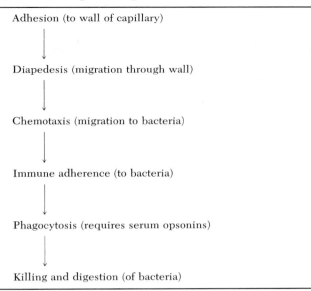

Adhesion (to wall of capillary)

↓

Diapedesis (migration through wall)

↓

Chemotaxis (migration to bacteria)

↓

Immune adherence (to bacteria)

↓

Phagocytosis (requires serum opsonins)

↓

Killing and digestion (of bacteria)

normal increase in oxidative metabolism of glucose after phagocytosis; this is reflected by an inability to reduce the dye nitroblue tetrazolium (NBT). This phenomenon has been used to advantage in the diagnosis of chronic granulomatous disease (Baehner and Nathan, 1968) and in the differentiation of bacterial from non-bacterial infection (Park et al., 1968). Another familial defect in neutrophil function has been traced to a deficiency of plasma opsonins, resulting in impaired phagocytosis and recurrent bacterial infections (Miller et al., 1968). A defect in chemotaxis has also been demonstrated in yet another group of children with persistent neutropenia—the so-called "lazy-leukocyte" syndrome (Miller et al., 1971).

It seems only natural that the methodology developed from the study of the above diverse clinical syndromes has been applied to the "normal" newborn who by accident of age has been plagued by an increased susceptibility to serious bacterial infection, the basis for which has only recently appeared within our understanding.

Neutrophil Function in the Newborn

Of the various phases in the neutrophil response to infection listed in Table 10–1, greatest attention has been directed in the newborn to the study of phagocytosis and bactericidal activity. Recently, chemotaxis and immune adherence have also been studied.

Chemotaxis. Comparing both cellular and humoral (serum) aspects of chemotaxis, Miller (1971) has shown a significant impairment in activity of both of these functions in normal term newborns compared to the adult. The cellular defect of chemotaxis was more striking than that of the serum. Failure of added serum IgM to correct the humoral deficiency suggested that it was not related to the low serum levels of IgM in the newborn. Complement factors in serum, however, seemed of some importance.

Immune adherence. In the same study as above, Miller found no difference in serum complement immune adherence activity between neonatal and adult sera.

Phagocytosis. A deficiency of phagocytosis by leukocytes at birth was observed as early as 1910 by Tunicliffe, and later confirmed by Bracco (1948) and Matoth (1952). Correction of the deficiency by the addition of normal adult serum in the latter study indicated the importance of separate consideration of humoral (opsonin) and cellular factors in phagocytosis. Moreover, the premature infant has been found to have a greater defect in phagocytic capacity than the term infant (Gluck and Silverman, 1957; Sato, 1959); in the former study this was also corrected by the addition of adult serum.

Since these early studies refinements in methodology and attention to the importance of both cellular and humoral aspects have led to a re-evaluation of the observed handicap in phagocytosis by the neutrophils of the newborn. Although no two workers have used identical techniques it is encouraging to note that most agree that the humoral (plasma opsonin) component of phagocytosis is deficient in the newborn (Miller, 1969; Dosset et al., 1969; McCracken and Eichenwald, 1971). Among the infants studied by Forman and Thiem (1969) only the low birth weight infants showed this defect. McCracken and Eichenwald found the defect in opsonization in both term and low birth weight infants; the degree of deficiency was greater, however, in the smaller infants. An important technical detail in these studies that may account for some of the conflicting results was brought out by Matoth (1952) and Miller (1969). They showed that when the concentration of plasma in the phagocytosis assay system was reduced from 10 per cent to 2.5 per cent the sensitivity of the assay was distinctly increased, and was sufficient to show a definite defect in the newborn. However, a subsequent refinement in which antibiotics were added to the phagocytosis assay revealed normal activity in the newborn (Coen et al. 1969); the validity of this technique has been criticized by Miller (1970).

In studies of the *cellular* component of phagocytosis by these workers only Miller (1969) was able to demonstrate a defect in the newborn. As discussed above this was attributed to his use of a lower concentration of plasma in the phagocytosis assay system. The unphysiologic nature of such concentrations raises questions of the relevance of these findings to the situation as it exists in the infant.

Bactericidal activity. Most workers have demonstrated normal killing of ingested bacteria by neutrophils of the newborn infant (Dossett et al., 1969; Forman and Thiem, 1969; Park et al., 1970; McCracken and Eichenwald, 1971). However, impaired killing has been demonstrated by Coen et al. (1971) in 9 of 25 term infants under 12 hours of age. Also among prematures, Cocchi and Marianelli (1967) found impaired killing of *Pseudomonas aeruginosa.*

As mentioned earlier, cell killing is preceded by metabolic changes in the neutrophil that are accompanied by reduction of the dye nitroblue tetrazolium (NBT). In the normal newborn NBT reduction by neutrophils is increased, both in the resting state and following phagocytosis (Park et al., 1970; Humbert et al., 1970). Similar results were obtained by Cocchi et al. (1971), who in addition compared term and premature infants and found no differences. This peculiar finding of increased NBT reduction limits the usefulness of the histochemical version of this test in the diagnosis of bacterial infection in the newborn infant.

Inflammatory cycle. Following abrasion of the skin there develops an inflammatory response which may be observed by serial application of coverslips to the involved skin—the "skin window" technique of Rebuck and Crowley (1955). In the normal adult there is exudation of polymorphonuclear neutrophils during the first few hours, followed by a shift within 12 hours to a predominance of mononuclear cells. Eitzman and Smith (1959) noted two essential differences between newborn infants and adults:

The first was that an inflammatory eosinophilia, averaging 19 per cent of the exudate cells, was seen in infants two to 21 days of age two hours after the initiation of the inflammation. This eosinophilic response was not observed in infants less than 24 hours of age or in older children and adults, regardless of their peripheral eosinophil count. The second difference observed by these investigators was that the shift from an early preponderance of granulocytes to a preponderance of mononuclear cells was slower and less intense in the infants. Sheldon and Caldwell (1963) also noted that this mononuclear cell response was less marked in the newborn. Twenty hours after initiation of the inflammatory cycle, mononuclear cells comprised 75 per cent of the cells in the exudate from adults but only 25 per cent in the infants. In more recent studies the early eosinophilia noted above was not consistently observed (Prindull, 1968; Bullock et al., 1969). Among the newborns studied by Bullock and co-workers eosinophilia was seen in only 13 of 61 infants, and was confined to those over 24 hours of age. The possibility that this group of infants may have had an allergic diathesis was suggested by positive family histories and follow-up studies. This chance inclusion of allergic infants might similarly explain the eosinophilia observed in the study of Eitzman and Smith (1959) and its absence in subsequent studies.

The Buffy Coat

The buffy coat from cord blood reveals many more nuclei and nuclear fragments of megakaryocytes, as well as metamyelocytes, myelocytes, and nucleated red blood cells than that from adult whole blood (Efrati et al., 1961). Rare blast forms have been seen in this type of preparation from neonates while they have never been observed in adults.

Chemical and Physical Properties of Leukocytes

White cell alkaline phosphatase activity is increased during the first week of life (Efrati et al., 1961; Leonard, 1965). Leonard found values four to nine times greater than those of the adult. The subsequent fall toward normal adult values and the high values observed during pregnancy and in women receiving oral contraceptive agents suggest that maternal estrogens and progesterone may be the cause of the increased leukocyte alkaline phosphatase activity found at birth (O'Kell, 1968.) The leukocytes of the newborn contain more glycogen (Brunelli and Flauto, 1963) and consume more glucose (Schuler et al., 1962) than do those of the adult.

Gelli and associates (1960) found the leukocytes of newborns to be more resistant to osmotic lysis than those of the adult, while Columbo and Castello (1961) reached the opposite conclusion.

CONGENITAL AND NEONATAL LEUKEMIA

Leukemia, or a disease indistinguishable from it by present diagnostic techniques, has been observed in infants at birth or has developed in the first few weeks of life. The term *congenital leukemia* is reserved for disease in infants that is apparent on the first day of life. Three essential criteria must be fulfilled before the diagnosis can be made — proliferation of immature cells of the myeloid or lymphoid series, infiltration of these cells into nonhematopoietic tissues, and absence of any other diseases such as erythroblastosis fetalis, congenital syphilis, or viral and bacterial infections that might result in diagnostic confusion.

Applying these criteria, at least 37 infants with congenital leukemia and 50 infants with neonatal leukemia have been recorded in the literature by 1966. These cases have been reviewed by Daalgaard and

Kass (1955), Pierce (1959), and Stransky and Sarcia (1964), and additional cases have been reported by Pridie et al. (1961), Bouton et al. (1961), Bernard et al. (1964), Cornet et al. (1965), DiPrati (1966), Iversen (1966) and Buhler and Landolt (1970). Some cases originally reported as instances of congenital leukemia were later found to be the result of other diseases (Bungeler, 1931; Kauffman and Hess, 1959). Bungeler (1954) and Kauffman and Hess (1962) urge that a high degree of skepticism be maintained before accepting a diagnosis of leukemia in the newborn. Because other neoplastic disorders have unequivocally been found in the newborn, there appears little reason to doubt that leukemia can and does occur in some infants. Most reported instances of the disease can be accepted until such time as more specific diagnostic criteria become available.

A disproportionately large number of cases have been observed in infants with Down's syndrome (trisomy 21). This aspect of the disease is discussed on page 321. Other conditions reported in association with congenital or neonatal leukemia include trisomy 13 (Schade et al., 1962), Turner's syndrome (Pridie et al., 1961) and a variant of the Ellis-van Creveld syndrome (Miller et al., 1969).

Clinical Manifestations

Congenital Form. In infants with the congenital form of leukemia, cutaneous manifestations are present and may be the first sign that attracts the attention of the physician. In addition to petechiae and ecchymoses, a characteristic nodular skin infiltration is seen in about 50 per cent of cases. The nodules may appear on the scalp, cheeks, ear lobes, nose, and trunk, and they vary from 0.2 to 3.0 cm. in diameter (Fortina and Petrocini, 1953). The nodules are palpated in the skin as firm, fibroma-like tumors of the deep corium that move freely over the subcutaneous tissues but appear well fixed to the skin. The overlying skin is bluish to slate gray. On occasion ulceration may develop. Such nodules have been observed in stillbirths with leukemia (Kock, 1922; Stransky, 1925). They may precede other manifestations of the disease by several weeks (Reimann et al., 1955).

In addition to the cutaneous manifestations of thrombocytopenia, bleeding may occur from the mucous membranes, gastrointestinal tract, and the umbilical stump.

At birth, respiratory difficulty may be observed. This is frequently a result of pulmonary infiltration by the leukemic process. Enlargement of the liver and spleen is usually evident, although occasionally the spleen may be of normal size. Lymphadenopathy and jaundice are uncommon.

Neonatal Form. The clinical manifestations of neonatal leukemia are not as well defined as those of congenital leukemia. These infants may show poor weight gain, unexplained fever, diarrhea, marked pallor, and petechiae. Nodular infiltration of the skin is unusual.

Physical findings include petechiae, purpura, jaundice, and hepatosplenomegaly. Again lymphadenopathy is uncommon.

Laboratory Findings

The essential feature of the disease is an elevated white cell count with a predominance of immature white cell forms. On occasion leukopenia has been observed (Hjelt et al., 1956), but in general, total white cell counts range from 30,000 to 500,000/cu. mm. Most cases seen in the neonatal period are examples of myeloblastic leukemia, in contrast to the usual lymphoblastic or stem cell leukemia of later infancy and childhood. The literature on congenital lymphoblastic leukemia has been reviewed by Wagner et al. (1968). The clinical and hematologic findings in the two types of leukemia are similar.

Thrombocytopenia is generally present. Anemia is unusual in the first few days of life in infants with the congenital form of the disease, but it is frequently profound in instances in which the disease is first diagnosed after this period.

Cirrhosis of the liver has been observed at autopsy (Daalgaard et al., 1955; Bouton et al., 1961; Mattelaer and Riley, 1964).

Chromosome analyses, aside from cases associated with Down's syndrome, Turner's syndrome and trisomy 13, have yielded results similar to those described in older children with acute leukemia. The karyotypes have been normal in some cases (Bouton et al., 1961; Campbell et al., 1962; Nowell, 1965), and in others they have shown a variety of abnormalities but with no uniform pattern (Zussman et al., 1967; Wagner et al., 1968; Bauke et al., 1970).

Treatment and Prognosis

In the congenital form of the disease, treatment has been unsatisfactory, and death usually occurs by two months of age.

Infants who develop leukemia after birth also do poorly, although survival may be longer. Cornet and associates (1965) have observed a 20 month remission in an infant in whom a thymectomy was performed at 68 hours of age. In this patient, no other specific antileukemic therapy was employed. DiPratti (1966) has observed a 22 month survival, despite repeated relapses, in an infant who was first treated at four weeks of age. Initial treatment consisted of methotrexate and maternal plasma. Subsequent relapses have responded to vincristine.

If recent experience with the treatment of acute myelocytic leukemia in older children and adults can be used as a model, the improved results of intensive combination chemotherapy merit such a trial in the newborn with this type of leukemia. Drugs found to be effective in such combinations include vincristine, cyclophosphamide, cytosine arabinoside and thioguanine (Freedman et al., 1971). Of equal importance in therapy are supportive measures such as transfusion of blood and platelet concentrates, and antibiotic therapy of infections. Since the above drug regimens require repeated intravenous infusions, one should carefully weigh the possible benefits of therapy against the problems of maintaining adequate veins and hematologic toxicity before committing an infant and its family to such a regimen.

Spontaneous remission, common in the leukemia-like disorder occurring in infants with Down's syndrome, has also been reported in an infant with congenital (myeloid) leukemia associated with normal karyotype (Van Eys and Flexner, 1969). The remission in this infant lasted until 9 months of age.

Differential Diagnosis

A variety of disorders in the neonatal period may mimic the signs of leukemia. Bacterial sepsis, erythroblastosis fetalis, congenital syphilis, cytomegalic inclusion disease, toxoplasmosis, many varieties of neonatal thrombocytopenia, congenital Letterer-Siwe disease and metastatic neuroblastoma may all cause some diagnostic confusion.

Infections with *Staphylococcus aureus* or gram-negative organisms may produce marked elevations in the white cell count, mild anemia, thrombocytopenia, purpura, hepatosplenomegaly, and jaundice. Generally, the peripheral smear shows all the transition forms from the promyelocyte to the mature granulocyte, in contrast to the characteristic gap, or leukemic hiatus, between the predominating blast form and the mature granulocyte. Infants with sepsis may on occasion also show a few blasts in the peripheral blood, even in the absence of appreciable leukocytosis (Holland and Mauer, 1963). The bone marrow shows a shift to the younger myeloid forms but is not dominated by blast cells. The jaundice of infection is generally accompanied by elevations of both the conjugated and unconjugated bilirubin fractions. Although the cellular response may be extreme, diffuse organ infiltration by immature cells is not observed. When leukemia and infection occur simultaneously, the diagnosis of leukemia becomes extremely difficult and can often be made only at autopsy.

Syphilis, cytomegalic inclusion disease, and toxoplasmosis have many distinctive features (see Chapter Two). These disorders should not cause a great deal of diagnostic confusion, provided they are considered in the differential diagnosis.

Kauffman and Hess (1962) have stressed the importance of excluding erythroblastosis fetalis. Although the severely affected erythroblastotic infant may manifest hepatosplenomegaly, purpura, and leukocytosis with some immature myeloid forms in the blood, the rapid onset of anemia and jaundice, normoblastemia, and the positive Coombs' test should be sufficient to exclude this possibility.

The purpuric lesions of congenital thrombocytopenia do not resemble the nodular infiltrates seen in leukemia. Hepatosplenomegaly is absent. In the form of congenital amegakaryocytic thrombocytopenia associated with absence of the radii, leukemoid reactions are frequent and should be kept in mind to avoid confusion of this syndrome with true leukemia. (See Chapter Nine, p. 299.)

A case of myeloid metaplasia masquerading as neonatal leukemia was described by Gordon (1969). This infant died at 12 days of age after a brief illness characterized by fever, hepatosplenomegaly, leukocytosis (total white cell count 86,000/cu.mm.; marked shift to the left and 30 per cent blasts), and thrombocytosis. At autopsy many of the organs showed infiltration with myeloid cells but there was no evidence of leukemia or fibrosis in the bone marrow. Although the author states that no evidence was uncovered to support sepsis or other cause of leukemoid reaction we find it hard to dismiss the possibility of an unrecognized infection as a basis for the findings in this case.

A nodular skin eruption has been observed in a stillborn infant in whom the histologic diagnosis of Letterer-Siwe disease was made (Ahnquist and Holyoke, 1960). The skin manifestations consisted of widely scattered circumscribed lesions consisting of intracutaneous and subcutaneous hemorrhagic nodules varying in size from 0.25 to 1.5 cm. in diameter. Some of the lesions showed superficial ulceration. Microscopically, there was a proliferation of reticuloendothelial cells in the skin and also in the lungs, liver, spleen, lymph nodes, thymus, and bone. This type of skin eruption could be confused with that of congenital leukemia, although histologically the two are dissimilar. Cohen et al. (1966) observed skin infiltrates and organ involvement in a premature who died immediately after birth. Letterer-Siwe disease was diagnosed at autopsy. A cutaneous eruption, present at birth, has been described in infants who over the first few weeks of life went on to develop evidence of Letterer-Siwe disease (Schafer, 1949; Batson et al., 1955).

Neonatal neuroblastoma frequently presents with extensive hepatic and subcutaneous metastases (Schneider et al., 1965; Shown and Durfee, 1970). The resulting hepatomegaly and bluish subcutaneous nodules, especially when associated with anemia, may suggest congenital leukemia. The skin nodules in metastatic neuroblastoma however are usually situated deeper in the subcutaneous tissue than those in leukemia, and the absence of marked leukocytosis or myelo-blasts in the bone marrow serve further to differentiate these two disorders.

CONGENITAL LEUKEMIA AND DOWN'S SYNDROME (MONGOLISM)

A disproportionately high number of cases diagnosed as con-genital leukemia have occurred in infants with Down's syndrome (Bernhard et al., 1951; Schunk and Lehman, 1954; O'Connor et al., 1954; Taylor and Geppert, 1950; Krivit and Good, 1957; Lee and Ciner, 1957; Honda et al., 1964; Mattelaer and Riley, 1964; Fischler and Farcy, 1960; Conen and Erkman, 1966; Wegelius et al., 1967; Gardais et al., 1969; Nagas et al., 1970). Recently, it has become apparent that in such infants this disease has one unique feature — a high incidence of apparently spontaneous remissions. Ross et al. (1963) reported a mongoloid infant in whom acute granulocytic leu-kemia was diagnosed soon after birth. The infant recovered completely, and on his death at age three years and nine months no evidence of leukemia could be found at autopsy. Engel and associates (1964) cite four similar cases from the literature and present three additional instances of the same phenomenon. In one instance, the infant re-mained free of leukemia until the time of his death at $6\frac{1}{2}$ years (Schunk and Lehman, 1954). Complete remissions have occurred within one month of birth (DeCarvalho, 1963), and autopsies per-formed at six weeks of life have shown no evidence of the original disease process (Mattelaer and Riley, 1964).

Behrman et al. (1966) observed two siblings with translocation mongolism who developed hemolytic anemia, increased erythro-poiesis, thrombocytopenia, and myeloid metaplasia in the newborn period. One infant died: infiltrative lesions resembling chronic myelocytic leukemia were evident. The other sibling, now aged two, shows gradual resolution of this unusual proliferative process.

In addition to the leukemia-like reactions described above, a number of cases have shown in addition polycythemia (Conen and Erkman, 1966; Wegelius et al., 1967; Gardais et al., 1969). Transient polycythemia without leukemia also occurs with increased frequency among newborns with Down's syndrome (Weinberger and Oleinick, 1970). Further broadening the spectrum of congenital marrow dys-function in Down's syndrome is a newborn reported by Miller et al. (1967) with thrombocythemia (platelet count 1,200,000 per cu. mm.) in association with a transient leukemia-like reaction.

It now appears that congenital leukemia is only one facet of a myeloproliferative disorder among newborns with Down's syndrome that includes a leukemia-like illness, erythrocytosis and thrombo-cytosis; in a number of cases, overlapping of the above hematologic abnormalities has been seen.

The leukemia-*like* disorder is generally characterized by hepatosplenomegaly, anemia, thrombocytopenia, skin infiltrates and a marrow and peripheral blood picture of acute granulocytic (myelocytic) leukemia. The occurrence of sepsis or blood group incompatibility in association with some of the earlier reports of this condition suggested that it may be a form of anaphylactoid reaction (Kauffman and Hess, 1959, 1962) or a result of labile granulopoiesis (Ross et al., 1963). Cases documented since then have not shown any consistent pattern of predisposing events. Evidence supporting abnormal granulopoiesis has been accumulated by Nagao et al. (1970), who demonstrated ultrastructural differences between the myeloblasts in the blood of their patient and those in the blood of patients with acute granulocytic leukemia, and also kinetic differences revealed by low labeling and mitotic indices in the bone marrow of their patient.

Engel and associates (1964) suggest instead that this disorder be regarded as true congenital leukemia, and they question why malignancy in these individuals has a higher incidence of spontaneous remission, or as Lahey and associates (1963) ask: "Can the Mongol recover from acute leukemia—and if so, why?"

Infants with Down's syndrome and congenital leukemia have also been observed to go into prolonged remissions and still die later of their original disease. Instances of such a course have been reported by Honda et al. (1964), Conen and Erkman (1966), Propp et al. (1966) and Gardais et al. (1969). In these cases the intervals from initial remission to death have varied from five to 30 months.

The literature suggests that most infants with Down's syndrome and congenital leukemia will go into spontaneous remission, and of these, the majority show no further relapse of the leukemic process. However, the greater tendency to report cases that pursue such a favorable course may give a falsely high impression of its incidence. Until a truer picture of this fascinating process emerges it would seem wise to observe such infants, reserving treatment for the appearance of serious symptoms. Although the likelihood of leukemic relapse appears to diminish as the child survives beyond two or three years of age, it is important that these children be followed for as long as possible.

NEUTROPENIA

Neutropenia—neutrophils numbering less than 5000/cu. mm. during the first few days of life, or less than 1000/cu. mm. by the end of the first week of life—appears to be an uncommon occurrence in the neonatal period. A variety of disorders are recognized as causing or being associated with a low white cell count during this period (Table

Table 10–2   Causes of Neutropenia in the Neonatal Period

1. Neonatal neutropenia associated with maternal neutropenia.
2. Neonatal neutropenia associated with maternal isoimmunization to fetal leukocytes.
3. Infantile genetic agranulocytosis (congenital neutropenia).
4. Benign chronic granulocytopenia of childhood.
5. Syndrome of neutropenia and pancreatic insufficiency.
6. Reticular dysgenesis (congenital aleukocytosis).
7. Maternal drug ingestion.
8. Infections.
9. Cyclic neutropenia.
10. Inborn errors of metabolism.

10–2). Because it is not customary to perform white blood cell counts and differentials on healthy newborns, the diagnosis of neutropenia has been made chiefly in symptomatic infants. How frequently neutropenia occurs in the absence of symptoms is not known. The recognized complications of neutropenia in the newborn period include omphalitis, skin infections, generalized sepsis, and meningitis.

This subject has been well reviewed by Kauder and Mauer (1966).

Neonatal Neutropenia Associated with Maternal Neutropenia

Stefanini and associates (1958) described neutropenia in three infants, two of whom were siblings, born to mothers with severe chronic neutropenia. The total neutrophils averaged approximately 1000/cu. mm. for the first two to four weeks of life and then returned to normal levels. Neutropenia in these infants was not accompanied by any sign of infection. Bone marrow aspirates revealed a maturation arrest at the myelocyte stage. In one of the two mothers, a leukocyte-agglutinating factor could be demonstrated in her sera and that of her offspring. The authors hypothesize that the transitory neutropenia in the infants was a consequence of the transplacental passage of a neutropenic factor. This situation is comparable to that seen in infants born of mothers with idiopathic thrombocytopenic purpura (see p. 280).

Seip (1962) observed neutropenia in the infant of a mother with neutropenia associated with disseminated lupus erythematosus.

Mild leukopenia was observed in a stillborn infant of a mother who developed aplastic anemia from arsenicals used in the treatment of syphilis (Browaeys and Pley, 1950), but mothers with aplastic anemia have given birth to infants with normal white cell counts (Rosner et al., 1964). An infant born at the height of severe vinblastine-induced leukopenia in a woman with Hodgkin's disease was found to have normal blood counts (Nordlund et al., 1968).

Neutropenia Associated with Maternal Isoimmunization to Leukocytes

Neutropenia and infection have been observed in infants born to mothers who have developed antibodies to their infant's leukocytes (Hitzig and Gitzelmann, 1959; Lalezari et al., 1960; Braun et al., 1960; Jensen, 1960; Rossi and Brandt, 1960). In contrast to the disorder described by Stefanini and associates in the preceding section, the white cell counts in these mothers have been normal. In several instances, more than one infant in a family has been affected. White cell counts as low as 1700/cu. mm., with complete absence of neutrophils, have been observed. Marrow aspirates reveal a paucity of the more mature white cell precursors, such as the metamyelocytes and the stab forms. Some of the infants died with infections in the neonatal period, while others took up to ten weeks to attain a normal white cell count.

Isoagglutinins to leukocytes are known to develop in nontransfused pregnant women. Approximately 20 to 25 per cent of gravid women show these antibodies (Payne, 1962; Abildgaard and Jensen, 1964). The stimulus for this antibody production is believed to be the passage of fetal leukocytes into the maternal circulation. Following the formation of leukocyte agglutinins, transfer from mother to child can occur (Jensen, 1962). It has been suggested that these antibodies might result in the destruction of the infant's leukocytes in a manner similar to that of the red cell destruction observed after maternal sensitization to fetal erythrocytes in erythroblastosis fetalis. Many of these antibodies cross-react with antigens on lymphocytes, platelets and various tissues.

Neither Abildgaard and Jensen (1964) nor Payne (1964) could demonstrate any correlation between leukocyte agglutinins in the mother and the white cell count or infection in the newborn. They conclude that the transplacental passage of leukocyte agglutinins to newborns does not induce significant leukopenia or neutropenia.

Rossi and Brandt (1960) have suggested that infection in these infants was the primary factor responsible for the neutropenia, and the presence of leukocyte agglutinins was a chance association. The appearance of this syndrome in more than one member of a family, however, makes the factor of mere coincidence seem unlikely. Possibly in the presence of leukocyte agglutinins alone the infant's marrow reserve may compensate for the increased leukocyte destruction with an increased production of cells, resulting in a normal white cell count. Thus, when confronted with the additional stress of infection this compensation fails.

The possibility that the reactivity of the antibody may be an important factor in determining whether or not neutropenia results is suggested by the studies of Lalezari and Bernard (1966). An antibody found in maternal sera in two unrelated families bearing successive infants with neonatal neutropenia was unusual in that it reacted only with neutrophils and not with other blood or tissue cells. The antibody was an IgG (7S) globulin and, therefore, capable of crossing the placenta. The relation between this monospecific antibody and neutropenia suggested that the absence of such correlation in the majority of cases may reflect an antibody of broad reactivity that is absorbed by various tissues to such a degree that its effects on neutrophils are negligible.

Infantile Genetic Agranulocytosis (Congenital Neutropenia)

Kostman (1956) applied the term *infantile genetic agranulocytosis* to a syndrome characterized by onset in early infancy, complete or almost complete absence of granulocytes in the peripheral blood, multiple infections, familial aggregation, and frequent early death.

Since the initial report of Kostman, which described 14 individuals in nine different families, other identical or quite similar reports have appeared (Luhby et al., 1957; Hedenberg, 1959; Aarskog, 1961; Andrews et al., 1960; Page, 1962; Krill and Mauer, 1966; Miller et al., 1968).

Infections are the first symptom of the disease and primarily involve the skin, although otitis media, pneumonia, meningitis, and generalized septicemia may occur during the course of the illness. Multiple furuncles, deep abscesses, and omphalitis have been observed during the first week of life.

The total white cell count may vary from 600 to 10,000/cu. mm. and the differential count reveals that 0 to 10 per cent of the cells are of the neutrophilic series. Monocytosis or eosinophilia may be present. In some patients, a mild normochromic normocytic anemia has been observed. The platelet count is normal.

Lymphadenopathy and hepatosplenomegaly are absent. No associated congenital abnormalities have been described.

Kostman believed the disease to be inherited as an autosomal recessive trait, and he was able to document a high incidence of consanguinity in his families. Other investigators have not been able to confirm this point.

The bone marrow was hypocellular in the patients described by Kostman, while other observers reported it to be of normal cellularity (Andrews et al., 1960). The striking feature of the marrow is the pronounced maturation arrest in myelopoiesis. The myeloid series is dominated by promyelocytes and myelocytes, with very few more mature cells present. In the patient of Page (1962), no neutrophil precursors were observed. The early myeloid elements may show vacuoles and multiple lobulations of the nuclei.

Many of the patients died during the first year of life from infections, while others survived to at least three years of age because of vigorous antibiotic therapy. No successful treatment for the neutropenia has been observed, although the results of testosterone therapy have not been reported.

Chronic Benign Granulocytopenia of Childhood

This disorder is generally not diagnosed in the newborn period because of the mildness of the associated infections, although it may manifest itself during the first few weeks of life (Stahlie, 1956; Zuelzer and Bajoghli, 1964). Infections include paronychiae, impetigo, gingivitis, subcutaneous abscesses, pneumonia, and ulcerations about the genitalia.

Although the total white cell count is generally depressed, on occasion it may be normal or slightly elevated. The granulocyte count always shows a marked depression, with the differential count showing that 0 to 20 per cent of the cells are of this series. Often the only granulocytes present in the peripheral blood are band forms. Anemia and thrombocytopenia are absent.

The bone marrow, in contrast to that in infantile genetic agranulocytosis, is cellular, and all but the most mature segmented neutrophils are present in normal to increased numbers. These segmented neutrophils are virtually absent.

Despite repeated trivial infections these patients do well, and many experience a spontaneous cure in later childhood.

Neutropenia and Pancreatic Insufficiency

In 1964, Schwachman and associates described five patients with neutropenia and bone marrow hypoplasia in association with pancreatic insufficiency, diarrhea, and failure to thrive. Cystic fibrosis was excluded by the finding of normal sweat electrolytes and the absence of pulmonary disease characteristic of that disorder. Similar cases had previously been observed (Hoyer, 1949; Wagner and Smith, 1962) and have subsequently been reported (Bodian et al., 1964; Burke et al., 1967).

Total white cell counts have ranged from 1115 to 26,500/cu. mm., 0 to 25 per cent of the cells being granulocytes. Recurrent infections have not accompanied the neutropenia.

In one of the patients described by Shwachman and associates (1964), a white cell count obtained on the first day of life was only 3670/cu. mm.; it therefore appears that this disorder must also be included among the causes of neutropenia during the first week of life.

Reticular Dysgenesia (Congenital Aleukocytosis)

In 1959, de Vaal and Seynhaeve described two newborn infants, male twins, in whom all leukocytes were absent, both from the peripheral blood and the bone marrow. Accompanying this aleukia, the red cell count and the platelet count were normal. One infant died at five days of age and the other at eight days of age, both of infection. At autopsy the bone marrow was found to be completely devoid of myeloid elements, and the spleen and thymus were devoid of lymphocytes. These authors suggested the term *reticular dysgenesia* for this disorder.

A similar case was reported subsequently by Gitlin and associates (1964). In this patient, pallor, and a hemoglobin of 10 gm./100 ml., was noted at 36 hours of age. The infant did poorly and developed diarrhea, conjunctivitis, and omphalitis. On the fifteenth day of life, the white cell count ranged from 200 to 600/cu. mm. At postmortem examination, no granulocytes or granulocyte precursors were identified in the bone marrow. The thymus was small and fibrotic and contained virtually no small lymphocytes. The lymph nodes, although in gross examination they appeared normal in size, were comprised of reticular cells and contained very few lymphocytes.

Drug-induced Neutropenia

The administration of thiazides to mothers near term has resulted in the appearance of neutropenia as well as thrombocytopenia in the infant (Rodriguez et al., 1964). Borrone (1961) observed pancytopenia in an infant born to a mother receiving Optalidon. Dilantin ingestion during pregnancy has been associated with transient bone marrow aplasia in a neonate (Pantarotto, 1965). Presumably, other medications known to induce leukopenia frequently in adults could be responsible for neutropenia in an infant if the mother received these medications near term. Such drugs include amidopyrine, thiouracil, propylthiouracil, trimethadione, sulfonamides, Pyribenzamine, phenothiazine, and tolbutamide. Occasionally drug-induced neutropenia in mothers is *not* associated with neutropenia in the infant; such a case was reported in a mother receiving vinblastine (Nordlund et al., 1968).

Neutropenia Secondary to Infection

Leukopenia may accompany severe infections in the newborn period (Dunham, 1933; Silverman and Homan, 1949; Nyhan and

Fousek, 1958). Dunham observed that death was more frequent in the leukopenic group of infants. Silverman and Homan recorded one instance of a white cell count of less than 5000 in the 24 infants they studied, and Nyhan and Fousek found five of 74 infants to have white cell counts below 3000/cu. mm. *Escherichia coli* was the infectious agent in one of these patients and Group A *Streptococcus* in four, with one of these latter infants having a white cell count of 500/cu. mm. The well recognized association between Shigella enteritis and neutropenia in older infants has also been observed in the newborn (Levin, 1967).

Cyclic Neutropenia

Symptoms attributable to cyclic neutropenia have not been observed in the neonatal period, but they have been observed as early as two to three and one-half months of age (Sutton, 1911; Leale, 1910; Vahlquist, 1946). The disease is characterized by regular fluctuations in the neutrophil count, each cycle lasting about 14 to 21 days. At the time of extreme neutropenia, fever, malaise, oral ulcers, and cutaneous infections may occur. The report by Leale in 1910 is probably the first documented case of neutropenia in infancy. This patient was studied for 34 years until his death from pneumonia. He developed diabetes insipidus in his teens and continued to demonstrate cyclic fluctuations in his neutrophil count until his death (Thompson, 1934), although the constitutional symptoms associated with the neutropenia had disappeared (Reiman and Di Bernardino, 1949).

Neutropenia with Inborn Errors of Metabolism

In 1961, Childs and co-workers described an infant who became ill shortly after birth with a syndrome consisting of lethargy, vomiting, ketosis, neutropenia and periodic thrombocytopenia. The finding of increased amounts of glycine in the plasma and urine led to the designation of this syndrome as idiopathic hyperglycinemia. An almost identical clinical syndrome, methylmalonic acidemia, was described later by Oberholzer et al. (1967); neutropenia and periodic thrombocytopenia were common among the cases reported subsequently (Morrow et al., 1969). Bone marrow aspirates in these cases revealed decreased numbers of myeloid precursors.

Iso-valericacidemia, a disorder presenting at birth with similar clinical manifestations along with a "sweaty foot" odor to the skin, may also be associated with neutropenia as part of a general bone marrow hypoplasia (Allen et al., 1969). The hematologic abnormality in this infant was corrected by a diet low in leucine.

LYMPHOCYTES IN THE NEWBORN

General

Lymphocytes serve an important immunologic function. They represent the *cellular* component of the immune response, in contrast to the *humoral* component which is mediated by antibodies. Such cell-mediated functions include delayed hypersensitivity, homograft rejection and immunologic memory. The circulating small lymphocyte originates from a precursor stem cell in the bone marrow and consists of two types of cells: (1) the thymus dependent "T-lymphocyte", and (2) the bone marrow(or bursa)-derived "B-lymphocyte." The T-lymphocytes are involved with the cellular immune functions described above, whereas the B-lymphocytes (largely through differentiation into plasma cells) are concerned with antibody production. Although the two types of lymphocytes are morphologically indistinguishable it has been demonstrated recently that the B-lymphocyte is coated heavily with immunoglobulin whereas the T-lymphocyte has little or none. By such a technique it has been shown that in the normal adult T-lymphocytes comprise about 66 per cent of the total number and B-lymphocytes about 34 per cent (Wilson and Nossal, 1971).

In the fetus, lymphoid development appears during the first trimester and is associated with increasing cellular immune function as pregnancy advances. Since much of the data on the ontogeny of immunologic development in the fetus is based on animal studies, the precise relationship between anatomic and functional expressions of the immunity in the human fetus must remain conjectural. The thymus plays an important role in the development of the immune system, as illustrated by the lymphoid hypoplasia seen in neonatally thymectomized animals and in infants born with an absent or hypoplastic thymus.

Lymphopenia

An absolute lymphocyte count in the newborn below 1500/cu. mm. constitutes definite lymphopenia and requires further investigation. During this age period the commonest causes of lymphopenia are the hereditary thymic dysplasias; this subject has been reviewed by Rosen (1968). These disorders include the following:

    (1) Reticular dysgenesia — associated with complete aleukocytosis, including agranulocytosis. (See p. 327.)

    (2) Lymphopenic agammaglobulinemia

        (a) Autosomal recessive

          — Swiss type (Hitzig et al., 1965)

   — associated with short-limbed dwarfism (Gatti et al.,
     1969)
  (b) Sex-linked recessive (thymic alymphoplasia)
 (3) Lymphopenia with dysgammaglobulinemia or normogamma-
     globulinemia (Nezelov et al., 1964).

These infants usually present in the first few months of life with
failure to thrive, diarrhea, persistent oral (and occasionally generalized) moniliasis, and a tendency to severe infection by viral, bacterial
and fungal organisms that are ordinarily considered benign. Most
infants with this disorder die within the first year or two of life.

The finding of lymphopenia in an infant with the above clinical
picture should lead to appropriate immunologic investigation for
defects of both cellular and humoral immune function, in particular,
skin tests for delayed hypersensitivity, serum immunoglobulins, and
in vitro lymphocyte response to phytohemagglutinin stimulation.
Because of physiological impairment of these responses in the normal
newborn, interpretation of these tests may be difficult and require a
repeat study at a few months of age.

Because infants with lymphopenia are unable to reject foreign
immunocompetent cells they are prone to the development of a
graft-versus-host reaction from transfusion of blood containing viable
lymphocytes (Hathaway et al., 1965). Such reactions are characterized
by retardation of growth, hepatosplenomegaly, lymphoid atrophy,
diarrhea, dermatitis and aplastic anemia. A possible example of
graft-versus-host reaction was reported by us in an infant who received intrauterine transfusions for Rh erythroblastosis fetalis (Naiman et al., 1969); immaturity rather than congenital immunologic
deficiency was felt to be the predisposing mechanism.

Interestingly, lymphopenia is generally not observed in infants
with congenital *aplasia* of the thymus and parathyroids (DiGeorge,
1965), even though severe impairment of cellular immunity and
susceptibility to infections are present in such infants.

CONGENITAL ANOMALIES OF THE LEUKOCYTES

Some generalized disturbances are associated with characteristic
alterations in leukocyte morphology. Some inherited variations of
leukocyte morphology may be observed that appear to have no associated pathologic significance. Table 10–3 lists the more common
leukocyte abnormalities and their significance. Most of these disturbances have not been recognized during the newborn period. This
is probably because examination of peripheral blood smears is uncommon during this period of life.

Table 10–3 Anomalies of the Leukocytes

ANOMALY	APPEARANCE	ASSOCIATED FINDINGS
Increased numbers of nuclear projections of the neutrophils	15 per cent or more of the neutrophils contain 2 or more nuclear projections.	Trisomy for one of the chromosomes of the D group. See p. 331 for complete list of associated congenital anomalies.
The Pelger-Huet anomaly	Virtual absence of leukocytes containing more than 2 lobes.	Autosomal dominant inheritance. No associated disease.
The May-Hegglin anomaly	Leukocytes containing Döhle bodies. Giant platelets.	Thrombocytopenia may be present. Autosomal dominant inheritance.
Hereditary hypersegmentation of the neutrophils	Most neutrophilic leukocytes contain 4 or more lobes.	Autosomal dominant inheritance (Undritz, 1939). Must be distinguished from the hypersegmentation of the leukocytes observed in pernicious anemia.
The Chediak-Higashi anomaly	Multiple refractile gray-green inclusions in the leukocytes. Large red or blue inclusions in the lymphocytes.	Multiple pyogenic infections, albinism, hepatosplenomegaly, mental retardation, increased incidence of lymphoma.
Jordans' anomaly	Vacuoles in cytoplasm of granulocytes	One family with muscular dystrophy, another with ichthyosis.
Alder's anomaly	Increased numbers of coarse, dark azurophilic granules in the cytoplasm of the neutrophils.	No pathologic significance. Must be distinguished from toxic granulation. Inherited as an autosomal recessive.
Reilly bodies	Same as Alder's anomaly.	Observed in patients with gargoylism. In these patients lymphocytic inclusions and bone marrow granules of acid mucopolysaccharide may also be seen.

Trisomy 13 (D₁ Trisomy)

Trisomy for one of the chromosomes of the D group (chromosome 13) is associated with multiple congenital anomalies. These anomalies include: congenital heart defects; flexion deformities of the wrist, hand, and fingers; malformed ears; rocker-bottom feet; simian creases; hairlip or cleft palate; microphthalmia; coloboma; cataracts; umbilical hernia or omphalocele; malrotation of the midgut; genital abnormalities; cutaneous hemangiomas; and arhinencephaly (Smith et al., 1963).

The polymorphonuclear leukocytes of these infants contain an increased number of nuclear projections (Huehns et al., 1964). Although normal newborns may have more of these projections than adults, Walzer et al. (1966) feel that the finding of two or more pro-

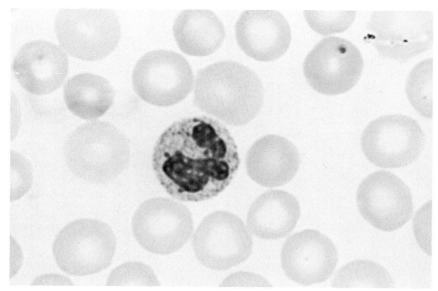

Figure 10–1 Neutrophils from patients with D₁ trisomy (× 5000). Neutrophils contain increased numbers of elongated projections.

jections in 15 per cent of the leukocytes is highly suggestive of D_1 trisomy (or D/D translocation). Figure 10–1 illustrates the numerous nuclear projections that may be observed in such patients. Such projections have also been described in patients with Turner's syndrome (Taylor, 1966) and partial C trisomy (Lutzner and Hecht, 1966), but not in children with trisomy 18 or trisomy 21 (Down's syndrome).

The Pelger-Huet Anomaly

The Pelger-Huet anomaly is a benign morphologic disorder that is inherited as an autosomal dominant. It is a defect in the process that normally results in the lobulation of the nuclei of the neutrophils. As a consequence, few, if any, of the mature neutrophils and none of the eosinophils have more than two lobes in their nuclei. The total leukocyte count, neutrophil count, neutrophil cell size, cytoplasm, and granular appearance are normal. It is world-wide in its distribution, and its incidence is estimated to vary between 1 in 1000 to 1 in 6000 (Davidson, 1961).

The anomaly persists throughout life and must be distinguished from a shift to the left with a predominance of metamyelocytes and myelocytes. It is easily distinguished from these more immature cells by the small size of its nucleus, the nature of the nuclear chromatin,

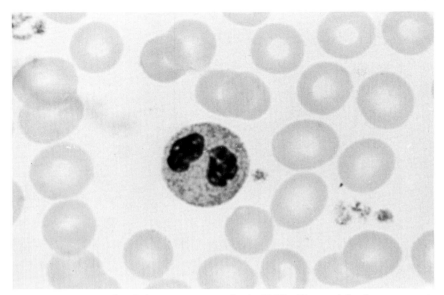

Figure 10–2 The Pelger-Huet anomaly (× 5000). Neutrophils do not contain more than two lobes despite their mature appearance.

and the appearance of the cytoplasmic granules (Fig. 10–2). When the disorder is suspected, it can easily be confirmed by demonstrating the same morphologic abnormality in one of the parents.

The May-Hegglin Anomaly

The May-Hegglin anomaly is characterized by Döhle bodies in the cytoplasm of the leukocytes in association with giant platelets. Thrombocytopenia may also be present. This disorder is inherited as an autosomal dominant.

With Wright's stain, Döhle bodies appear as sky blue areas in the leukocyte cytoplasm (Fig. 10–3). They are usually 1 to 2 μ in diameter. There is generally only one in a cell, but occasionally there may be more. These bodies are composed largely of ribonucleic acid. They may be observed transiently in patients with septicemia or burns, but when they are persistent and associated with giant platelets, May-Hegglin anomaly may be suspected. Diagnosis is confirmed by demonstrating similar morphologic abnormalities in one of the parents or in siblings. Döhle bodies are not to be confused with the cytoplasmic granules observed in the Chediak-Higashi syndrome (for comparative color photos, see Oski et al., 1962).

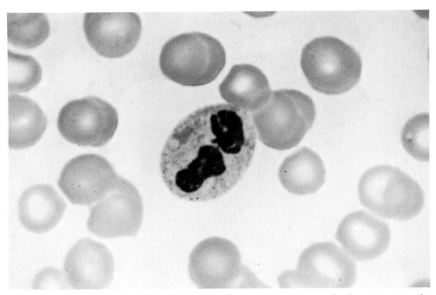

Figure 10–3 Döhle body in neutrophil of a patient with the May-Hegglin anomaly (× 5000). Döhle body is dark area in the cytoplasm.

The Chediak-Higashi Syndrome

In the Chediak-Higashi anomaly (Chediak, 1952; Higashi, 1954), the leukocytes contain bizarre giant peroxidase-positive granules. These granules appear refractile and stain greenish-gray with Wright's stain (Fig. 10–4). The lymphocytes may contain inclusions as well, generally single, and staining red or the color of the nuclear chromatin. The eosinophil granules are very large.

This disorder appears to be inherited as an autosomal recessive, and it is characterized by progressive impairment in the resistance to infection, partial or complete albinism, hepatosplenomegaly, lymphadenopathy, terminal leukopenia and thrombocytopenia, and varying degrees of mental retardation. These patients have an increased tendency to succumb to a peculiar form of lymphoma (Page and associates, 1962).

Jordans' Anomaly

The occurrence of lipid-containing vacuoles in the cytoplasm of the leukocytes of two brothers with muscular dystrophy was described by Jordans in 1953. Subsequently, similar vacuoles were described by Rozenszajn et al. (1966) in two sisters affected with ichthyosis. The significance of these associations remains unclear.

Vacuoles in the cytoplasm of neutrophils are common among

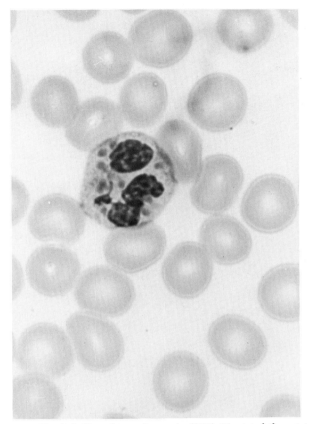

Figure 10–4   Chediak-Higashi syndrome (× 5000). Neutrophil contains numerous refractile inclusions in the cytoplasm.

patients with septicemia, presumably reflecting the end result of bacterial phagocytosis and digestion.

The Alder-Reilly Anomaly

This anomaly of the leukocytes, which makes the granules more prominent, was discovered independently by Alder (1939) and Reilly (1941). Reilly reported this disturbance in four of eight patients with gargoylism (Hurler-Pfaundler syndrome). This disorder of acid mucopolysaccharides results in the increased urinary excretion of chondroitin sulfuric acid B and heparin monosulfuric acid (Dorfman and Lorincz, 1957). It is associated with grotesque facies, hepatosplenomegaly, cardiac abnormalities, cloudy corneas, clawlike changes in the hands, and mental retardation.

Patients with Hurler's syndrome and other mucopolysaccharide storage diseases may demonstrate Reilly bodies in their leukocytes

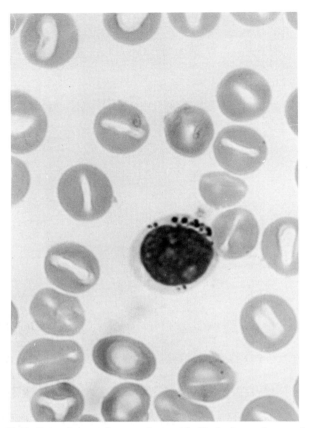

Figure 10–5   Lymphocyte from patient with Hurler's syndrome, demonstrating presence of cytoplasmic inclusions (× 5000).

(neutrophils and monocytes) or inclusions in their lymphocytes (Mittwoch, 1961); the latter are a more consistent finding in this group of disorders (Fig. 10–5). The mucopolysaccharide nature of these granules and inclusions may be demonstrated by a metachromatic stain such as toluidine blue. Pearson and Lorincz (1964) were able to demonstrate the presence of these mucopolysaccharide granules in the bone marrow of 17 of 18 patients with Hurler-Pfaundler syndrome after simple Wright-Giemsa staining, and they feel that this is the most reliable method for demonstrating the presence of this abnormality.

If the peripheral blood films of newborn infants are carefully examined, many of these disturbances may possibly be diagnosed before the infant leaves the nursery. Careful examination may also disclose presently unrecognized defects. The chances of finding something new in medicine are small, but they become infinitely smaller if one doesn't look.

Bibliography

AARSKOG, D.: Infantile congenital aneutrocytosis. Arch. Dis. Child., 36:511, 1961.

AASE, J. M., and SMITH, D. W.: Congenital anemia and triphalangeal thumbs. A new syndrome. J. Pediatrics, 74:471, 1969.

ABALLI, A.: The action of vitamin K in the neonatal period. South. Med. Jour., 58:48, 1965.

ABALLI, A. J., and DELAMERENS, S.: Coagulation changes in neonatal period and early infancy. Ped. Clin. North Am., 9:785, 1962.

ABALLI, A. J., LOPEZ BANUS, V., DELAMERENS, S., and ROZENGVAIG, S.: Coagulation studies in the newborn period. I. Alterations of thromboplastin generation and effects of vitamin K on full-term and premature infants. Am. J. Dis. Child., 94: 594, 1957.

ABALLI, A. J., PUAPONDH, Y., and DESPOSITO, F.: Platelet counts in thriving premature infants. Pediatrics, 42:685, 1968.

ABELSON, N. M., and RAWSON, A. J.:Studies of blood group antibodies. V. Fractionation of examples of anti-B, anti-A, B, anti-M, anti-P, anti-JK^a, anti-Le^a, anti-D, anti-CD, anti-K, anti-Fy^a, anti-S and anti-Good. Transfusion, 1:116, 1961.

ABILDGAARD, C. F.: Recognition and treatment of intravascular coagulation. J. Pediatrics, 74:163, 1969.

ABILDGAARD, H., and JENSEN, K. G.: The influence of maternal leucocyte antibodies on infants. Scand. J. Haemat., 1:47, 1964.

ABLIN, A. R., KUSHNER, J. H., MURPHY, A., and ZIPPIN, C.: Platelet enumeration in the newborn period. Pediatrics, 28:822, 1961.

ABRAHAMOV, A., and DIAMOND, L. K.: Reduction of oxygen-carrying capacity of Rh-positive erythrocytes coated with anti-D antibodies. Am. J. Dis. Child., 97:380, 1959.

ABRAHAMOV, A., and DIAMOND, L. K.: Erythrocyte glycolysis in erythroblastotic newborns. Am. J. Dis. Child., 99:202, 1960.

ABRAHAMOV, A., SALZBERGER, M., and BROMBERG, Y. M.: Fetal hemoglobin in postmature newborn infants. Am. J. Clin. Path., 26:146, 1956.

ABT, L., and DOWNEY, W. S., JR.: Melena neonatorum: the swallowed blood syndrome. J. Pediat., 47:6, 1955.

ACEVEDO, G., and MAUER, A. M.: The capacity for removal of erythrocytes containing Heinz bodies in premature infants and patients following splenectomy. J. Pediat., 63:61, 1963.

ACKERMAN, B. D.: Infantile pyknocytosis in Mexican-American infants. Am. J. Dis. Child., 117:417, 1969.

ACKERMAN, B. D., DYER, G. Y., and TAYLOR, P. M.: Decline in serum bilirubin concentration coincident with clinical onset of kernicterus. Pediat., 48:647, 1971.

ADLER, A.: Über konstitutionell bedingte Granulationsveränderungen der Leukozyten. Dtsch. Arch. Klin. Med., 183:372, 1939.

337

ADNER, M. M., FISCH, G. R., STAROBIN, S. G., and ASTER, R. H.: Use of "compatible" platelet transfusions in treatment of congenital isoimmune thrombocytopenia purpura. New Eng. J. Med., 280:244, 1969.

AGER, J. A. M., and LEHMANN, H.: Observations on some "fast" haemoglobins: K, J, N and "Bart's." Brit. Med. J., 1:929, 1958.

AGRESS, H., and DOWNEY, H.: Blood picture of human newborns, with special reference to lymphocytes. Folia Haemat., 55:207, 1936.

AHNQUIST, G., and HOLYOKE, J. B.: Congenital Letterer-Siwe disease (reticuloendotheliosis) in a term stillborn infant. J. Pediat., 57:897, 1960.

ALLEN, D. M., NECHELES, T. F., RIEKER, R., and SENIOR, B.: Reversible neonatal pancytopenia due to isovaleric acidemia. Abstract, Soc. Pediat. Res., Atlantic City, May, 1969, p. 156.

ALLEN, D. W., and JANDL, J. H.: Oxidative hemolysis and precipitation of hemoglobin. II. Role of thiols in oxidant drug action. J. Clin. Invest., 40:454, 1961.

ALLEN, D. W., SCHROEDER, W. A., and BALOG, J.: Observations on the chromatographic heterogeneity of normal adult and fetal hemoglobin. J. Amer. Chem. Soc., 80:1628, 1958.

ALLEN, D. W., WYMAN, J., JR., and SMITH, C. A.: The oxygen equilibrium of fetal and adult hemoglobin. J. Biol. Chem., 203:81, 1953.

ALLEN, F. H., JR.: Attempts at prevention of intrauterine death in erythroblastosis fetalis. New Eng. J. Med., 269:1344, 1963.

ALLEN, F. H., JR., and DIAMOND, L. K.: Erythroblastosis Fetalis. Boston, Little, Brown and Company, 1957.

ALLEN, F. H., JR., DIAMOND, L. K., and JONES, A. R.: Erythroblastosis fetalis. IX. Problems of stillbirth. New Eng. J. Med., 251:453, 1954.

ALLEN, F. H., JR., DIAMOND, L. K., and VAUGHAN, V. C., III.: Erythroblastosis fetalis. VI. Prevention of kernicterus. Am. J. Dis. Child., 80:779, 1950.

ALLISON, A. C.: Acute haemolytic anemia with distortion and fragmentation of erythrocytes in children. Brit. J. Haemat., 3:1, 1957.

ALTHOFF, H., DAHM, P., and WERNER, H.: Presence of erythropoetin in umbilical cord blood. Arch. Kindherh., 157:238, 1958.

ANDERSON, G. W.: Studies on nucleated red cell count in chorionic capillaries and cord blood of various ages of pregnancy. Am. J. Obst. Gynec., 42:1, 1941.

ANDERSON, J., MARKS, V., TOMLINSON, R. W. S., and WALKER, W.: Changes in the blood concentration of glucose, α-oxyglutarate, pyruvate and citrate during exchange transfusion in haemolytic disease of the newborn. Arch. Dis. Child., 38:481, 1963.

ANDRE, R., DUCAS, P., VERGOZ, D., and MAYER, M.: Purpura thrombopenique neonatal thrombopenie maternelle cliniquement latente. Arch. Franç. de Pediat., 22:167, 1965.

ANDREWS, B. F., and FALKNER, F.: Fetal hemoglobin synthesis in fraternal and identical twins. Biol. neonat., 12:23, 1968.

ANDREWS, B. F., and THOMPSON, J. W.: Materno-fetal transfusion. A common phenomenon. Pediatrics, 29:500, 1962.

ANDREWS, B. F., and WILLET, G. P.: Fetal hemoglobin concentration in the newborn. Am. J. Obst. Gynec., 91:85, 1965.

ANDREWS, J. P., McCLELLAN, J. T., and SCOTT, C. H.: Lethal congenital neutropenia with eosinophilia occurring in two siblings. Am. J. Med., 29:358, 1960.

ANSELMINO, K. T., and HOFFMAN, F.: Die ursachen des icterus neonatorum. Arch. Gynäk., 143:477, 1930.

ANTHONY, B., and KRIVIT, W.: Neonatal thrombocytopenic purpura. Pediatrics, 30: 776, 1962.

APPLEYARD, W. J., and BRINTON, A.: Venous platelet counts in low birth weight infants. Biol. Neonate 17:30, 1971.

ARCILLA, R. A., OH, W., LIND, J., and BLANKENSHIP, W.: Portal and atrial pressures in the newborn period. Acta Paed. Scand., 55:615, 1966.

ARIAS, I. M., WOLFSON, S., LUCEY, J. F., and McKAY, R. J.: Transient familial neonatal hyperbilirubinemia. J. Clin. Invest., 44:1442, 1965.

ARMSTRONG, D. H., SCHROEDER, W. A., and FENNINGER, W. D.: A comparison of the percentage of fetal hemoglobin in human umbilical cord blood as determined by chromatography and by alkali denaturation. Blood, 22:554, 1963.

ASCARI, W. Q., LEVINE, P., and POLLOCK, W.: Incidence of maternal Rh immunization by ABO compatible and incompatible pregnancies. Brit. Med. J., 1:399, 1967.

ASTER, R. H., and JANDL, J. H.: Platelet sequestration in man. II. Immunological and clinical studies. J. Clin. Invest., 43:856, 1964.

ATA, M., FISHER, O. D., and HOLMAN, C. A.: Inherited thrombocytopenia. Lancet, 1:119, 1965.

AUSSANNAIRE, M., JOLY, C., and POHLMANN, A.: Méthémoglobinémie acquise du nourrisson par cau de canalisation urbaine. La presse med., 76:1723, 1968.

AUSTIN, R. F., and DESFORGES, J. F.: Hereditary elliptocytosis: An unusual presentation of hemolysis in the newborn associated with transient morphologic abnormalities. Pediatrics, 44:196, 1969.

AVERY, M. E., OPPENHEIMER, E. H., and GORDON, H. H.: Renal-vein thrombosis in newborn infants of diabetic mothers. New Eng. J. Med., 256:1134, 1957.

BAAR, H. S.: Foetal haemoglobin and erythroblastosis. Nature, 162:190, 1948.

BAAR, H. S., BAAR, S., ROGERS, K. B., and STRANSKY, E.: *Disorders of Blood and Blood-Forming Organs in Childhood.* New York, Hafner Publishing Co., 1963.

BAEHNER, R. L., and NATHAN, D. G.: Quantitative nitroblue tetrazolium test in chronic granulomatous disease. New Eng. J. Med., 278:971, 1968.

BAEHNER, R. L., and STRAUSS, H. S.: Hemophilia in the first year of life. New Eng. Jour. Med., 275:524, 1966.

BAIN, A. D., BOWIE, J. H., FLINT, W. F., BEVERLEY, J. K. A., and BEATTIE, C. P.: Congenital toxoplasmosis simulating haemolytic disease of the newborn. J. Obst. Gynaec. Brit. Emp., 63:826, 1956.

BAIN, G. O., WANG, G. C., and MISANIK, L. F.: Giant cell hepatitis associated with hereditary spherocytosis. J. Pediat., 51:549, 1957.

BAJPAI, P. C., SUGDEN, D., STERN, L., and DENTON, R. L.: Serum ionic magnesium in exchange transfusion. J. Pediat., 70:193, 1967.

BAKER, H., FRANK, O., PASTER, E., ZIFFER, H., and SOBOTKA, H.: Pantothenic acid, thiamine and folic acid levels at parturition. Proc. Soc. Exp. Biol. Med., 103:321, 1960.

BAKER, H., ZIFFER, H., PASKER, I., and SOBOTKA, H.: A comparison of maternal and foetal folic acid and vitamin B_{12} at parturition. Brit. Med. J., 1:978, 1958.

BAKKEN, A. F.: Effects of unconjugated bilirubin on bilirubin-UDP-glucuronyl transferase activity in liver of newborn rats. Pediat. Res., 3:205, 1969.

BAKKEN, A. F., and FOG, J.: Bilirubin conjugation in the newborn. Lancet, 1:1280, 1967.

BAKWIN, H., and MORRIS R.: The leukocyte count in the new-born with dehydration fever. Am. J. Dis. Child., 26:23, 1923.

BALDINI, M., KIM, B., STEINER, M., KURAMOTO, A., OKUMA, M., and OTRIDGE, B. W.: Metabolic platelet defect in the Wiskott-Aldrich syndrome. Pediat. Res., 3:377, 1969.

BANATVALA, J. E., HORSTMANN, D. M., PAYNE, M. C., and GLUCK, L.: Rubella syndrome and thrombocytopenic purpura in newborn infants: clinical and virologic observations. New Eng. J. Med., 273:474, 1965.

BANTON, A. H.: The development of Mediterranean anaemia. Arch. Dis. Child., 26:235, 1951.

BARD, H., MAKOWSKI, E. L., MESCHIA, G., and BATTAGLIA, F. C.: The relative rates of synthesis of hemoglobins A and F in immature red cells of newborn infants. Pediatrics, 45:766, 1970.

BARRETT, C. T., and OLIVER, T. K., JR.: Hypoglycemia and hyperinsulinism with erythroblastosis fetalis. New Eng. J. Med., 278:1260, 1968.

BARRIE, H.: pH changes in exchange transfusion (letter). Lancet, 2:476, 1964.

BARRIE, H.: Acid-base control during exchange transfusion. Lancet, 2:712, 1965.

BARRY, A., and DELAGE, J. M.: Congenital deficiency of fibrin stabilizing factor: observation of a new case. New Eng. J. Med., 272:943, 1965.

BAR-SHANY, S., and HERBERT, V.: Transplacentally acquired antibody to intrinsic factor with vitamin B_{12} deficiency. Blood, 30:777, 1967.

BARTOS, H. R., and DESFORGES, J. F.: Erythrocyte DPNH dependent diaphorase levels in infants. Pediatrics, 37:991, 1966.

BATSON, R., SHAPIRO, M., and CHRISTIE, A.: Acute non-lipid disseminated reticuloendotheliosis. Am. J. Dis. Child., 90:323, 1955.

BAUER, C., LUDWIG, I., and LUDWIG, M.: Different effects of 2,3-diphosphoglycerate and adenosine triphosphate on oxygen affinity of adult and fetal human hemoglobin. Life Sci., 7:1339, 1968.

BAUGHAN, M. A., VALENTINE, W. N., PAGLIA, D. E., WAYS, P. O., SIMONS, E. R., and DeMARSH, Q. B.: Hereditary hemolytic anemia associated with glucosephosphate isomerase (GPI) deficiency—a new enzyme defect of human erythrocytes. Blood, 32:236, 1968.

BAUKE, J., CREMER, H. J., and HEIMPEL, H.: Kongenitale myelo-monocytäre leukämie mit aneuploider stammlinie. Z. Kinderheilk., 108:288, 1970.

BAUM, R. S.: Hyperviscous blood and perinatal pathology. Program Amer. Ped. Society, 1967, p. 1.

BAYER, W. L., SHERMAN, F. E., MICHAELS, R. H., SZETO, I. L. F., and LEWIS, J. H.: Purpura in congenital and acquired rubella. New Eng. J. Med., 273:1362, 1965.

BEAVEN, G. H., ELLIS, M. J., and WHITE, J. C.: Studies on human foetal haemoglobin. I. Detection and estimation. Brit. J. Haemat., 6:1, 1960.

BEAVEN, G. H., ELLIS, M. J., and WHITE, J. C.: Studies on human foetal haemoglobin. II. Foetal haemoglobin levels in healthy children and adults and in certain haematologic disorders. Brit. J. Haemat., 6:201, 1960.

BEAZLEY, J. M.: Maternal complications of Rhesus iso-immunization. Brit. Med. J., 2:919, 1965.

BECK, J. S., and ROWELL, N. R.: Transplacental passage of antinuclear antibody. Lancet, 1:134, 1963.

BECKER, A. H., and GLASS, H.: Twin to twin transfusion syndrome. Am. J. Dis. Child., 106:624, 1963.

BECKETT, R. S., and FLYNN, F. J., JR.: Toxoplasmosis: report of two new cases, with a classification and with a demonstration of the organisms in the human placenta. New Eng. J. Med., 249:345, 1953.

BEHRMAN, R. E., and HSIA, D. Y. Y.: Summary of a symposium on phototherapy for hyperbilirubinemia. J. Pediat., 75:718, 1969.

BEHRMAN, R. E., SIGLER, A. T., and PATCHEFSKY, A. S.: Abnormal hematopoiesis in 2 of 3 siblings with mongolism. J. Pediat., 68:569, 1966.

BELL, A. D., MOLD, J. W., OLIVER, R. A., and SHAW, S.: Study of transfused platelets in a case of congenital hypoplastic thrombocytopenia. Brit. Med. J., 2:692, 1956.

BENCZE, G., KOVÁCS, J., and CSERHÁTI, J.: Two types of lupus erythematosus cell factor shown by induced L.D. cell phenomenon in man. Brit. Med. J., 2:864, 1959.

BENESCH, R. E., and BENESCH, R.: Relation between erythrocyte integrity and sulfhydryl groups. Arch. Biochem., 48:38, 1954.

BENESCH, R., and BENESCH, R. E.: The effect of organic phosphates from the human erythrocyte on the allosteric properties of hemoglobin. Biochem. Biophys. Res. Commun., 26:162, 1967.

BENESCH, R., BENESCH R. E., and YU, C. I.: Reciprocal binding of oxygen and diphosphoglycerate by human hemoglobin. Proc. Nat. Acad. Sci., 59:526, 1968.

BENIRSCHKE, K.: Accurate recording of twin placenta. Obst. Gynec., 18:334, 1961.

BENTLEY, H. P., JR., ALFORD, C. A., JR., and DISEKER, M.: Erythrocyte glucose consumption in the neonate. J. Lab. Clin. Med., 76:311, 1970.

BERGE, T., BRUNNHAGE, F., and NILSSON, L. R.: Congenital hypoplastic thrombocytopenia in rubella embryopathy. Acta Paediat., 52:349, 1963.

BERGHINZ, G.: Lymphosarcomatosis of mother and metastases in fetus (abstract). J.A.M.A., 34:1588, 1900.

BERGSTEDT, J.: Monozygotic twins, one with high erythrocyte values and jaundice, the other with anemia neonatorum and no jaundice. Acta Paediat., 46:201, 1957.

BERGSTRAND, C. G., CZAR, B., TARUKOSKI, P. H., and FIIRST, P.: Factors influencing the serum haptoglobin level in infancy. Acta Paediat., Suppl. 135:21, 1962.

BERNARD, J., CHAVELET, F., and JACQUILLAT, C.: Leucémies du nouveau—né (À propos de 4 observations). Nouv. Rev. Franc. Hémat., 4:125, 1964.

BERNARD, J., JACQUILLAT, C., CHAVALET, F., BOIRON, M., STOITCHKOV, Y., and TANZER, J.: Leucémie aiguë d'une enfant de 5 mois née d'une mère atteinte de leucémie aiguë au moment de l'accouchement. Nouv. Rev. Franc. Hémat., 4:140–146, 1964.

BERNARD, J., SELIGMANN, M., CHASSIGNEUX, J., and DRESCH, C.: Anémie de Blackfan-Diamond. Nouv. Rev. Franc. Hémat., 2:721, 1962.

BERNHARD, W. G., GORE, I., and KILBY, R. A.: Congenital leukemia. Blood, 6:990, 1951.

BERNSTEIN, J., and BROWN, A. K.: Sepsis and jaundice in early infancy. Pediatrics, 29:873, 1962.

BERNSTEIN, R. E.: Alterations in metabolic energetics and cation transport during aging of red cells. J. Clin. Invest., 38:1572, 1959.

BERTLES, J. F.: Sodium transport across the surface membrane of red blood cells in hereditary spherocytosis. J. Clin. Invest., 36:816, 1957.

BERTOYE, A., CARRON, R., FREDERICK, A., HORTEMANN, E., COTTE, M. F., and COTTON, J. B.: Polyglobulie neonatale et hypernatremie transitoire. Pediatrie, 19:703, 1964.

BETKE, K.: Vergleichende Untersuchung der Oxydation von Fetalem und Erwach-senen-Oxyhämoglobin durch Natriumnitrit. Naturwissenschaften, 40:60, 1953.

BETKE, K., BALTZ, A., and MAAS, V.: Utilisation von Galaktose durch Erythrocyten minochilcher Neugelborener. Ztschr. Kinderh., 84:226, 1960.

BETKE, K., DIEBEL, R., and SCHLICHT, I.: Anemia neonatorum bei einem Zwelling durch Blutverschiebung in den anderen Zwelling. Mschr. Kinderh., 106:468, 1958.

BETKE, K., KLEIHAUER, E., GÄRTNER, C., and SCHIEBE, G.: Verminderung von Methämoglobinreduktion, Diaphorasektivität und Flavinen in Erythrozyten junger Säuglinge. Arch. Kinderh., 170:66, 1964.

BEUTLER, E.: A series of new screening procedures for pyruvate kinase deficiency, glucose-6-phosphate dehydrogenase deficiency, and glutathione reductase de-ficiency. Blood, 28:553, 1966.

BEUTLER, E.: Drug-induced hemolytic anemia. Pharmacol. Rev., 21:73, 1969.

BEUTLER, E. (ED.): Hereditary Disorders of Erythrocyte Metabolism. New York, Grune & Stratton, 1969.

BEUTLER, E., and BALUDA, M. C.: The separation of glucose-6-phosphate dehydro-genase—deficient erythrocytes from the blood of heterozygotes for glucose-6-phosphate dehydrogenase deficiency. Lancet, 1:189, 1964.

BEVIS, D. C. A.: Blood pigments in haemolytic disease of the newborn. J. Obst. Gynaec. Brit. Emp., 63:68, 1956.

BIGGS, R., and DOUGLAS, A. S.: The thromboplastin generation test. J. Clin. Path., 6:23, 1953.

BIGGS, R., and MACFARLANE, R. G.: Human Blood Coagulation. 4th Ed., Oxford, Blackwell, 1966.

BILLING, B. H., and LATHE, G. H.: The excretion of bilirubin as an ester glucuronide, giving the direct van den Bergh reaction. Biochem. J., 63:6p, 1956.

BIRDSONG, M., SMITH, D. E., MITCHELL, F. N., and COREY, J. H.: Generalized cyto-megalic inclusion disease in newborn infants. J.A.M.A., 162:1305, 1956.

BIRNBAUM, G., LYNCH, J. I., MARGILETH, A. M., LONERGAN, W. M., and SEVER, J. L.: Cytomegalovirus infections in newborn infants. J. Pediatrics, 75:789, 1969.

BITHELL, T. C., DIDISHEIM, P., CARTWRIGHT, G. E., and WINTROBE, M. M.: Throm-bocytopenia inherited as an autosomal dominant trait. Blood, 25:231, 1965.

BLEYER, W. A., and BRECKENRIDGE, R. T.: Studies in the detection of adverse drug reactions in the newborn. II. The effects of prenatal aspirin on newborn hemos-tasis. J.A.M.A., 213:2049, 1970.

BLEYER, W. A., AU, W. Y., LANGE, W. A., SR., and RAISZ, L. G.: Studies on the detection of adverse drug reactions in the newborn. I. Fetal exposure to maternal medication. J.A.M.A., 213:2046, 1970.

BLEYER, W. A., HAKAMI, N., and SHEPARD, T. H.: The development of hemostasis in the human fetus and newborn infant. J. Pediat. 79:838, 1971.

BLONDHEIM, S. H.: The relationship between albumin concentration of serum and its dye-binding capacity. J. Lab. Clin. Med., 45:740, 1955.

BLOOM, G. E., WARNER, S., GERALD, P. S., and DIAMOND, L. K.: Chromosome abnor-malities in constitutional aplastic anemia. New Eng. J. Med., 274:8, 1966.

BLOOM, W., and BARTELMEZ, G. W.: Hematopoiesis in young human embryos. Am. J. Anat., 67:21, 1940.

BLUM, S. F., and OSKI, F. A.: Red cell metabolism in the newborn infant. IV. Trans-membrane potassium flux. Pediatrics, 43:396, 1969.

BODIAN, M., SHELDON, W., and LIGHTWOOD, R.: Congenital hypoplasia of the exocrine pancreas. Acta Paediat., 53:282, 1964.

BOGER, W. P., BAYNE, G. M., WRIGHT, L. D., and BECK, G. D.: Differential serum vitamin B_{12} concentrations in mothers and infants. New Eng. J. Med., 256:1085, 1957.

BOGGS, T. R., JR.: Proper place of intrauterine transfusions in management of fetuses with Rh hemolytic disease. Clin. Pediat., 9:636, 1970.

BOGGS, T. R., JR.: Survival rates in Rh sensitizations. 140 interrupted versus 141 uninterrupted pregnancies. Pediatrics, 33:758, 1964.

BOGGS, T. R., JR., and JOHNSON, L.: Unpublished observations. Personal communication, 1971.

BOGGS, T. R., and WESTPHAL., M. C.: Mortality of exchange transfusion. Pediatrics, 26:745, 1960.

BOINEAU, F. G. and HALLOCK, J. A.: Two examples of severe fetal disease due to ABO incompatibility. Clin. Pediat., 10:180, 1971.

BOIVIN, P., and GALAND, C.: Recherche d'une anomalie moléculaire lors des déficits en pyruvate kinase érythrocytaire. Nouv. Rev. Franç. d'Hemat., 8:201, 1968.

BOIVIN, P., GALAND, C., ANDRE, R., and DEBRAY, J.: Anémies hémolytiques congénitales avec déficit isolé en glutathion réduct par déficit en glutathion synthétase. Nouv. Rev. Franç. Hemat., 6:859, 1966.

BOIVIN, P., GALAND, C., HAKIM, J., and BLERY, M.: Déficit en glutathion-peroxydase erythrocytaire et anémie hémolytique médicamenteuse. La Presse Med., 78:171, 1970.

BOIVIN, P., GALAND, C., HAKIM, J., ROGE, J., and GUEROULT, N.: Anémie hémolytique avec déficit en glutathion-peroxydase chez un adulte. Enzymol. Biol. Clin., 10:68, 1969.

BOIVIN, P., GALAND, C., HAKIM, J., SIMONY, D., and SELIGMAN, M.: Anémie hémolytique congénitale non sphérocytaire et déficit héréditaire en adénylate-kinase érythrocytaire. La Presse Med., 79:215, 1971.

BOOKER, C. R., SCOTT, R. B., and FERGUSON, A. D.: Clinical manifestations of sickle cell anemia during the first two years of life. Clin. Pediat., 3:111, 1964.

BORRONE, C.: Porpora trombopenica associata a leucopenia e anemia in prematuro. Probabili rapporti con l'abuso di Optalidon in gravidanza. Minerva Pediat., 13:132, 1961.

BORST-EILERS, E.: The foetal origin of red cells staining with Kleihauer's technique, as established by the application of the "mixed agglutination" reaction on those cells. Vox Sang., 6:451, 1961.

BOSMA, J. F.: Autotransfusion between two twins. Am. J. Dis. Child., 88:509, 1954.

BOSSU, M., DACHÀ, M. and FORNAINI, G.: Neonatal hemolysis due to a transient severity of inherited pyruvate kinase deficiency. Acta Haem., 40:166, 1968.

BOUND, J. P., HARVEY, P. W., and BAGSHAW, H. B.: Prevention of pulmonary syndrome of the newborn. Lancet, 1:1200, 1962.

BOUTON, M. J., PHILLIPS, H. J., SMITHELLS, R. W., and WALKER, S.: Congenital leukemia with parental consanguinity. Case report with chromosome studies. Brit. Med. J., 2:866, 1961.

BOWDLER, A. J., and PRANKERD, T. A. J.: Studies in congenital non-spherocytic haemolytic anaemias with specific enzyme defects. Acta Haemat., 31:65, 1964.

BOWIE, E. J. W., THOMPSON, J. H., JR., and OWEN, C. A., JR.: The blood platelet (including a discussion of the qualitative platelet diseases). Proc. Mayo Clin., 40:625, 1965.

BOWMAN, H. S., and PROCOPIO, F.: Hereditary non-spherocytic hemolytic anemia of pyruvate kinase deficient type. Ann. Int. Med., 58:567, 1963.

BOWMAN, J. D., and FRIESEN, R. F.: Hemolytic disease of the newborn, in Gellis, S. S. and Kagan, B. M., eds., Current Pediatric Therapy, Vol. 4, Philadelphia, W. B. Saunders Co., 1970, p. 405.

BOWMAN, J. M.: Rh prevention, Manitoba, 1969. Manitoba Medical Review (Oct. 1969), 14.

BOWMAN, J. M., and FRIESEN, R. F.: Multiple intraperitoneal transfusions of the fetus for erythroblastosis fetalis. New Eng. J. Med., 271:703, 1964.

BOWMAN, J. M., and POLLACK, J. M.: Amniotic fluid spectrophotometry and early delivery in the management of erythroblastosis fetalis. Pediatrics, 35:815, 1965.

BOWMAN, J. M., CHOWN, B., LEWIS, M., KAITA, H., PEDDLE, L. J., and POLLOCK, J. M.: Rh immunization of primigravidae. Abstract, Amer. Pediat. Soc., Atlantic City, May, 1969, p. 20.

Bowman, J. M., Friesen, R. F., Bowman, W. D., McInnis, A. C., Barnes, P. H., and Grewar, D.: Fetal transfusion in severe Rh isoimmunization. J.A.M.A., 207:1101, 1969.

Bracci, R.: Il deficit de glutatione-perossidasi eritrocitaria nel neonate con malattia emolitica. Minerva Pediat., 20:2692, 1968.

Bracci, R., Corvaglia, E., Princi, P., Bettini, F., and Pindinelli, C.: The role of GSH-peroxidase deficiency in the increased susceptibility to Heinz body formation in the erythrocytes of newborn infants. Ital. J. Biochem., 18:100, 1969.

Bracci, R., Seeler, R., Rudolph, N., Kochen, J. A., and Gross, R. T.: Erythrocyte glutathione peroxidase activity and hydrogen peroxide sensitivity: mechanism for drug induced hemolysis in newborn. Society for Pediatric Research, Philadelphia, May, 1965.

Bracco, G.: Potere fagocitario del sangue placentare fetali. Gior. Balleriol. Immunol., 38:449, 1948.

Bratlid, D. and Fog, J.: The binding capacity of human albumin for bilirubin and its significance in the pathogenesis of kernicterus. Scand. J. Clin. Lab. Invest., 25:257, 1970.

Bratteby, L. E.: Studies on erythrokinetics in infancy. Acta Paediat. Scand., 57:125, 1968.

Bratteby, L. E., Garby, L., and Wadman, B.: Studies on erythrokinetics in infancy. XII. Acta Paediat. Scand., 57:305, 1968.

Braun, E. H., Buckwold, A. E., Emson, H. E., Russell, A. V.: Familial neonatal neutropenia with maternal leucocyte antibodies. Blood, 16:1745, 1960.

Brazie, J. V., Bowes, W. A., Jr., and Ibbot, F. A.: An improved, rapid procedure for the determination of amniotic fluid bilirubin and its use in the prediction of the course of Rh-sensitized pregnancies. Am. J. Obst. Gynec., 104:80, 1969.

Breathnach, C. S.: Red cell diameters in human cord and neonatal blood. Quart. J. Exp. Physiol., 47:148–56, 1962.

Brecher, G., and Cronkite, E. P.: Morphology and enumeration of human blood platelets. J. Appl. Physiol., 3:365, 1950.

Brecher, G., Schneiderman, M., and Cronkite, E. P.: Reproducibility and constancy of platelet count. Am. J. Clin. Path., 23:15, 1953.

Brewer, G. J., Tarlov, A. R., and Alving, A. S.: Methemoglobin reduction test: a new simple, in vitro test for identifying primaquine sensitivity. Bull. W.H.O., 22:633, 1960.

Brewer, G. J., Tarlov, A. R., and Kellermeyer, R. W.: The hemolytic effect of primaquine: XII. Shortened erythrocyte life span in primaquine sensitive male Negroes in the absence of drug administration. J. Lab. Clin. Med., 58:217, 1961.

Bridge, R. G., and Foley, F. E.: Placental transmission of the lupus erythematosus factor. Am. J. Med. Sci., 227:1, 1954.

Bridges, J. M., and Carré, I. J.: Congenital thrombocytopenia purpura treated by exchange transfusion. Arch. Dis. Child., 36:210, 1961.

Brin, M., and Yonemoto, R. H.: Stimulation of glucose oxidative pathway in human erythrocytes by methylene blue. J. Biol. Chem., 230:307, 1958.

Brines, J. K., Gibson, J. G., Jr., and Kunkel, P.: Blood volume in normal infants and children. J. Pediat., 18:447, 1941.

Brinkhous, K. M., Smith, H. P., and Warner, E. D.: Plasma prothrombin level in normal infancy and in hemorrhagic disease of the newborn. Am. J. Med. Sci., 193:475, 1937.

Britten, A. F. H.: Congenital deficiency of Factor XIII (fibrin-stabilizing factor). Am. J. Med., 43:751, 1967.

Brizel, H. E., and Raccuglia, G.: Giant hemangioma with thrombocytopenia: radioisotopic demonstration of platelet sequestration. Blood, 26:751, 1965.

Brodsky, I., Baren, M., Kahn, S. B., Lewis, G., Jr., and Tellum, M.: Metastatic malignant melanoma from mother to fetus. Cancer, 18:1048, 1965.

Brody, N. I., Walker, J. G., and Siskind, G. W.: Studies on the control of antigenic competition and suppression of antibody formation by passive antibody on the immune response. J. Exp. Med., 126:81, 1967.

Brody, S.: Further studies on the reliability of a new method for the determination of the duration of pregnancy. J. Obst. Gynaec. Brit. Emp., 67:819, 1960.

BRODY, S., and ENGSTROM, L.: Foetal and adult haemoglobin in newborn infants with erythroblastosis fetalis. Acta Paediat., 49: 868, 1960.

BRODY, S., and NILSSON, B.: Foetal and adult haemoglobin mass in relation to foetal development. J. Obst. Gynaec. Brit. Emp., 67:827, 1960.

BROMBERG, Y. M.: Serial determinations of foetal haemoglobin; method and value of determination during replacement transfusions. Obst. Gynec., 6:604, 1955.

BROMBERG, Y. M., ABRAHAMOV, A., and SALZBERGER, M.: The effect of maternal anoxemia on the foetal haemoglobin of the newborn. J. Obst. Gynaec. Brit. Emp., 63: 875, 1956.

BROWAEYS, J., and PLEY, J.: Hématologie d'un prématuré agranulocytose maternelle. Sang, 21:826, 1950.

BROWN, A. K.: Bilirubin metabolism with special reference to neonatal jaundice. Adv. Pediat., 12:121, 1962.

BROWN, A. K.: Erythrocyte metabolism and hemolysis in the newborn. Ped. Clin. N. A., 13:879, 1966.

BROWN, A. K., and ZUELZER, W. W.: Studies on the neonatal development of the glucuronide conjugating system. J. Clin. Invest., 37:332, 1958.

BROWN, C. M., and NATHAN, B. J.: Maternal rubella and congenital defects. Lancet, 1:975, 1954.

BROWN, W. R., and WONG, H. B.: Ethnic group differences in plasma bilirubin levels of full-term healthy Singapore infants. Pediatrics, 41:1055, 1965.

BRUNELLI, A., and FLAUTO, U.: Contributo alla conoscenza del contenuto polisaccaridico leucocitario nel neonato normale. Minerva Pediat., 15:445, 1963.

BRUNETTI, P., and NENCI, G.: A screening method for the detection of erythrocyte pyruvate kinase deficiency. Enzymol. Biol. Clin., 4:51, 1964.

BUCHANAN, D. I., BELL, R. E., BECK, R. P., and TAYLOR, W. C.: Use of different doses of anti-Rh IgG in the prevention of Rh isoimmunization. Lancet, 2:288, 1969.

BUHLER, M., and LANDOLT, R.: Kongenitale Leukämie. Helv. Paediat. Acta, 25:176, 1970.

BULLOCK, J. D., ROBERTSON, A. F., BODENBENDER, J. G., KONTRAS, S. B., and MILLER, C. E.: Inflammatory response in the neonate re-examined. Pediat., 44:58, 1969.

BÜNGELER, W.: Angeborene leukämie. Frankfurt. Ztschr. Path., 41:257, 1931.

BÜNGELER, W.: Verh. Dtsch. Ges. Path., 37:231, 1954 (Cited by Kauffman, H. J., and Hess, R. Brit. Med. J., 1:867, 1962).

BURKE, V., COLEBATCH, J. H., ANDERSON, C. M., and SIMONS, M. J.: Association of pancreatic insufficiency and chronic neutropenia of childhood. Arch. Dis. Childh., 42:147, 1967.

BURMAN, D.: Congenital spherocytosis in infancy. J. Pediat., 50:446, 1957.

BURMAN, D.: Red cell cholinesterase in infancy and childhood. Arch. Dis. Child., 36: 362, 1961.

BURRELL, J. M.: A comparative study of the circulating eosinophil levels in babies. Arch. Dis. Child., 27:337, 1952.

BUTLER, E. A., FLYNN, F. V., and HUEHNS, E. R.: The haemoglobin of foetal blood. Clin. Chim. Acta, 5:571, 1960.

CADE, J. F., HIRSH, J., and MARTIN, M.: Placental barrier to coagulation factors: Its relevance to the coagulation defect at birth and to haemorrhage in the newborn. Brit. Med. J., 1:281, 1969.

CALLADINE, M., and GAIRDNER, D.: pH changes in exchange transfusion. Lancet, 2:477, 1964.

CALLAHAN, W. P., RUSSELL, W. O., and SMITH, M. G.: Human toxoplasmosis. Medicine, 25:343, 1946.

CAMPBELL, W. A. B., MACAFEE, A. L., and WADE, W. G.: Familial neonatal leukemia. Arch. Dis. Child., 37:93, 1962.

CANALES, L., and MAUER, A. M.: Sex-linked hereditary thrombocytopenia as a variant of Wiskott-Aldrich syndrome. New Eng. J. Med., 277:899, 1967.

CAPPS, F. P. A., GILLES, H. M., and WORLLEDGE, S. M.: Glucose-6-phosphate dehydrogenase deficiency and neonatal jaundice in Nigeria. Lancet, 2:379, 1963.

CARSON, P. E., and FRISCHER, H.: Glucose-6-phosphate dehydrogenase deficiency and related disorders of the pentose phosphate pathway. Amer. J. Med., 41:744, 1966.

CARSON, P. E., BREWER, G. J., and ICKES, C.: Decreased glutathione reductase with susceptibility to hemolysis (abstract). J. Lab. Clin. Med., 58:804, 1961.

CARSON, P. E., FLANAGAN, C. L., ICKES, C. E., and ALVING, A. S.: Enzymatic deficiency in primaquine-sensitive erythrocytes. Science, 124:484, 1956.

CARSON, P. E., and TARLOV, A. R.: Biochemistry of hemolysis. Ann. Rev. Med., 13: 105, 1962.

CARUSO, P., CONTI, F., and LONDRILLO, A.: Diagramma delle attività Enzimaticke endoeritrocitarie nel neonato, nel lattante, nel bambino. Minerva Pediat., 15: 1136, 1963.

CASSADY, G.: Plasma volume studies in low birth weight infants. Pediatrics, 38:1020, 1966.

CATHIE, I. A. B.: Apparent idiopathic Heinz-body anemia. Gt. Ormond St. J., 3:43, 1952.

CAUCHI, M. N., CLEGG, J. B., and WEATHERALL, D. J.: Haemoglobin F (Malta): a new foetal haemoglobin variant with a high incidence in Maltese infants. Nature, 223: 311, 1969.

CAVELL, B.: Transplacental metastasis of malignant melanoma. Acta Paediat. Suppl., 146:37, 1963.

CAVILES, A. P., SONLEY, M., and HAMMOND, D.: Negative antiglobulin tests in hemolytic disease of the newborn. Proc. 9th Congr. Int. Soc. Blood Trans., 1962, p. 363 (1964).

CHAN, A. C., CHUNG, F., and KEITEL, H. G.: ABO hemolytic disease. J. Pediat., 61: 405, 1962.

CHANUTIN, A., and CURNISH, R. R.: Effect of organic and inorganic phosphates on the oxygen equilibrium of human erythrocytes. Arch. Biochem., 121:96, 1967.

CHAPLIN, H., JR.: Cited by Mollison, P. L.: in Blood Transfusion in Clinical Medicine. 3rd Ed., Springfield, Ill., Charles C Thomas, 1961, p. 581.

CHEDIAK, M.: Nouvelle anomalie leucocytaire de caractère constitutionnel familial. Rev. Hémat., 7:362, 1952.

CHERNOFF, A. I., and SINGER, K.: Studies on abnormal hemoglobins. IV. Persistence of fetal hemoglobin in the erythrocytes of normal children. Pediatrics, 9:469, 1952.

CHERRY, S. H., KOCHWA, S., and ROSENFIELD, R. E.: Bilirubin-protein ratio in amniotic fluid as an index of the severity of erythroblastosis fetalis. Obst. Gynec., 26:826, 1965.

CHERRY, S. H., ROSENFIELD, R. E., and KOCHWA, S.: Mechanism of accumulation of amniotic fluid pigment in erythroblastosis fetalis. Am. J. Obstet. Gynec., 106:297, 1970.

CHESSELLS, J. M., and PITNEY, W. R.: Fibrin split products in serum of newborn. (Letter to the Editor) Pediatrics, 45:155, 1970.

CHESSELLS, J. M., and WIGGLESWORTH, J. S.: Haemostatic failure in babies with Rhesus isoimmunization. Arch. Dis. Childh., 46:38, 1971.

CHOREMIS, K. B., ZERVOS, N., TSEVRENIS, H., APOSTOLOPOULAU, E., and MANDALAKI, T.: Hémophilie A chez une felle âgée de deux ans. Helvet. Paediat. Acta, 11:305, 1956.

CHOWN, B.: Anaemia from bleeding of the fetus into the maternal circulation. Lancet, 1:1213, 1954.

CHOWN, B.: The fetus can bleed. Am. J. Obst.Gynec., 70:1298, 1955.

CHOWN, B.: On a search for Rhesus antibodies in very young foetuses. Arch. Dis. Child., 30:232, 1955.

CHOWN, B., and BOWMAN, W. D.: The place of early delivery in the prevention of foetal death from erythroblastosis fetalis. Ped. Clin. North Am., May, 1958.

CLARKE, C. A.: Prevention of Rhesus iso-immunisation. Lancet, 1:1, 1968.

CLARKE, C. A., DONOHUE, W. T. A., McCONNELL, R. B., WOODROW, J. C., FINN, R., KREVANS, J. R., KULKE, W., LEHANE, D., and SHEPPARD, P. M.: Further experimental studies on the prevention of Rh haemolytic disease. Brit. Med. J., 1:979, 1963.

CLARKE, C. A., and SHEPPARD, P. M.: Prevention of Rhesus haemolytic disease (letter). Lancet, 2:343, 1965.

CLAYTON, E. M., HYUN, B. H., PALUMBO, V. N., and DEAN, V. M.: Penicillin induced positive Coombs' test in a newborn. Am. J. Clin. Path., 52:370, 1969.

CLAYTON, E. M., PRYOR, J. A., WIERDSMA, J. G., and WHITACRE, F. E.: Fetal and maternal components in third-trimester obstetric hemorrhage. Obst. Gynec., *24*: 56, 1964.

CLIFFORD, J. H., MATHEWS, P., REIQUAM, C. W., and PALMER, H. D.: Screening for hemolytic disease of the newborn by cord blood Coombs' testing. Clin. Pediat., 7:465, 1968.

CLIMIE, C. R., McLEAN, S. STARMER, G. A., and THOMAS, J.: Methaemoglobinaemia in mother and foetus following continuous epidermal analgesia with prilocaine. Brit. J. Anaesth., *39*:155, 1967.

CLOUTIER, M. D., and BURGERT, E. O., JR.: Congenital nonspherocytic hemolytic disease secondary to glucose-6-phosphate dehydrogenase deficiency: Report of three cases. Mayo Clin. Proc., *41*:316, 1966.

COCCHI, P., and MARIANELLI, L.: Phagocytosis and intracellular killing of *Pseudomonas aeruginosa* in premature infants. Helvet. Paediat. Acta, *22*:110, 1967.

COEN, R. W., and SUTHERLAND, J. M.: Placental vascular communications between twin fetuses. Am. J. Dis. Child., *120*:332, 1970.

COEN, R., GRUSH, O., and KAUDER, E.: Studies of bacterial activity and metabolism of the leukocyte in full-term neonates. J. Pediat., 75:400, 1969.

COHEN, A.: Maternal syndrome in Rh isoimmunization. J. Obst. Gynaec. Brit. Emp., 67:325, 1960.

COHEN, D. M., MITCHELL, C. B., and ALEXANDER, J. W.: Letterer-Siwe disease in a newborn. Arch. Path., *81*:347, 1966.

COHEN, F., and ZUELZER, W. W.: Mechanisms of isoimmunization. II. Transplacental passage and postnatal survival of fetal erythrocytes in heterospecific pregnancies. Blood, *30*:796, 1967.

COHEN, F., and ZUELZER, W. W.: The transplacental passage of maternal erythrocytes into the fetus. Am. J. Obst. Gynec., *93*:566, 1965.

COHEN, F., ZUELZER, W. W., and COHEN, S.: Maternal Rh antibody and delayed neonatal expression of Rh antigen. Transfusion, *10*:247, 1970.

COHEN, F., ZUELZER, W. W., and EVANS, M. M.: Identification of blood group antigens and minor cell populations by the fluorescent antibody method. Blood, *15*:884, 1960.

COHEN, F., ZUELZER, W. W., GUSTAFSON, D. C., and EVANS, M. M.: Mechanisms of isoimmunization. I. The transplacental passage of fetal erythrocytes in homospecific pregnancies. Blood, *23*:621, 1964.

COHEN, G., and HOCHSTEIN, P.: Glucose-6-phosphate dehydrogenase and detoxification of hydrogen peroxide in human erythrocytes. Science, *134*:1756, 1961.

COHEN, S. M., MILLER, B. M., and ORRIS, H. W.: Fatal sickle cell anemia in a one-month-old infant. J. Pediat., *30*:468, 1947.

COHEN, S. N., SCHWARTZ, S. A., and FERN, L. M.: The influence of penicillins on the protein-binding of other drugs. Abstract. Soc. Pediat. Research, Atlantic City, May, 1971, p. 183.

COLLINS, M., OSKI, F. A., and BARNES, L.: Unpublished observations (1966).

COLOMBO, M. L., and CASTELLO, D.: Rapporto fia resistenza osmotica leucocitaria ed immaturanza. Minerva Pediat., *13*:479, 1961.

COLOZZI, A. E.: Clamping of the umbilical cord; its effect on the placental transfusion. New Eng. J. Med., *250*:629, 1954.

COMBINED STUDY: Prevention of Rh-haemolytic disease: final results of the "high-risk" clinical trial. A combined study from centres in England and Baltimore. Brit. Med. J., 2:607, 1971.

COMLEY, A. and WOOD, B.: Albumin administration in exchange transfusion for hyperbilirubinemia. Arch. Dis. Childh., *43*:151, 1968.

COMMITTEE ON FETUS AND NEWBORN, AMERICAN ACADEMY OF PEDIATRICS: Recommendations on a uniform bilirubin standard. Pediatrics, *31*:878, 1963.

COMMITTEE ON NUTRITION, AMERICAN ACADEMY OF PEDIATRICS: Vitamin K compounds and the water-soluble analogues: use in therapy and prophylaxis in pediatrics. Pediatrics, *28*:501, 1961.

CONEN, P. E., and ERKMAN, B.: Combined mongolism and leukemia. Am. J. Dis. Child., *112*:429, 1966.

COOK, C. D., BRODIE, H. R., and ALLEN, D. W.: Measurement of fetal hemoglobin in newborn infants. Correlation with gestational age and intrauterine hypoxia. Pediatrics, 20:272, 1957.

COOPER, L. Z., GREEN, R. H., KRUGMAN, S., GILES, J. P., and MIRICK, G. S.: Neonatal thrombocytopenic purpura and other manifestations of rubella contracted in utero. Am. J. Dis. Child., 110:416, 1965.

CORBY, D. G., and SCHULMAN, I.: The effects of antenatal drug administration on aggregation of platelets of newborn infants. J. Pediat., 79:307, 1971.

CORN, M., and UPSHAW, J. D., JR.: Evaluation of platelet antibodies in idiopathic thrombocytopenic purpura. Arch. Int. Med., 109:157, 1962.

CORNEY, G., and AHERNE, W.: The placental transfusion syndrome in monozygous twins. Arch. Dis. Childh., 40:264, 1965.

CORNBLATH, M., and HARTMANN, A. F.: Methemoglobinemia in young infants. J. Pediat., 33:421, 1948.

CORNBLATH, M., KRAMER, I., and KELLY, A. B.: Rh isoimmunization associated with regurgitation jaundice beginning in utero: A report of two patients. Am. J. Dis. Child., 90:628, 1955.

CORNET, J. A., ABILDGAARD, C., SCHULMAN, I., and SMITH, R. T.: Thymectomy for leukemia in a 68 hour old infant: 20 month follow-up of hematologic and immunologic status. Prog. Soc. Ped. Res., Philadelphia, May, 1965, p. 75.

CORTÉS, L.: Caúdruples contransfusions de feto a feto un producto con anemia y otro con policitemia. Rev. Méd. Costa Rica, 21:89, 1964.

COTTE, J., KISSIN, C., MATHIEU, M., PONCET, J., MONNET, P., SALLE, B., and GERMAIN, D.: Observation d'un cas de déficit partiel en ATPase intraérythrocytaire. Rev. Franç. Études Clin. et Biol., 13:284, 1968.

COTTE, J., NIVELON, J. L., CUIVRÉ, M., KISSIN, C., GESSEN-CAMPOS, J., BÉTHENOD, M., and MATHIEU, M.: Les enzymes de la glycolyse intra-érythrocytaire chez le prématuré. Ann. de Pédiatrie, 43:3158, 1967.

COTTER, J., and PRYSTOWSKY, H.: Fetal blood studies. XIX. Adult and fetal hemoglobin levels of human fetal blood in term pregnancy and in prolonged pregnancy. Obst. Gynec., 22:745, 1963.

COTTOM, D. G.: Foetal haemoglobin and postmaturity. J. Obst. Gynaec. Brit. Emp., 62:945, 1955.

CRACCO, J. B., DOWER, J. C., and HARRIS, L. E.: Bilirubin metabolism in the newborn. Proc. Mayo Clin., 40:868, 1965.

CRAIG, J. M.: Sequences in the development of cirrhosis of the liver in cases of erythroblastosis fetalis. Arch. Path., 49:665, 1950.

CRAMBLATT, H. G., FRIEDMAN, J. L., and NAJJAR, S.: An infant born to a mother with leukemia. New Eng. J. Med., 259:727, 1958.

CRAWFORD, H., CUTBUSH, M., and MOLLISON, P. L.: Hemolytic disease of newborn due to anti-A. Blood, 8:620, 1953.

CREMER, R. J., PERRYMAN, P. W., and RICHARDS, D. H.: Influences of light on the hyperbilirubinemia of infants. Lancet, 1:1094, 1958.

CROWLEY, J., WAYS, P., and JONES, J. W.: Human fetal erythrocyte and plasma lipids. J. Clin. Invest., 44:989, 1965.

CRUVEILLER, J., HARPEY, J. P., VERON, P., CANNAT, A., DELATTRE, A., HERVET, E., LAFOURCADE, J., and TURPIN, R.: Lupus erythemateux systemique. Arch. Franç., Péd., 27:195, 1970.

CURTIS, J. C., DODGE, W. F., and DAESCHNER, C. W.: Cytomegalic inclusion disease associated with hypothyroidism. Pediatrics, 29:52, 1962.

CZAPEK, E. E., BARRY, D., and GRYBOSKI, J. D.: Malaria in an infant, transmitted by an exchange transfusion. J.A.M.A., 204:549, 1968.

DAAMEN, C. B. F., BLOEM, G. W. D., and WESTERLEEH, A. G.: Chorionepithelioma in mother and child. J. Obst. Gynaec. Brit. Emp., 68:144, 1961.

DACIE, J. V., MOLLISON, P. L., RICHARDSON, N., SELWYN, J. G., and SHAPIRO, L.: Atypical congenital hemolytic anaemia. Quart. J. Med., 22:79, 1953.

DALGAARD, J. B., and KASS, A.: Congenital leukemia with cirrhosis of the liver. Acta Path. Microbiol. Scand., 37:465, 1955.

DAM, H., DYGGVE, H., LARSEN, H., and PLUM, P.: Vitamin K and hemorrhagic disease of the newborn. Adv. Pediat., 5:129, 1952.

DAM, H., GLAVIND, J., LARSEN, H., and PLUM, P.: Investigations into the cause of physiological hypoprothrombinemia in newborn children. IV. The vitamin K content of woman's milk and cow's milk. Acta Med. Scand., *112*:210, 1942.

DAM, H., TAGE, H. E., and PLUM, P.: K-Avitaminose hos spaede born som aarag til hemorrhagisk diathese. Vgesk. Laeger, *101*:896, 1939.

DANIEL, S. J., and CASSADY, G.: Non-immunologic hydrops fetalis associated with a large hemangioendothelioma. Pediatrics, *42*:829, 1968.

DANKS, D. M.: Childhood hypoglycemia, as a sequel of erythroblastosis foetalis. Acta Pediat. Scand., *58*:369, 1969.

DANKS, D. M., and STEVENS, L. H.: Neonatal respiratory distress associated with a high hematocrit reading. Lancet, *1*:499, 1964.

DANON, Y., KLEINMAN, A., and DANON, D.: The osmotic fragility and density distribution of erythrocytes in the newborn. Acta Haemat., *43*:242, 1970.

DAVIDSON, R. G., NITOWSKY, H. M., and CHILDS, B.: Demonstration of two populations of cells in the human female heterozygous for glucose-6-phosphate variants. Proc. Nat. Acad. Sci., *50*:481, 1963.

DAVIDSON, W. M.: Inherited variations in leucocytes. Brit. Med. Bull., *17*:190, 1961.

DAVIS, J. W., and WILSON, S. J.: Platelet survival in the May-Hegglin anomaly. Brit. J. Haemat., *12*:61, 1966.

DEBRÉ, R., MOZZICONACCI, P., CAMIS, M.: L'infection générale à bacille pyocyanique du nourisson. Semaine Hôp. Paris, *26*:1918, 1950.

DeBRUIJNE, J. I., VAN CREVELD, S. V., and HOO, L. K.: Clotting factors in haemolytic disease of the newborn. II. Thrombocytopenia after replacement transfusion. Étud. Néo-natal., *5*:109, 1956.

DeCARVALHO, S.: Preliminary experimentations with specific immunotherapy of neoplastic disease in man. I. Immediate effects of hyperimmune equine gamma globulin. Cancer, *16*:311, 1963.

DE GIER, J., VAN DEENAN, L. L. M., GEERDINK, R. A., PUNT, K., and VERLOOP, M. C.: Phosphatide patterns of normal, spherocytic and elliptocytic red blood cells. Biochim. Biophys. Acta, *50*:383, 1961.

deLEEUW, N. K. M., LOWENSTEIN, L., and HSIEH, Y-S.: Iron deficiency and hydremia in normal pregnancy. Medicine, *45*:291, 1966.

DE LOECKER, W. C., PRANKERD, T. A.: Factors influencing the hexose monophosphate shunt in red cells. Clin. Chim. Acta, *6*:641–7, 1961.

DELIVORIA-PAPADOPOULOS, M., MORROW, G., and OSKI, F. A.: Exchange transfusion in the newborn with fresh and "old" blood: Effects on oxygen release. J. Pediat., *78*:898, 1971a.

DELIVORIA-PAPADOPOULOS, M., RONCEVIC, N. P., and OSKI, F. A.: Postnatal changes in oxygen transport of term, premature, and sick infants: The role of red cell 2, 3-diphosphoglycerate and adult hemoglobin. Pediat. Res., *5*:235, 1971.

DELTA, B. G., EISENSTEIN, E. M., and ROTHENBERG, A. M.: Rupture of a normal spleen in the newborn: Report of a survival and review of the literature. Clin. Ped., *7*: 373, 1968.

DE LUCA, C., STEVENSON, J. H., JR., and KAPLAN, E.: Simultaneous multiple-column chromatography: its application to the separation of the adenine nucleotides of human erythrocytes. Anal. Biochem., *4*:39, 1962.

DeLUCA, S., ZORCOLO, G., and ANGIONI, G.: Sull' incidenza dell' emoglobina Bart's nei neonati Sardi. Riv. Ital. Ginec., *52*:601, 1968.

DeMARSH, Q. B., ALT, H. L., and WINDLE, W. F.: Factors influencing the blood picture of the newborn: studies on sinus blood on the first and third days. Am. J. Dis. Child., *75*:860, 1948.

DeMARSH, Q. B., WINDLE, W. F., and ALT, H. L.: Blood volume of newborn infant in relation to early and late clamping of umbilical cord. Am. J. Dis. Child., *63*:1123, 1942.

DERN, R. J., WEINSTEIN, I. M., LeROY, G. V., TALMAGE, D. W., and ALVING, A. S.: The hemolytic effect of primaquine: 1. The localization of the drug induced hemolytic defect in primaquine sensitive individuals. J. Lab. Clin. Med., *43*:303, 1954.

DERRIEN, Y.: Studies on the heterogeneity of adult and fetal haemoglobins by salting-out, alkali denaturation and moving boundary electrophoresis. Conference on Hemoglobin, National Academy of Sciences, National Research Council, Washington, D. C., 1958.

DERVICHIAN, D., FOURNET, C., GUINIER, A., and PONDER, E.: Structure submicroscopique des globules rouges contenant des hémoglobines abnormales. Rev. Hématol., 7:567, 1952.

DESAI, R. G., McCUTCHEON, E., LITTLE, B., and DRISCOLL, S. G.: Fetomaternal passage of leukocytes and platelets in erythroblastosis fetalis. Blood. 27:858, 1966.

DESFORGES, J.: Comment in *Yearbook of Pediatrics 1964-65* (S. S. Gellis, ed.), Chicago, Year Book Medical Publishers, 1965, p. 338.

DESMOND, M.: Coxsackie septicemia in newborn with intravascular coagulation. Clinical Pathologic Conference. J. Pediat., 73:283, 1968.

DE VAAL, O. M., and SEYNHAEVE, V.: Reticular dysgenesia. Lancet. 2:1123, 1959.

DE VRIES, A., MATOTH, P., and SHAMIR, Z. S.: Familial congenital labile factor deficiency with syndactylism; investigation on the mode of action of the labile factor. Acta Haemat., 5:129, 1951.

DIAMOND, I.: Bilirubin binding and kernicterus. Adv. Pediat., 16:99, 1969. (Yearbook Med. Publishers, Chicago, Ill.)

DIAMOND, L. K.: Erythroblastosis fetalis or hemolytic disease of the newborn. Proc. Roy. Soc. Med., 40:546, 1947.

DIAMOND, L. K.: Personal communication (1961).

DIAMOND, L. K., ALLEN, D. M., and MAGILL, F. B.: Congenital (erythroid) hypoplastic anemia. Am. J. Dis. Child., 102:149, 1961.

DIAMOND, L. K., BLACKFAN, K. D., and BATY, J. M.: Erythroblastosis fetalis and its association with universal edema of fetus, icterus gravis neonatorum, and anemia of the newborn. J. Pediat., 1:269, 1932.

DIAMOND, L. K., McELFRESH, A. E., SAY, B., and DiGEORGE, A. M.: Turner's phenotype in children with congenital hypoplastic anemia. Program of the American Soc. Hematology, 30th Ann. Meeting, 1970, p. 132.

DIAMOND, M. P., COTGROVE, I., and PARKER, A.: Case of intrauterine death due to α-thalassaemia. Brit. Med. J., 2:278, 1965.

DIAMANDOPOULOS, G. T., and HERTIG, H. T.: Transmission of leukemia and allied diseases from mother to fetus. Obst. Gynec., 21:150, 1963.

DIDISHEIM, P., and LEWIS, J. H.: Congenital disorders of the mechanism for coagulation of blood. Pediatrics, 22:478, 1958.

DiGEORGE, A. M.: Discussion of Cooper, M. D., Peterson, R D. A., and Good, R. A. New concept of cellular basis of immunity. J. Pediat., 67:907, 1965.

DIGNAN, P. ST. J., MAUER, A. M., and FRANTZ, C.: Phocomelia with congenital hypoplastic thrombocytopenia and myeloid leukemoid reactions. J. Pediat., 70:561, 1967.

DIMMICK, J. E., HARDWICK, D. F., and HO-YUEN, B.: A case of renal necrosis and fibrosis in the immediate newborn period. Association with the twin-to-twin transfusion syndrome. Amer. J. Dis. Child. 122:345, 1971.

DINE, M. S.: Congenital methemoglobinemia in the newborn period. Am. J. Dis. Child., 92:15, 1956.

DIPPEL, A. L.: Hematomas of umbilical cord. Surg. Gynec. Obst., 70:51, 1940.

DiPRATTI, V.: Personal communication (1966).

DITTMER, D. (ed.): *Blood and Other Body Fluids.* Washington, D. C., Federation of American Societies for Experimental Biology, 1961, pp. 109, 114, 125, 132, 140.

DOCHAIN, J., LEMAGE, L., and LAMBRECHTS, A.: Principales données hématologiques chez le nouveau-né normal. Arch. Franc. Pediat., 9:274, 1952.

DODD, B. E., and WILKINSON, P. C.: A study of the distribution of incomplete Rhesus antibodies among the serum immunoglobulin fractions. J. Exp. Med., 120:45, 1964.

DONOHUE, W. L., and WAKE, E. J.: Effect of ABO incompatibility on pregnancy-induced Rh isoimmunization. Canad. M.A.J., 90:1, 1964.

DONOVAN, J. C., and LUND, C. J.: Transplacental passage of maternal erythrocytes. Am. J. Obstet. Gynec., 95:834, 1966.

DORFMAN, A., and LORINCZ, A. E.: Occurrence of urinary acid mucopolysaccharides in the Hurler syndrome. Proc. Nat. Acad. Sci., 43:443, 1957.

DORROS, G., KLEINER, G. J., and ROMNEY, S. L.: Fetal leukocyte pattern in premature rupture of amniotic membranes and in normal and abnormal labor. Am. J. Obst. Gynec., 105:1269, 1969.

DOSSET, J. H., WILLIAMS, R. C., JR., and QUIE, P. G.: Studies on interaction of bacteria, serum factors and polymorphonuclear leukocytes in mothers and newborns. Pediatrics, 44:49, 1969.

Douglas, A. S., and Davies, P. L.: Hypoprothrombinaemia in the newborn. Arch. Dis. Child., *30*:509, 1955.

Douglas, H.: Haemorrhage in the newborn (Letter to the Editor). Lancet, *1*:816, 1966.

Doxiadis, S. A., Fessas, P., Valaes, T., and Mastrokalos, N.: Glucose-6-phosphate dehydrogenase deficiency; a new aetiological factor of severe neonatal jaundice. Lancet, *1*:297, 1961.

Doxiadis, S. A., and Valaes, T.: The clinical picture of glucose-6-phosphate dehydrogenase deficiency in early infancy. Arch. Dis. Child., *39*:545, 1964.

Drescher, H., and Künzer, W.: Der Blutfarbstoff des Menschlichen Feten. Klin. Wschr., *32*:92, 1954.

Duckert, F., Jung, E., and Shmerling, D. H.: Hitherto undescribed congenital haemorrhagic diathesis probably due to fibrin stabilizing factor deficiency. Thromb. Diath. Haemorrh., 5:179, 1960.

Duhring, J. L., Smith, K., Greene, J. W., Jr., Rochlin, D. B., and Blakemore, W. S.: Placental transfer of maternal erythrocytes into the fetal circulation. Surg. Forum, *10*:720–22, 1959.

Duncan, W., and Halnan, K. E.: Giant hemangioma with thrombocytopenia. Clin. Radiol., *15*:224, 1964.

Dunham, E. C.: Septicemia in the newborn. Am. J. Dis. Child., *45*:229, 1933.

Dunn, I., Ibsen, K. H., Coe, E. L., Schneider, A. S., and Weinstein, I. M.: Erythrocyte carbohydrate metabolism in hereditary spherocytosis. J. Clin. Invest., *42*:1535, 1963.

Dunn, P. M.: Obstructive jaundice and haemolytic disease of the newborn. Arch. Dis. Child., *38*:54, 1963.

Dunn, P. M.: The unnecessary exchange transfusion: A study of Rh hemolytic disease of the newborn. J. Pediat., *69*:829, 1966.

Dyer, N. C., Brill, A. B., Glasser, S. R., and Goss, D. A.: Maternal-fetal transport and distribution of ^{59}Fe and ^{131}I in humans. Am. J. Obst. Gynec., *103*:290, 1969.

Dyggve, H.: Prophylactic treatment with vitamin K of 11,000 newborn infants compared to 22,000 untreated infants. Sixth Internat. Congr. of Pediatrics, 1950.

Dyggve, H.: Prothrombin and proconvertin in the newborn and during the first year of life. Acta Paediat., *47*:251, 1958.

Dyggve, H.: Hydrops foetalis without blood group incompatibility but associated with hydramnios. Acta Paediat., *49*:437, 1960.

Earle, R., Jr.: Congenital salicylate intoxication: report of a case. New Eng. J. Med., *265*:1003, 1961.

Earn, A. A.: The effect of congenital abnormalities of the umbilical cord and placenta on the mother and newborn. J. Obst. Gynaec. Brit. Emp., *58*:456, 1951.

East, W. R., and Lumpkin, L. R.: Lupus erythematosus in an infant. Minnesota Med., *52*:477, 1969.

Eastman, N. J.: In *Williams' Obstetrics.* 10th Ed., New York, Appleton, 1950, p. 555.

Eckstein, H. B., and Jack, B.: Breast feeding and anticoagulant therapy. Lancet, *1*: 672, 1970.

Efrati, P., Rozenszajn, L., and Shapira, E.: The morphology of buffy coat from cord blood of normal human newborns. Blood, *17*:497, 1961.

Egan, W. A. II, Julius, R. L., and Gessner, I. H.: Neonatal hyperbilirubinemia associated with ingestion of maternal blood. Pediatrics, *43*:894, 1969.

Ehrlich, P.: De- und regeneration rotor blutscheiben. Verhandl. Gesellsch. Charité Ärzte, 10 Juni and 9 Dezember, 1880.

Eichenwald, H. F.: Congenital toxoplasmosis. A study of 150 cases. A.M.A. J. Dis. Child., *94*:411, 1957.

Eichenwald, H. F., and Shinefield, H.: Viral infections of the fetus and of the premature and newborn infant. Adv. Pediat., *12*:249, 1962.

Eisenstein, E. M.: Congenital amegakaryocytic thrombocytopenic purpura. Clin. Pediat., 5:143, 1966.

Eitzman, D. V., and Smith, R. T.: The nonspecific inflammatory cycle in the neonatal infant. A.M.A. J. Dis. Child., *97*:326, 1959.

Ekelund, H., Hedner, V., and Nilsson, I. M.: Fibrin split products in serum of newborn. (Letter to the Editor.) Pediatrics, *45*:156, 1970.

Ekelund, H., Hedner, V., and Nilsson, I. M.: Fibrinolysis in newborns. Acta Paediat. Scand., *59*:33, 1970.

EKERT, H. and MATHEW, R. Y.: Platelet counts and plasma fibrinogen levels in erythroblastosis foetalis. Med. J. Austr., 2:844, 1967.

ELDER, H. A., and MORTENSEN, R. A.: The incorporation of labeled glycine into erythrocyte glutathione. J. Biol. Chem., 218:261, 1956.

ELDJARN, L., and BREMER, J.: The reduction of disulphides by human erythrocytes. Biochem. J., 82:192, 1962.

ELSAS, L. J., WHITTEMORE, R., and BURROW, G. M.: Maternal and neonatal Grave's Disease. J.A.M.A., 200:250, 1967.

EMANUEL, B., and SCHOENFELD, A.: Favism in a nursing infant. J. Pediat., 58:263, 1961.

EMBIL, J. A., OZERE, R. L., and HALDANE, E. V.: Congenital cytomegalovirus infection in two siblings from consecutive pregnancies. J. Pediatrics, 77:417, 1970.

EMERY, J. L., GORDON, R. R., RENDLE-SHORT, J., VARADI, S., and WARRACK, A. J. N.: Congenital amegakaryocytic thrombocytopenia with congenital deformities and a leukemoid blood picture in the newborn. Blood, 12:567, 1957.

ENGEL, R. R., HAMMOND, D., EITZMAN, D. V., PEARSON, H., and KRIVIT, W.: Transient congenital leukemia in 7 infants with mongolism. J. Pediat., 65:303, 1964.

ENGSTRÖM, L., and KAGER, L.: Changes in plasma fibrinolytic activity of newborn infants during first hour after birth. Acta Paediat., 53:326, 1964.

EPSTEIN, H. C., and LITT, J. Z.: Discoid lupus erythematosus in a newborn infant. New Eng. J. Med., 265:1106, 1961.

EPSTEIN, R. D., LOZNER, E. L., LOBBEY, T. S., and DAVIDSON, C. S.: Congenital thrombocytopenic purpura. Purpura hemorrhagica in pregnancy and in the newborn. Am. J. Med., 9:44, 1950.

ERDEM, S., and AKSOY, M.: The increase of hemoglobin A₂ to its adult level. Israel J. Med. Sci., 5:427, 1969.

ERLANDSON, M. E., and HILGARTNER, M.: Hemolytic disease in the neonatal period and early infancy. J. Pediat., 54:566, 1959.

ERLANDSON, M. E., SCHULMAN, I., WALDEN, B., and SMITH, C. H.: Chromium⁵¹ elution from hemoglobin and erythrocytes of adults, infants and patients with Cooley's anemia. Proc. Soc. Exp. Biol. Med., 99:173, 1958.

ESHAGHPOUR, E., OSKI, F. A., and NAIMAN, J. L.: Iron deficiency in a newborn infant. J. Pediat., 68:806, 1966.

ESHAGHPOUR, E., OSKI, F. A., and WILLIAMS, M.: The relationship of erythrocyte glucose-6-phosphate dehydrogenase deficiency to hyperbilirubinemia in Negro premature infants. J. Pediat., 70:595, 1967.

ESKIN, B. A., and FRUMIN, A. M.: Transplacental transfer of maternal cold agglutinins in pregnancy. Am. J. Obst. Gynec., 86:848, 1963.

ESTREN, S., and DAMESHEK, W.: Familial hypoplastic anemia of childhood. Am. J. Dis. Child., 73:671, 1947.

EVANS, R. S., and DUANE, R. T.: Acquired hemolytic anemia: relation of erythrocyte antibody production to activity of disease; significance of thrombocytopenia and leukopenia. Blood, 4:1196, 1949.

EVELYN, K. A., and MALLOY, G. T.: Microdetermination of oxyhemoglobin, methemoglobin and sulfhemoglobin in a single sample of blood. J. Biol. Chem., 126:655, 1938.

FAIRWEATHER, D. V. I., MURRAY, S., PARKIN, D., and WALKER, W.: Possible immunological implications of amniocentesis. Lancet. 2:1190, 1963.

FALBE-HANSEN, I.: The composition of the alkali-resistant haemoglobin fraction in blood from normal adults. Brit. J. Haemat., 7:187, 1961.

FARMER, M. B., LEHMANN, H., and RAINE, D. N.: Two unrelated patients with congenital cyanosis due to haemoglobinopathy M. Lancet, 2:786, 1964.

FARQUHAR, J. W.: The evaluation of the eosinopenic response to corticotrophin and cortisone in the newborn infant. Arch. Dis. Child., 30:133, 1955.

FARRAR, J. F., and BLOMFIELD, J.: Alkali-resistant haemoglobin content of blood in congenital heart disease. Brit. J. Haemat., 9:278, 1963.

FAXEN, N.: Red blood picture in healthy infants. Acta Paediat., 19:1, 1937.

FELDMAN, H. A.: Toxoplasmosis. Pediatrics, 22:559, 1958.

FESSAS, P. H.: Haemoglobin H and Barts. In *Haemoglobin Colloquium* (Lehmann, H., and Betke, K., eds.). Stuttgart, Georg Thieme Verlag, 1961, p. 90.

FESSAS, P. H., DOXIADIS, S. A., and VALAES, T.: Neonatal jaundice in glucose-6-phosphate dehydrogenase deficient infants. Brit. Med. J., 2:1359, 1962.

FESSAS, P. H., KARAKLIS, A., and GNAFAKIS, N.: A further abnormality of foetal haemoglobin. Acta Haemat., 25:62, 1961.

FESSAS, P. H., and MASTROKALOS, N.: Demonstration of small components in red cell hemolysates by starch gel electrophoresis. Nature, 183:1261, 1959.

FESSAS, P. H., MASTROKALOS, N., and FOSTIROPOULOS, G.: New variant of human foetal haemoglobin. Nature, 183:30, 1959.

FETTERMAN, G. H.: New laboratory acid in clinical diagnosis of inclusion disease of infancy. Am. J. Clin. Path., 22:424, 1952.

FIKENTSCHER, R., SCHMIDT, D., and STICH, W.: Untersuchungen über den fetalen hamstoffwechsel. III. Das hämpräcursoren-muster des menschlichen neugeborenblutes. Klin. Wschr., 47:919, 1969.

FILLMORE, S. J., and McDEVITT, E.: Effects of coumarin compounds on the fetus. Ann. Int. Med., 73:731, 1970.

FINN, R., CLARKE, C. A., DONOHUE, W. T. A., McCONNELL, R. B., SHEPPARD, P. M., LEHANE, D., and KULKE, W.: Experimental studies on the prevention of Rh haemolytic disease. Brit. Med. J., 1:1486, 1961.

FINNE, P. H.: Erythropoietin levels in the amniotic fluid, particularly in Rh-immunized pregnancies. Acta Paediat., 53:269, 1964.

FINNE, P. H.: Erythropoietin levels in cord blood as an indicator of intrauterine hypoxia. Acta Paediat. Scand., 55:478, 1966.

FINNE, P. H.: Erythropoietin production in fetal hypoxia and in anemic uremic patients. Ann. New York Acad. Sci., 149:497, 1968.

FINNE, P. H.: On placental transfer of erythropoietin. Acta Paed. Scand., 56:233, 1967.

FISCH, R. O., BERGLUND, E. B., BRIDGE, A. G., FINLEY, P. R., AND RAILE, R.: Methemoglobinemia in a hospital nursery. A search for causative factors. J.A.M.A., 185:124, 1963.

FISCHLER, E., AND FARCHY, R.: Mongolism associated with congenital leukemia. Report of a case. Helv. Paediat. Acta, 15:253, 1960.

FISHER, S., RIKOVER, M., AND NAOR, S.: Factor 13 deficiency with severe hemorrhage diathesis. Blood, 28:34, 1966.

FLATZ, G., SRINGAM, S., AND KOMKRIS, V.: Neonatal jaundice in glucose-6-phosphate dehydrogenase deficiency. Lancet, 1:1382, 1963.

FLESSA, H. C., KAPSTROM, A. B., and GLUECK, H. I.: Placental transport of heparin. Clin. Res., 12:346, 1964.

FOCONI, S., and SJÖLIN, S.: Survival of Cr^{51}-labelled red cells from new-born infants. Acta Paediat., 48:18, 1959.

FOGEL, B. J., ARIAS, D., and KUNG, F.: Platelet counts in healthy premature infants. J. Pediat., 73:108, 1968.

FOIS, A., BIAGOLI, M. L., and CONTU, L.: Comportamento della glucosio-6-fosfato deidrogenase e del glutathione redotto negli eritrociti dei neonate a termine e dei prematuri. Haematologica, 46:178, 1961.

FONG, S. W., QUQUNDAH, B. Y., and TAYLOR, W. F.: Normal patterns of isoagglutinins. Prog. Soc. Pediatric Research, 1970, p. 214.

FORMAN, M. L., and STIEHM, E. R.: Impaired opsonic activity but normal phagocytosis in low-birth-weight infants. New Eng. J. Med., 281:926, 1969.

FORTINA, A., and PETROCINI, S.: Contributo alto studio della manifestazoni cutanee nelle leucemie dell'infanzia. Pediatrica, 61:199, 1953.

FOST, N. C., and ESTERLY, N. B.: Successful treatment of juvenile hemangiomas with prednisone. J. Pediat., 72:351, 1968.

FRAGA, J. R., REICHELDERFER, T. E., SCOTT, R. B., and SARD, D. M.: Giant cell hepatitis associated with hereditary spherocytosis. Clin. Pediat., 7:364, 1968.

FRASER, I. D., and RAPER, A. B.: Observations on the change from foetal to adult erythropoiesis. Arch. Dis. Child., 37:289, 1962.

FRAZIER, C. A., and RICE, C. E.: Neonatal sickle cell anemia. J.A.M.A., 143:1065, 1950.

FREDA, V. J., GORMAN, J. G., and POLLACK, W.: Successful prevention of experimental Rh sensitization in man with an anti-Rh γ_2-globulin antibody preparation. Transfusion, 4:26, 1964.

FREDA, V. J., GORMAN, J. G., and POLLACK, W.: Rh factor: prevention of isoimmuniza-
tion and clinical trial on mothers. Science, *151*:828, 1966.
FREEDMAN, W. L., and MCMAHON, F. J.: Placental metastasis. Review of the literature
and report of a case of metastatic melanoma. Obst. Gynec., *16*:550, 1960.
FREIMAN, I., and SUPER, M.: Thrombocytopenia and congenital syphilis in South
African Bantu infants. Arch. Dis. Childh., *41*:87, 1966.
FRESH, J. W., FERGUSON, J. H., and LEWIS, J.: Blood clotting studies in parturient
women and the newborn. Obst. Gynec., 7:117, 1956.
FRESH, J. W., FERGUSON, J. H., STAMEY, C., MORGAN, F. M., and LEWIS, J. H.: Blood
prothrombin, proconvertin and proacceterin in normal infancy: questionable
relationships to vitamin K. Pediatrics, *19*:241, 1957.
FRIEDENTHAL, H.: Über Säuglingsernährung nach physiologischen Grundsätzen mit
Friedenthal schwer Kindermilch und Gemüsepulvern. Berliner Klin. Woch.,
1:727, 1914.
FROELICH, L. A., and HOUSLER, M.: Neonatal thrombocytopenia and chorangioma.
J. Pediat., 78:516, 1971.
FULLERTON, H. W.: The iron-deficiency anemia of late infancy. Arch. Dis. Child.,
12:91, 1937.
GABURRO, D., VOLPATO, S., and GIAQUINTO, M.: Ictère nucleaire du nouveau-né par
defaut de la G-6-PD. Semaine Hôp. Paris, Suppl. to Ann. Pédiat., 37:69, 1961.
GABURRO, D., VOLPATO, S., and VIGI, V.: Diagnosis of beta thalassemia in the newborn
by means of haemoglobin synthesis. Acta Paediat. Scand., 59:523, 1970.
ÇAIRDNER, D.: *Recent Advances in Paediatrics*. Boston, Little, Brown and Co., 1958,
Chapter 2.
GAIRDNER, D., MARKS, J., and ROSCOE, J. D.: Blood formation in infancy; normal
erythropoiesis. Arch. Dis. Child., 27:214, 1952.
GAIRDNER, D., MARKS, J., ROSCOE, J. D., and BRETTELL, R. O.: The fluid shift from the
vascular compartment immediately after birth. Arch. Dis. Child., 33:489, 1958.
GALANT, S. P.: Accidental heparinization of a newborn infant. Am. J. Dis. Child.,
114:313, 1967.
GAMBINO, S. R., and FREDA, V. J.: The measurement of amniotic fluid bilirubin by the
method of Jendrassik and Grof. Am. J. Clin. Path., 46:198, 1966.
GARBY, L., SJÖLIN, S., and VUILLE, J.-C.: Studies of erythro-kinetics in infancy. II. The
relative rate of synthesis of haemoglobin F and haemoglobin A during the first
months of life. Acta Paediat., 51:245, 1962.
GARBY, L., SJÖLIN, S., and VUILLE, J.-C.: Studies of erythro-kinetics in infancy. IV. The
long-term behavior of radioiron in circulating foetal and adult haemoglobin, and
its faecal excretion. Acta Paediat., 53:33, 1964.
GARBY, L., SJÖLIN, S., and VUILLE, J.-C.: Studies on erythro-kinetics in infancy. V.
Estimation of the life span of red cell in the newborn. Acta Paediat., 53:165, 1964.
GARCIA, A. G. P.: Congenital toxoplasmosis in two successive sibs. Arch. Dis. Childh.,
43:705, 1968.
GARDAIS, J., LARGET-PIET, L., LEROUX, J.-P., and VIDAL, J.-L.: Leucoblastose néo-
natale transitoire puis leucose aiguë chez un trisomique 21. Ann. Pédiat., *16*:780,
1969.
GARG, S. K., AMOROSI, E. L., and KARPATKIN, S.: Use of the megathrombocyte as an
index of megakaryocyte number. New Eng. J. Med., *284*:11, 1971.
GARTNER, L. M., and ARIAS, I. M.: Formation, transport, metabolism and excretion of
bilirubin. New Eng. J. Med., *280*:1339, 1969.
GARTNER, L. M., and LANE, D.: Hepatic metabolism and transport of bilirubin during
physiologic jaundice in the newborn Rhesus monkey. Abstract, Soc. Pediat. Re-
search, Atlantic City, May, 1971, p. 100.
GARTNER, O. T., GILBERT, R., JR., MCDERMOT, M., BENOVITZ, S., and WOLF, A. M.:
Anti-A and anti-B antibodies in children. J.A.M.A., *201*:206, 1967.
GASSER, C.: Die hämolytischen Frühgeburtenanämie mit spontaner Innenkörper-
bildung; ein neue Syndrom, beobachtet an 14 Fälle. Helv. Paediat. Acta, 8:491,
1953.
GASSER, C.: Heinz body anemia and related phenomena. J. Pediat., *54*:673, 1959.
GATTI, R. A.: Hematocrit values of capillary blood in the newborn infant. J. Pediat.,
70:117, 1967.

GATTI, R. A., MUSTER, A. J., COLE, R. B., and PAUL, M. H.: Neonatal polycythemia with transient cyanosis and cardiorespiratory abnormalities. J. Pediat., 69:1063, 1966.

GATTI, R. A., PLATT, N., POMERANCE, H. H., HONG, R., LANGER, L. O., KAY, H. E. M., and GOOD, R. A.: Hereditary lymphopenic agammaglobulinemia associated with a distinctive form of short-limbed dwarfism and ectodermal dysplasia. J. Pediat., 75:675, 1969.

GELLI, G. D., and DELLA SANTA, L.: Le resistenze osmotche leucocitarie nel neonato, nel lattante e nel bambino normali. Aggiorn. Pediat., 11:219, 1960.

GELLIS, S. S., and LYON, R. A.: The influence of diet of the newborn infant on the prothrombin index. J. Pediat., 19:495, 1941.

GELSTON, C. F.: On the etiology of hemorrhagic disease of the newborn. Am. J. Dis. Child., 22:361, 1921.

GERALD, P. S.: The electrophoretic and spectroscopic characterization of hemoglobin M. Blood, 12:936, 1958.

GERALD, P. S., and EFRON, M. L.: Chemical studies of several varieties of hemoglobin M. Proc. Nat. Acad. Sci., 47:1758, 1961.

GERBIE, A. B., DeCOSTA, E. J., and REIS, R. A.: Fetal hemoglobin as an index of maturity. Am. J. Obst. Gynec., 78:57, 1959.

GERLACH, E., DUHM, J., and DEUTICKE, B.: Metabolism of 2,3-diphosphoglycerate in red blood cells under various experimental conditions. In Red Cell Metabolism and Function, Brewer, G., ed. Plenum Press, New York, 1970, p. 155.

GIBLETT, E.: Cited by Mollison, P. L.: Blood Transfusion in Clinical Medicine. 3rd ed., Springfield, Ill., Charles C Thomas, 1961, p. 167.

GIBSON, J. G., JR., and EVANS, W. A.: Clinical studies of the blood volume. I. Clinical application of a method employing the blue azo-dye 'Evans blue' and the spectro-photometer. J. Clin. Invest., 16:301, 1937.

GILARDI, VON, A., and MIESCHER, P.: Die Lebensdauer von autolagen und homologen Erythrocyten bei frühgeboremen und älteren Kindern. Schweiz. med. Wschr., 87:1456, 1957.

GILES, C.: An account of 335 cases of megaloblastic anemia of pregnancy and the puerperium. J. Clin. Path., 19:1, 1966.

GILL, F. M., and SCHWARTZ, E.: Platelet transfusion as a diagnostic and therapeutic aid in the newborn. Abstract, Soc. Pediat. Res., Atlantic City, May 1971, p. 92.

GILLESPIE, A., DORMAN, D., WALKER-SMITH, J. A., and YU, J. S.: Neonatal hepatitis and Australia Antigen. Lancet, 2:1081, 1970.

GILMOUR, J. R.: Normal haemopoieses in intra-uterine and neo-natal life. J. Path. Bact., 52:25, 1941.

GILON, E., RAMOT, B., and SHEBA, C.: Multiple hemangiomata associated with thrombo-cytopenia: remarks on the pathogenesis of the thrombocytopenia in this syndrome. Blood, 14:74, 1959.

GITHENS, J. H., and FERRIER, P. E.: Changing concepts in the etiology and treatment of bleeding diseases of the newborn. Quart. Rev. Pediat., 14:141, 1959.

GITLIN, D., VAWTER, G., and CRAIG, J. M.: Thymic alymphoplasia and congenital aleukocytosis. Pediatrics, 33:184, 1964.

GLAUN, B. P., WEINBERG, E. G., and MALAN, A. F.: Peripheral gangrene in a newborn. Arch. Dis. Childh. 46:105, 1971.

GLUCK, L., and SILVERMAN, W. A.: Phagocytosis in premature infants. Pediatrics, 20:951, 1957.

GMÜR, J., VON FELTEN, A., and STRAUB, W.: Gerinnungsuntersuchungen an Nabel-venenblut: fetales Fibrinogen? Schweiz Med. Wochen., 100:299, 1970.

GOLD, A. P., and MICHAEL, A. F., JR.: Congenital adrenal hyperplasia associated with polycythemia. Pediatrics, 23:727, 1959.

GOLDBERG, A., and RIMINGTON, C.: Diseases of Porphyrin Metabolism. Springfield, Ill., Charles C Thomas, 1962.

GOLDBERG, L. S., BARNETT, E. V., and DESAR, R.: Effect of transplacental transfer of antibody to intrinsic factor. Pediatrics, 40:851, 1967.

GOLDBERG, S. J., and FONKALSRUD, E.: Successful treatment of hepatic hemangioma with corticosteroids. J.A.M.A., 208:2473, 1969.

GOLDBLOOM, R. B., FISCHER, E., REINHOLD, J., and HSIA, D. Y. Y.: Studies on the mechanical fragility of erythrocytes. I. Normal values for infants and children. Blood, 8:165, 1953.

GOLDFARB, D. L., GINSBERG, V., KAUFMAN, M., ROBINSON, M. G., and WATSON, R. J.: Hemolytic disease of the newborn due to ABO incompatibility: a study of the use of group O erythrocytes in AB plasma. Pediatrics, *34*:664, 1964.

GOLDITCH, I. M., and BOYCE, N. E.: Management of abruptio placentae. J.A.M.A., *212*:288, 1970.

GOLUBOFF, N., and WHEATON, R.: Methylene blue induced cyanosis and acute hemolytic anemia complicating the treatment of methemoglobinemia. J. Pediat., *58*:86, 1961.

GOODALL, H. B., GRAHAN, F. S., MILLER, M. C., and CAMERON, C.: Transplacental bleeding from the fetus. J. Clin. Path., *11*:251, 1958.

GOODALL, J. R., ANDERSON, F. O., ALTIMUS, G. T., and MACPHAIL, F. L.: An inexhaustible source of blood for transfusion and its preservation. Surg. Gynec. Obst., 66:176, 1938.

GOODHUE, P. A., and EVANS, T. S.: Idiopathic thrombocytopenic purpura in pregnancy. Obst. Gynec. Surv., *18*:671, 1963.

GORDON, H. W.: Myeloid metaplasia masquerading as neonatal leukemia. Am. J. Dis. Child., *118*:932, 1969.

GORDON, R. R., and DEAN, I.: Fetal deaths from antenatal anticoagulant therapy. Brit. Med. J., *2*:719, 1955.

GREENWALT, T. J., and AYERS, V. E.: The phosphate partition of the erythrocytes of normal newborn infants and of infants with hemolytic disease. J. Clin. Invest., 35:1404, 1956.

GREENWALT, T. J., AYERS, V. E., and MORELL, S. A.: Phosphate partition in the erythrocytes of normal newborn infants and infants with erythroblastosis fetalis. III. P^{32} uptake and incorporation. Blood, *19*:468, 1962.

GREGG, G. S., and HUTCHINSON, D. L.: Developmental characteristics of infants surviving fetal transfusion. J.A.M.A., *209*:1059, 1969.

GRIMES, A. J., MEISLER, A., and DACIE, J. V.: Congenital Heinz-body anaemia: further evidence of the cause of Heinz-body production in red cells. Brit. J. Haemat., *10*:281, 1964.

GROSS, G. P., and HATHAWAY, W. E.: Fetal erythrocyte deformability – physiologic, rheologic and clinical considerations. Prog. Soc. Pediat. Res., 1971, p. 87.

GROSS, R. T., and HURWITZ, R. E.: The pentose phosphate pathway in human erythrocytes; relationship between the age of the subject and enzyme activity. Pediatrics, *22*:453, 1958.

GROSS, R. T., and SCHROEDER, E. A. R.: The relationship of triphosphopyridine nucleotide content to abnormalities in the erythrocytes of premature infants (abstract). J. Pediat., *63*:823, 1963.

GROSS, R. T., SCHROEDER, E. A. R., and BROUNSTEIN, S. A.: Energy metabolism in the erythrocytes of premature infants compared to full term newborn infants and adults. Blood, *21*:755, 1963.

GROSS, S., and MELHORN, D. K.: Exchange transfusion with citrated whole blood for disseminated intravascular coagulation. J. Pediatrics, 78:415, 1971.

GROSSMAN, A., RAMANATHAN, K., JUSTICE, P., GORDON, J., SHALIDI, N. T., and HSIA, D.: Congenital nonspherocytic hemolytic anemia associated with erythrocyte glucose-6-phosphate dehydrogenase deficiency in a Negro family. Pediatrics, *37*:624, 1966.

GROSSOWICZ, N., ARONOVITCH, J., RACHMILEWITZ, M., IZAK, G., SADOVSKY, A., and BERCOVICI, B.: Folic acid and folinic acid in maternal and foetal blood. Brit. J. Haemat., 6:296, 1960.

GROSSOWICZ, N., IZAK, G., and RACHMILEWITZ, M.: The effect of anemia on the concentration of folate derivatives in paired fetal-maternal blood. Israel J. Med. Sci., *2*:510, 1966.

GUEST, G. M., and BROWN, E. W.: Erythrocytes and hemoglobin of the blood in infancy and childhood. Am. J. Dis. Child., *93*:486, 1957.

GUEST, G. M., BROWN, E. W., and WING, M.: Erythrocytes and hemoglobin of blood in infancy and in childhood; variability in number, size and hemoglobin content of erythrocytes during first five years of life. Am. J. Dis. Child., *56*:529, 1938.

GUNSON, H. H.: Combined Rh and AB hemolytic disease of the newborn. Am. J. Clin. Path., *27*:35, 1957.

GUNSON, H. H.: An evaluation of the immunohematological tests used in the diagnosis of AB hemolytic disease. Am. J. Dis. Child., 94:123, 1957.

GUNSON, H. H.: Neonatal anaemia due to fetal hemorrhage into the maternal circulation. Pediatrics, 20:3, 1957.

GUNTHER, M.: The transfer of blood between baby and placenta in the minutes after birth. Lancet, 1:1277, 1957.

GUYTON, T. B., EHRLICH, F., BLANC, W. A., and BECKER, M. H.: New observations in generalized cytomegalic inclusion disease of newborn: report of case with chorioretinitis. New Eng. J. Med., 257:803, 1957.

HABERMAN, S., BLANTON, P., and MARTIN, J.: Some observations on the ABO antigen sites of the erythrocyte membranes of adults and newborn infants. J. Immun., 98:150, 1967.

HABERMAN, S., KRAFFT, J., LUECKE, P. E., JR., and PEACH, R. O.: ABO isoimmunization: the use of the specific Coombs and heat elution tests in the detection of hemolytic disease. J. Pediat., 56:471, 1960.

HAGBERG, B.: The iron-binding capacity of serum in infants and children. Acta Paediat., 42:589, 1953.

HAGGARD, M. E., and SCHNEIDER, R. G.: Sickle cell anemia in the first two years of life. J. Pediat., 58:785, 1961.

HALBRECHT, I.: Role of hemagglutinins anti-A and anti-B in pathogenesis of jaundice of the newborn (icterus neonatorum precox). Am. J. Dis. Child., 64:248, 1944.

HALBRECHT, I., and KLIBANSKI, C.: Identification of a new normal embryonic haemoglobin. Nature, 178:794, 1956.

HALBRECHT, I., KLIBANSKI, C., and BAR ILAN, F.: Co-existence of the embryonic (third normal) haemoglobin fraction with erythroblastosis in the blood of the two full-term newborn babies with multiple malformations. Nature, 183:327, 1959.

HALL, E. G., HAY, J. D., MOSS, P. D., and RYAN, M. M. P.: Congenital toxoplasmosis in the newborn. Arch. Dis. Child., 28:117, 1953.

HALL, J. G., LEVIN, J., KUHN, J. P., OTTENHEIMER, E. J., VAN BERKUM, K. A. P., and McKUSICK, V. A.: Thrombocytopenia with absent radius. Medicine, 48:411, 1969.

HALVORSEN, S.: Plasma erythropoietin levels in cord blood and in blood during the first weeks of life. Acta Paediat., 52:425, 1963.

HANEL, H. K., and BRANDT, N. J.: Haemolytic anemia due to abnormal pyruvate kinase. Lancet, 2:113, 1968.

HARDWICKE, S. H.: Studies on the minimum effective dose of a water soluble vitamin K substitute in the prevention of hypoprothrombinemia in newborn infants. J. Pediat., 24:259, 1941.

HARLEY, J. D., and CELERMAJER, J. M.: Neonatal methaemoglobinaemia and the "red-brown" screening test. Lancet, 2:1223, 1970.

HARLEY, J. D., ROBIN, H., and ROBERTSON, S. E. J.: Thiazide induced neonatal haemolysis? Brit. Med. J., 1:696–697, 1964.

HARPER, M. A., ROBIN, H., and HARLEY, J. D.: Transient infantile cyanosis in a diaphorase-deficient male. Aust. Paediat. J., 4:44, 1968.

HARRINGTON, W. J., SPRAGUE, C. C., MINNICH, V., MOORE, C. V., AULVIN, R. C., and DUBACH, R.: Immunologic mechanisms in idiopathic and neonatal thrombocytopenic purpura. Am. Int. Med., 38:433, 1953.

HARRIS, E. J., and PRANKERD, T. A. J.: The rate of sodium extrusion from human erythrocytes. J. Physiol., 121:470, 1953.

HARRIS, I. M., McALISTER, J. M., and PRANKERD, T. A. J.: Relationship of abnormal red cells to the normal spleen. Clin. Sci., 16:223, 1957.

HARRIS, J. W., and KELLERMEYER, R. W.: The Red Cell. Cambridge, Mass., Harvard University Press, 1970.

HARRIS, L. E., FARRELL, F. J., SHORTER, R. G., BANNER, E. A., and MATHIESON, D. R.: Conjugated serum bilirubin in erythroblastosis fetalis: an analysis of 38 cases. Mayo Clin. Proc., 37:574, 1962.

HARTMANN, J. R., and DIAMOND, L. K.: Haemophilia and related haemorrhagic disorders. Practioner, 178:179, 1957.

HARTMANN, J. R., HOWELL, D. A., and DIAMOND, L. K.: Disorders of blood coagulation during the first weeks of life. A.M.A. Am. J. Dis. Child., 90:594, 1955.

HARVALD, B., HANEL, K. H., SQUIRES, R., and TRAP-JENSEN, T.: Adenosinetriphosphatase deficiency in patients with nonspherocytic haemolytic anemia. Lancet, 2:18, 1964.

HARVEY, B., REMINGTON, J. S., and SULZER, A. J.: IgM malaria antibodies in a case of congenital malaria in the United States. Lancet, 1:333, 1969.

HARWIN, M., and ANGRIST, A.: Neonatal toxoplasmic encephalitis. Case presentation. Arch. Pediat., 65:124, 1948.

HASSELHORST, G., and ALLMELING, A.: Die Gewichtszunahme von Neugeboren infolge postnataler Transfusion. Ztschr. Geburtsh. Gynäk., 98:103, 1930.

HATHAWAY, W. E.: Coagulation problems in the newborn infant. Pediat. Clin. N.A., 17:929, 1970.

HATHAWAY, W. E.: Fibrin split products in serum of newborn. (Letter to the Editor.) Pediatrics, 45:154, 1970.

HATHAWAY, W. E., GITHENS, J. H., BLACKBURN, W. R., FULGINITI, V., and KEMPE, C. H.: Aplastic anemia, histiocytosis and erythrodermia in immunologically deficient children; probable human runt disease. New Eng. J. Med., 273:953, 1965.

HATHAWAY, W. E., MULL, M. M., and PECHET, G. S.: Disseminated intravascular coagulation in the newborn. Pediat., 43:233, 1969.

HAUPT, H.: Zur vitamin K: dosieren bei neu und Fruhgeborenen. Dtsch. Med. Wschr., 85:474, 1960.

HAYES, K., and GIBAS, H.: Placental cytomegalovirus infection without fetal involvement following primary infection in pregnancy. J. Pediat. 79:401, 1971.

HAZELTINE, F. G.: Hypoglycemic and Rh erythroblastosis fetalis. Pediatrics, 39:696, 1967.

HECHT, F., JONES, R. T., and KOLER, R. D.: Newborn infants with Hb Portland I, an indicator of α-chain deficiency. Ann. Hum. Genet., 31:215, 1967.

HECHT, F., MOTULSKY, A. G., LEMIRE, R. J., and SHEPARD, T. E.: Predominance of hemoglobin Gower I in early embryonic development. Science, 152:91, 1966.

HEDENBERG, F.: Infantile agranulocytosis of probably congenital origin. Acta Paediat., 48:77, 1959.

HEDENSTEDT, S., and NAESLUND, J.: Investigations of permeability of placenta with help of elliptocytes. Acta Med. Scand., 170:390, 1946.

HEISSEN, A., and SCHALLOER, R.: Über die Grossenverhältnisse der roten Blutkörperchen bein Neugeborenen und Säugling. Ztschr. Kinderh., 46:105, 1928.

HELDRICH, F. J., JR.: Sickle-cell anemia: report of a case in a newborn infant. J. Pediat., 39:90, 1951.

HELLER, P., YAKULIS, V. J., and JOSEPHSON, A. M.: Immunologic studies of human hemoglobins. J. Lab. Clin. Med., 59:401, 1962.

HELLMAN, L. M., and SHETTLES, L. B.: Factors influencing plasma prothrombin in the newborn infant: prematurity and vitamin K. Bull. Johns Hopkins Hosp., 63:138, 1939.

HELZ, M. K., and MENTEN, M. L.: Elliptocytosis, a report of two cases. J. Lab. Clin. Med., 29:185, 1944.

HENDERSON, J. L.: Hepatic haemorrhage in stillborn and newborn infants; clinical and pathological study of 47 cases. J. Obst. Gynaec. Brit. Emp., 48:377, 1941.

HENDRICKSE, R. G., BOYO, A. E., FITZGERALD, P. A., and KUTI, S. R.: Studies on the haemoglobin of newborn Nigerians. Brit. Med. J., 1:611, 1960.

HERLITZ, G.: Zur Kenntnis der anämischen und polyzytämischen Zustände bei Neugeborenen, soivie des Icterus gravis neonatorum. Acta Paediat., 29:211, 1942.

HEY, E. N., KOHLINSKY, S., and O'CONNELL, B.: Heat-losses from babies during exchange transfusion. Lancet, 1:335, 1969.

HEYS, R. F.: Steroid therapy for idiopathic thrombocytopenic purpura during pregnancy. Obst. Gynec., 28:532, 1966.

HIGASHI, O.: Congenital gigantism of peroxidase granules. First case ever reported by qualitative abnormality of peroxidase. Tohoku J. Exp. Med., 59:315, 1954.

HILGARTNER, M. W.: Transient functional thrombasthenia in the newborn. Abstr., Soc. Pediat. Res., Atlantic City, May, 1968, p. 120.

HILLMAN, R. S., and PHILLIPS, L. L.: Clotting-fibrinolysis in a cavernous hemangioma. Am. J. Dis. Child., 113:649, 1967.

HIRSCH, A.: Die physiologische Ikterusbereitschaft des Neugeborenen. Ztschr. Kinderh., 9:196, 1913.

Hitzig, W. H., and Gitzelmann, R.: Transplacental transfer of leukocyte agglutinins. Vox Sang., 4:445, 1959.

Hitzig, W. H., Kay, H. E. M., and Cottier, H.: Familial lymphopenia with agammaglobulinemia. Lancet, 2:151, 1965.

Hjelt, L., and Wegelius, R.: Congenital leukemia. Ann. Paediat. Fenn., 2:206, 1956.

Hobel, C. J.: The value of fetal scalp blood hemoglobin determination in Rh erythroblastosis fetalis. J. Pediat., 77:460, 1970.

Hodapp, R. V.: The case of the red and white Minnesota twins. J. Lancet, 82:413, 1962.

Hollan, S. R., Szelényi, J. G., Breuer, J. H., Medgyesi, G. A., and Söter, V. N.: Structural and functional differences between human foetal and adult erythrocytes. Haematol. 4:409, 1967.

Holland, E.: A case of transplacental metastases of malignant melanoma from mother to fetus. J. Obst. Gynaec. Brit. Emp., 56:529, 1949.

Holland, P., and Mauer, A. M.: Myeloid leukemoid reactions in childhood. Am. J. Dis. Child., 105:568, 1963.

Hollenberg, M. D., Kaback, M. M., and Kazazian, H. H.: Adult hemoglobin synthesis by reticulocytes from the human fetus at midtrimester. Science, 174:698, 1971.

Hollingsworth, J. W.: Lifespan of fetal erythrocytes. J. Lab. Clin. Med., 45:469, 1955.

Holmberg, E.: Rupture of liver in new-born observed at General Lying-In Hospital in Helsingfors from 1924 to 1932. Finska Läk.-Sällsk. Handl., 75:1067, 1933.

Holroyde, C. P., Oski, F. A., and Gardner, F. H.: The "pocked" erythrocyte. New Eng. J. Med., 281:516, 1969.

Honda, F., Punnett, H. H., Charney, E., Miller, G., and Thiede, H. A.: Serial cytogenetic and hematologic studies on a mongol with trisomy-21 with acute congenital leukemia. J. Pediat., 65:880, 1964.

Honig, G. R., Lacson, P. S., and Maurer, H. S.: A new familial disorder with abnormal erythrocyte morphology and increased permeability of the erythrocytes to sodium and potassium. Pediat. Res., 5:159, 1971.

Horley, J. F.: Congenital tuberculosis. Arch. Dis. Child., 27:167, 1952.

Horton, B. F., Thompson, R. B., Dozy, A. M., Nechtman, C. M., Nichols, E., and Huisman, T. H. J.: Inhomogeneity of hemoglobin. VI. The minor hemoglobin components of cord blood. Blood, 20:302, 1962.

Hosoi, T., Kashiwabara, S., and Nakamura, V.: The survival time of transfused erythrocytes of the newborn as determined by serological method. Yokohama Med. Bull., 10:71, 1959.

Høyer, A.: Lipomatosis pseudohypertrophy of the pancreas with complete absence of exocrine tissue. J. Path. Bact., 61:93, 1949.

Hoyeraal, H. M., Lamvik, J., and Moe, P. J.: Congenital hypoplastic thrombocytopenia and cerebral malformations in two brothers. Acta Paediat. Scand. 59:185, 1970.

Hrodek, O.: Blood platelets in the newborn. Acta Univ. Carol. Med., Monograph 22, 1966.

Hryniuk, W., Foerster, J., Shojania, M., Bercovitch, L., and Chow, C.: Disseminated herpes zoster infections controlled with low doses of cytosine arabinoside. Prog. Amer. Soc. Hemat. p. 30, 1971.

Hsia, D. Y., Allen, F. H., Jr., Gellis, S. S., and Diamond, L. K.: Erythroblastosis fetalis. VIII. Studies of serum bilirubin in relation to kernicterus. New Eng. J. Med., 247:668, 1952.

Hsia, D. Y., and Walker, F. A.: Variability in clinical manifestation of galactosemia. J. Pediat., 59:872, 1961.

Huehns, E. R., Dance, N., Beaven, G., Keil, J. V., Hecht, F., and Motulsky, A. G.: Human embryonic haemoglobins. Nature, 201:1095, 1964.

Huehns, E. R., Hecht, F., Keil, J. V., and Motulsky, A. G.: Developmental hemoglobin anomalies in a chromosomal triplication: D_1-trisomy syndrome. Proc. Nat. Acad. Sci., 51:89, 1964.

Huehns, E. R., Lutzner, M., and Hecht, F.: Nuclear abnormalities of the neutrophils in D (13-15) trisomy syndrome. Lancet, 1:589, 1964.

Huehns, E. R., and Shooter, E. M.: Polypeptide chains of haemoglobin A_2. Nature, 189:918, 1961.

Huehns, E. R., and Shooter, E. M.: Review article: human haemoglobins. J. Med. Genet., 2:48, 1965.

HUENNEKENS, F. M., CAFFREY, R. W., and GABRIO, B. W.: Electron transport sequence of methemoglobin reductase. Ann. N. Y. Acad. Sci., 75:167, 1958.

HUGHES, D. W. O'G., and DIAMOND, L. K.: A new type of constitutional aplastic anemia without congenital anomalies presenting as thrombocytopenia in infancy. J. Pediat., 65:1060, 1964.

HUGHES-JONES, N. C., HUGHES, M. I. J., and WALKER, W.: The amount of anti-D on red cells in haemolytic disease of the newborn. Vox Sang., 12:279, 1967.

HUGH-JONES, K., MANFIELD, P. A., and BREWER, H. F.: Congenital thrombocytopenic purpura. Arch. Dis. Child., 35:146, 1960.

HUISMAN, T. H. J.: Genetic aspects of two different minor haemoglobin components found in cord blood samples of Negro babies. Nature, 188:589, 1960.

HUISMAN, T. H. J., DOZY, A. M., HORTON, B. E., and WILSON, J. B.: A fetal hemoglobin with abnormal γ-polypeptide chains: hemoglobin Warren. Blood, 26:668, 1965.

HUISMAN, T. H. J., SCHROEDER, W. A., ADAMS, H. R., SHELTON, J. R., SHELTON, J. B., and APELL, G.: A possible subclass of the hereditary persistence of fetal hemoglobin. Blood, 36:1, 1970.

HUMBERT, J. R., ABELSON, H., HATHAWAY, W. E., and BATTAGLIA, F. C.: Polycythemia in small for gestational age infants. J. Pediat., 75:812, 1969.

HUMBERT, J. R., KURTZ, M. L., and HATHAWAY, W. E.: Increased reduction of nitro-blue tetrazolium by neutrophils of newborn infants. Pediatrics, 45:125, 1970.

HUMES, J. J., and HARMELING, J. G.: Identification of antibodies in erythroblastosis fetalis. In Clinical Pathology in Infancy, seminar prepared by the Institute for Clinical Science, Inc., for the Association of Clinical Scientists, Washington, D. C., 1965.

HUNT, J. A.: Identity of the α-chains of adults and foetal haemoglobin. Nature, 183: 1373, 1959.

HUNT, J. A., and LEHMANN, H.: Haemoglobin Bart's: a foetal haemoglobin without α-chains. Nature, 184:872, 1959.

HUNTER, W. C.: A further study of a white family showing elliptical erythrocytes. Ann. Intern. Med., 6:775, 1932.

HYMAN, C. B., KEASTER, J., HANSON, V., HARRIS, I., SEDGWICK, R., WURSTEN, H., and WRIGHT, A. R.: CNS abnormalities after neonatal hemolytic disease or hyperbilirubinemia. Am. J. Dis. Child., 117:395, 1969.

INALL, J. A., BLUHM, M. M., KERR, M. M., DOUGLAS, T. A., HOPE, C. S., and HUTCHISON, J. H.: Blood volume and haematocrit studies in respiratory distress syndrome of the newborn. Arch. Dis. Child., 40:480, 1965.

INGRAM, V. M., and STRETTON, A. O. W.: Human haemoglobin A_2. I. Comparison of haemoglobins A_2 and A. Biochim. Biophys. Acta, 62:456, 1962.

IOB, V., and SWANSON, W. W.: Mineral growth of the human fetus. Am. J. Dis. Child., 47:302, 1934.

IRANI, P. K.: Haematoma of the umbilical cord. Brit. Med. J., 2:1436, 1964.

IRLE, V.: Acute haemolytic anaemia due to naphthalene inhalation in two premature and one full-term infant. German Med. Monthly, 10:59, 1965.

IVERSEN, T.: Leukemia in infancy and childhood. A material of 570 Danish cases. Acta Paed. Scand., Suppl. 167, 1966.

JACKSON, D. P., SCHMID, H. J., ZIEVE, P. D., LEVIN, J., and CONLEY, C. L.: Nature of a platelet-agglutination factor in serum of patients with idiopathic thrombocytopenic purpura. J. Clin. Invest., 42:383, 1963.

JACKSON, R.: Discoid lupus in a newborn infant of a mother with lupus erythematosus. Pediatrics, 33:425, 1964.

JACOB, H. S., and JANDL., J. H.: Increased cell membrane permeability in the pathogenesis of hereditary spherocytosis. J. Clin. Invest., 43:1704, 1964.

JADHAV, M., WEBB, J. K. G., VAISHNAVA, S., and BAKER, S. J.: Vitamin B_{12} deficiency in Indian infants. Lancet, 2:903, 1962.

JAFFÉ, E. R.: Clinical profile: Hereditary hemolytic disorders and enzymatic deficiencies of human erythrocytes. Blood, 35:116, 1970.

JAMES, G. W., III, RUDOLPH, S. G., and ABBOTT, L. D., JR.: Delta-aminolevulinic acid, porphobilinogen, and porphyrin excretion throughout pregnancy in a patient with acute intermittent porphyria with "passive porphyria" in the infant. J. Lab. Clin. Med., 58:437, 1961.

JANDL, J. H., JONES, A. R., and CASTLE, W. B.: The destruction of red cells by anti-bodies in man. I. Observations on the sequestration and lysis of red cells altered by immune mechanisms. J. Clin. Invest., 36:1428, 1957.

JAVERT, C. T.: The occurrence and significance of the nucleated erythrocytes in the fetal vessels of the placenta. Am. J. Obst. Gynec., 37:184, 1939.

JEGIER, W., BLANKENSHIP, W., and LIND, J.: Venous pressure in the first hour of life and its relationship to placental transfusion. Acta Paed., 52:485, 1963.

JEGIER, W., MACLAURIN, J., BLANKENSHIP, W., and LIND, J.: Comparative study of blood volume estimation in the newborn infant using I^{131} labeled human serum albumen (IHSA) and T-1824. Scand. J. Clin. Lab. Invest., 16:125, 1964.

JENKINS, G. C., BEALE, D., BLACK, A. J., HUNTSMAN, R. G., and LEHMANN, H.: Hemo-globin F Texas I: a variant of haemoglobin F. Brit. J. Haemat., 13:252, 1967.

JENNISON, R. F., and WALKER, A. H. C.: Amniocentesis (letter). Lancet, 2:1387, 1963.

JENSEN, K. G.: Transplacental passage of leucocyte agglutinins occurring on account of pregnancy. Dan. Med. Bull., 7:55, 1960.

JENSEN, K. G.: Leucocyte antibodies in serums of pregnant women. Vox Sang., 7:454, 1962.

JESIONEK, A., and KIOLEMENOGLOV, B.: Über einen befund von protozönartigen Gebilden in den Organen eines hereditärleutischen Fötus. Münch. Med. Wschr., 51:1905, 1904.

JIM, R. T. S., and CHU, F. K.: Hyperbilirubinemia due to glucose-6-phosphate dehy-drogenase deficiency in a newborn Chinese infant. Pediatrics, 31:1046, 1963.

JOHNSON, A. B., and MARKS, P. A.: Glucose metabolism and oxygen consumption in normal and glucose-6-phosphate dehydrogenase deficient human erythrocytes. Clin. Res., 6:187, 1958.

JOHNSON, L.: Personal communication (1965).

JOHNSTON, W. H., ANGARA, V., BAUMAL, R., HAWKE, W. A., JOHNSON, R. H., KEET, S., and WOOD, M.: Erythroblastosis fetalis and hyperbilirubinemia. A five-year follow-up with neurological, psychological and audiological evaluation. Pediatrics, 39: 88, 1967.

JONES, B., and KLINGBERG, W. G.: A study of erythropoietin in 2 types of hemolytic anemia—erythroblastosis fetalis and sickle cell anemia. J. Pediat., 56:752–8, 1960.

JONES, E. R.: The application of the Kleihauer technique to fetal blood. Aust. N. Z. J. Obstet. Gynaec., 9:33, 1969.

JONES, J. E., and REED, J. F., JR.: Renal vein thrombosis and thrombocytopenia in a newborn infant. J. Pediat., 67:681, 1965.

JONES, P., McNAY, A., and WALKER, W.: Association between foeto-maternal bleeding and hypertension in pregnancy. Brit. Med. J., 2:738, 1969.

JONES, P. E. H., and McCANCE, R. A.: Enzyme activities in the blood of infants and adults. Biochem. J., 45:464, 1949.

JONES, R. A., and SILVER, S.: The detection of minor erythrocyte population by mixed agglutinates. Blood, 13:763, 1958.

JONXIS, J. H. P.: Foetal haemoglobin and erythroblastosis. Nature, 161:850, 1948.

JOPE, E. M.: The ultra-violet spectral absorption of haemoglobin inside and outside the red blood cell. In Haemoglobin. (Barcroft memorial volume, Roughton, F. J. W., and Kendrew, J. C., eds.). London, Butterworth, 1949, p. 205.

JORDANS, G. H.: The familial occurrence of fat containing vacuoles in the leukocytes diagnosed in two brothers suffering from dystrophia musculorum progressiva. Acta Med. Scand., 145:419, 1953.

JORGENSEN, J.: Rhesus antibody development after abortion. Lancet, 2:1253, 1969.

JOSEPHS, H. W.: Iron metabolism and the hypochromic anemia of infancy. Medicine, 32:125, 1953.

KAISER, I. H., and GOODLIN, R. C.: Alterations of pH, gases and hemoglobin in blood and electrolytes in plasma of fetuses of diabetic mothers. Pediatrics, 22:1097, 1958.

KALPAKTSOGLOU, P. K., and EMERY, J. L.: The effect of birth on the haemopoietic tissue of the human bone marrow. Brit. J. Haemat., 11:453, 1965.

KALPAKTSOGLOU, P. K., and EMERY, J. L.: Human bone marrow during the last 3 months of intrauterine life. Acta Haemat., 34:228, 1965.

KAN, Y. W., and NATHAN, D. G.: Beta thalassemia trait: detection at birth. Science, 161:589, 1968.

KAN, Y. W., ALLEN, A., and LOWENSTEIN, L.: Hydrops fetalis with alpha thalassemia. New. Eng. J. Med., 276:18, 1967.

KAN, Y. W., FORGET, B. G., and NATHAN, D. G.: Gamma-beta thalassemia as a cause of hemolytic disease of the newborn. New Eng. J. Med., 286:129, 1972.

KAN, Y. W., SCHWARTZ, E., and NATHAN, D. G.: Globin chain synthesis in the alpha thalassemia syndromes. J. Clin. Invest., 47:2515, 1968.

KAPLAN, E., HERZ, F., and HSU, K. S.: Erythrocyte acetylcholinesterase activity in ABO hemolytic disease of the newborn. Pediatrics, 33:205, 1964.

KAPLAN, E., HERZ, F., SCHEYE, E., and ROBINSON, L., JR.: Phototherapy in ABO hemolytic disease of the newborn. J. Pediat., 79:911, 1971.

KAPLAN, E., and HSU, K. S.: Determination of erythrocyte survival in newborn infants by means of Cr51-labeled erythrocytes. Pediatrics, 27:354, 1961.

KAPLAN, E., and KLEIN, S. W.: Thrombocytopenia and intestinal bleeding in premature infants. J. Pediat., 61:17, 1962.

KAPLAN, N. D., SWARTZ, M. H., FRECH, M. E., and CIOTTI, M. M.: Phosphorylative and nonphosphorylative pathways of electron transfer in rat liver mitochondria. Proc. Nat. Acad. Sci., 42:481, 1956.

KARPATKIN, M.: Diagnosis and management of disseminated intravascular coagulation. Pediat. Clin. N.A., 18:23, 1971.

KARPATKIN, M.: Fibrin split products in serum of newborn. (Letter to the Editor.) Pediatrics, 45:157, 1970.

KASABACH, H. H., and MERRITT, K. K.: Capillary hemangioma with extensive purpura. Report of a case. Am. J. Dis. Child., 59:1063, 1940.

KASDON, S. C.: Pregnancy and Hodgkin's disease. Am. J. Obst. Gynec., 57:282, 1949.

KATO, K.: Physiological variations in reticulocytes in new born; study of 219 cases. Folia Haemat., 46:377, 1932.

KATO, K.: Leucocytes in infancy and childhood; statistical analysis of 1081 total and differential counts from birth to 15 years. J. Pediat., 7:7, 1935.

KATTAMIS, C.: Favism in breast-fed infants. Arch. Dis. Childh. 46:741, 1971.

KATZ, J.: Transplacental passage of fetal red cells in abortion; increased incidence after curettage and effect of oxytocic drugs. Brit. Med. J., 4:84, 1969.

KATZ, S., and KIBRICK, S.: Nonbacterial infections of the newborn. Ped. Clin. North Am., 8:493, 1961.

KAUDER, E. and MAUER, A. M.: Neutropenias of childhood. J. Pediat., 69:147, 1966.

KAUFFMANN, H. J., and HESS, R.: Kasuestescher Beitrag zur Problematek der kongenitalen Leukämie. Schweiz. Med. Wschr., 89:1053, 1959.

KAUFFMANN, H. J., and HESS, R.: Does congenital leukemia exist? Brit. Med. J., 1: 867, 1962.

KEENAN, W. J., JEWETT, T., and GLUECK, H. I.: Role of feeding and Vitamin K in hypoprothrombinemia of the newborn. Am. J. Dis. Child., 121:271, 1971.

KEITT, A. S.: Hemolytic anemia with impaired hexokinase activity. Clin. Res., 16: 306, 1969; J. Clin. Invest., 48:1997, 1969.

KELLERMEYER, R. W., TARLOV, A. R., SCHRIER, S. L., CARSON, P. E., and ALVING, A. S.: The hemolytic effect of primaquine: XIII. Gradient susceptibility to hemolysis of primaquine sensitive erythrocytes. J. Lab. Clin. Med., 58:225, 1961.

KEVY, S.: Clinical pathologic conference. J. Pediat., 60:304, 1962.

KHALIL, M.: Haptoglobin level in normal infants and children. Alexandria Med. J., 13:1, 1967.

KIBRICK, S., and BENIRSCHKE, K.: Severe generalized disease (encephalohepatomyocarditis) occurring in the newborn period and due to infection with Coxsackie virus Group B. Pediatrics, 27:857, 1958.

KILLANDER, A.: On the use of exchange transfusion in neonatal thrombocytopenic purpura; report of a case. Acta Paediat., 48:29, 1959.

KILLANDER, A., and VAHLQUEST, B.: B12 vitamin koncentrationen serum från fullgångna och prematurt födda barn. Nord. Med., 51:777, 1954.

KIRKMAN, H. N., and RILEY, H. D., JR.: Posthemorrhagic anemia and shock in the newborn. A review. Pediatrics, 24:97, 1959.

KIRSCHBAUM, T. H.: Fetal hemoglobin content of cord blood determined by column chromatography. Am. J. Obst. Gynec., 84:1375, 1962.

KITCHEN, W. H.: Birth weight of infants with Rhesus incompatibility. Aust. N. Z. J. Obstet. Gynaec., 10:30, 1970.

KITTERMAN, J. A., PHIBBS, R. H., and TOOLEY, W. H.: Catheterization of umbilical vessels in newborn infants. Pediat. Clin. N. Amer., 17:895, 1970.

KLEIHAUER, E., and BRANDT, G.: Survival time of fetal erythrocytes in maternal circulation. Klin. Wschr., 42:458, 1964.

KLEIHAUER, E., BRAUN, H., and BETKE, K.: Demonstration von fetalem Hämoglobin in den Erythrocyten eines Blutausstrichs. Klin. Wschr., 35:637, 1957.

KLEIHAUER, E., HILDEGARD, B., and BETKE, K.: Demonstration von fetalem Hämoglobin in den Erythrocyten eines Blutausstrichs. Klin. Wschr., 35:637, 1957.

KLEIHAUER, E. F., TANG, T. E., and BETKE, K.: Die intrazelluläre verteilung von embryonalem hämoglobin in roten blutzellen menschlicher embryonen. Acta Haemat., 38:264, 1967.

KLEIN, R.: Cited by Kirkman, H. N., and Riley, H. D., Jr.: Posthemorrhagic anemia and shock in the newborn. A review. Pediatrics, 24:97, 1959.

KLEIN, R., and HANSON, J.: Adrenocortical function in the newborn infant as measured by adrenocorticotropic hormone eosinophil response. Pediatrics, 6:192, 1950.

KLEMPERER, M. R., OSTHOLD, M., VASQUEZ, D., and DIAMOND, L. K.: The incidence of complete complement-fixing platelet antibodies in pregnant women. Vox Sang., 11:124, 1966.

KLUGE, R. C., WICKSMAN, R. S., and WELLER, T. H.: Cytomegalic inclusion disease of the newborn. Report of a case with persistent viruria. Pediatrics, 25:35, 1960.

KNOLL, W.: Der Gang der Erythropoese beim menschlichen Embryo. Acta Haemat., 2:369, 1949.

KNOX, E. G.: Obstetric determinants of Rhesus immunization. Lancet, 1:433, 1968.

KOCH, F. R.: Bluteweissuntersuchungen bei in Neugeborenen unter Berücksichtigung der Gerinnungsstorungen. Z. Geburtsh. Beilageheft., Bd. 159, 1962.

KOCH, M. I.: Zur Frage du kongenitalen Leukämie. Zbl. Allg. Pathol., 33:7, 1922.

KOCHWA, S., ROSENFIELD, R. E., TALLAL, L., and WASSERMAN, L. R.: Isoagglutinins associated with ABO erythroblastosis. J. Clin. Invest., 40:874, 1961.

KOHLER, H. G.: Haemorrhage in the newborn of epileptic mothers (Letter to the Editor). Lancet, 1:267, 1966.

KOJ, A.: Biosynthesis of glutathione in human blood. Acta Biochim. Pol., 9:11, 1962.

KONRAD, P. N., RICHARDS, F., VALENTINE, W. N., and PAGLIA, D. E.: γ-Glutamyl-cysteine synthetase deficiency—a new cause of hereditary hemolytic anemia. Blood, 38:808, 1971.

KONTRAS, S. B., BODENBENDER, J. G., SOMMER, A., and CRAENEN, J.: Viscosity studies in neonatal polycythemia. Program, Soc. Pediat. Res., 1970, p. 223.

KONTRAS, S. B., GREEN, O. C., KING, L., and DURAN, R. J.: Giant hemangioma with thrombocytopenia; case report with survival and sequestration studies of platelets labeled with chromium 51. Am. J. Dis. Child., 105:188, 1963.

KÖRBER, E.: Cited by Bischoff, H.: Inaugural dissertations, Dorpat. Ztschr. Exp. Med., 48:472, 1926.

KORN, D.: Congenital hypoplastic thrombocytopenia. Am. J. Clin. Path., 37:405, 1962.

KORONES, S. B., AINGER, L. E., MONIF, G. R. G., ROANE, J., SEVER, J. L., and FUSTE, F.: Congenital rubella syndrome: New clinical aspects with recovery of virus from affected infants. J. Pediat., 67:166, 1965.

KOSOWER, N. S., VANDERHOFF, G. A., JAFFE, E. R., and LONDON, I. M.: Metabolic changes in normal and glucose-6-phosphate dehydrogenase-deficient erythrocytes induced by acetylphenylhydrazine. J. Clin. Invest., 42:1025, 1963.

KOSTINAS, J. E., CANTOW, E. F., and WETZEL, R. A.: Autohemolysis of cord blood in congenital spherocytosis and ABO incompatibility. J. Pediat., 70:273, 1967.

KOSTMAN, R.: Infantile genetic agranulocytosis. Acta Paediat., 45:105, 1956.

KOZINN, P. J., RITZ, N., and HOROWITZ, A. W.: Scalp hemorrhage as an emergency in the newborn. J.A.M.A., 194:567, 1963.

KRAUS, A. P., LANGSTON, M. F., JR., and LYNCH, B. L.: Red cell phosphoglycerate kinase deficiency. A new cause of nonspherocytic hemolytic anemia. Biochem. Biophys. Res. Commun., 30:173, 1968.

KRAVITZ, H., ELEGANT, L. D., KAISER, E., and KAGAN, B. M.: Methemoglobin values in premature and mature infants and children. Am. J. Dis. Child., 91:1, 1956.

KRAVKOVA, E.: Morphological picture of the blood of the human foetus in pregnancy complicated by heart disease. Akush. Ginek., 5:49, 1962.

KRESKY, B.: Transplacental transfusion syndrome. Clin. Pediat., 3:600, 1964.

KRILL, C. E., JR., and MAUER, A. M.: Congenital agranulocytosis. J. Pediat., 68:361, 1966.

KRIVIT, W., and GOOD, R. A.: Simultaneous occurrence of leukemia and mongolism. Report of a nationwide survey. A.M.A. J. Dis. Child., *94*:289, 1957.

KRUEGER, H. C. and BURGERT, E. O., JR.: Hereditary spherocytosis in 100 children. Mayo Clin. Proc., *41*:821, 1966.

KÜNZER, W., and SAVELSBERG, W.: Der Hämiglobingehalt kindlichen Blutes. Klin. Wschr., *29*:648, 1951.

KURKCOUGLU, M., and McELFRESH, A. E.: The Hageman factor. Determination of the concentration during the neonatal period and presentation of a case of Hageman factor deficiency. J. Pediat., *57*:61, 1960.

KURTH, D., DEISS, A., and CARTWRIGHT, G. E.: Circulating siderocytes in human subjects. Blood, *34*:754, 1969.

LACHHEIN, L., GRUBE, E., JOHNIGK, C., MATTHIES, H.: Der Verbrauch an Glucose, Galaktose, Ribose und Inosin von Erwachsenen—und Nabelschnur—Erythrocyten. Klin. Wschr., *39*:875, 1961.

LAFER, C. Z. and MORRISON, A. N.: Thrombocytopenic purpura progressing to transient hypoplastic anemia in a newborn with rubella syndrome. Pediatrics, *38*:499, 1966.

LAHEY, M. E., BEIER, F. R., and WILSON, J. F.: Leukemia in Down's syndrome (editor's column). J. Pediat., *63*:189, 1964.

LALEZARI, P., NUSSBAUM, M., GELMAN, S., and SPAET, T. H.: Neonatal neutropenia due to maternal isoimmunization. Blood, *15*:236, 1960.

LAMPKIN, B. C., SHORE, N. A., and CHADWICK, D.: Megaloblastic anemia of infancy secondary to maternal pernicious anemia. New England J. Med., *274*:1168, 1966.

LANG, D. J. and NOREN, B.: Cytomegaloviremia following congenital infection. J. Pediatrics, *73*:812, 1968.

LANZKOWSKY, P.: Effects of early and late clamping of umbilical cord on infant's haemoglobin level. Brit. Med. J., *2*:1777, 1960.

LANZKOWSKY, P.: The influence of maternal iron deficiency on the haemoglobin of the infant. Arch. Dis. Child., *36*:205, 1961.

LARKIN, I. L. M., BAKER, T., LORKIN, P. A., LEHMANN, H., BLACK, A. J., and HUNTSMAN, R. G.: Haemoglobin F Texas II, the second of the haemoglobin F Texas variants. Brit. J. Haemat., *14*:23, 1968.

LASCARI, A. D.: Christmas disease in a girl. Am. J. Dis. Child., *117*:585, 1969.

LASCARI, A. D., and WALLACE, P. D.: Disseminated intravascular coagulation in the newborn. Clin. Pediat., *10*:11, 1971.

LAURELL, C. B.: Studies on the transportation and metabolism of iron in the body. Acta Physiol. Scand., *14*:1, 1947.

LEALE, M.: Recurrent furunculosis in an infant showing an unusual blood picture. J.A.M.A., *54*:1854, 1910.

LEAPE, L. L., and BORDY, M. D.: Neonatal rupture of the spleen. Report of a case successfully treated after spontaneous cessation of hemorrhage. Pediatrics, *47*:101, 1971.

LEE, C. L., and CINER, E.: Congenital leukemia associated with mongolism. J. Pediat., *51*:303, 1957.

LEE, R. E., and VAZQUEZ, J. J.: Immunocytochemical evidence for transplacental passage of erythrocytes. Lab. Invest., *11*:580, 1962.

LEES, M. H., and JOLLY, H.: Severe congenital methaemoglobinaemia in an infant. Lancet, *2*:1147, 1957.

LEHMANN, H.: Different types of alpha-thalassaemia and significance of haemoglobin Bart's in neonates. Lancet, *2*:78, 1970.

LEIKIN, S. L., and McCOO, J. W.: Sickle-cell anemia in infancy. Am. J. Dis. Child., *96*:51, 1958.

LEISSRING, J. C., and VORLICKY, L. N.: Disseminated intravascular coagulation in a neonate. Am. J. Dis. Child., *115*:100, 1968.

LELONG, M., ALAGILLE, D., HABIB, E.-C., and STEINER, A.: L'Hémangiome géant du nourrisson avec thrombopenie. Arch. Franc. Pediat., *21*:769, 1964.

LELONG, M., ALAGILLE, D., and ODIÈVRE, M.: Les anomalies hémolytiques du nouveau-né, à l'exception des incompatibilités sanguines. Nouv. Rev. Franc. Hémat., *4*:110, 1964.

LELONG, M., ROSSIER, A., ALAGILLE, D., and MARCHAND, E.: Étude functionelle du foie chez le prémature aide du complexe prothrombinique et de l'electro-phorèse. Rev. Int. Hépat., 5:1129, 1955.

LEMBERG, R., and LEGGE, J. W.: Hematin Compounds and Bile Pigments. New York, Interscience Publishers, 1949.

LEONARD, J. G.: White cell alkaline phosphatase in the developing foetus. Arch. Dis. Child., 40:450, 1965.

LEONARD, S., and ANTHONY, B.: Giant cephalohematoma of newborn. Am. J. Dis. Child., 101:170, 1961.

LESTER, R., BEHRMAN, R. E., and LUCEY, J. F.: Transfer of bilirubin-C^{14} across monkey placenta. Pediatrics, 32:416, 1963.

LETTS, H. W., and KREDENSTER, B.: Thrombocytopenia, hemolytic anemia and two pregnancies. Report of a case. Am. J. Clin. Path., 49:481, 1968.

LETTS, H. W., and KREDENSTER, B. K.: Thrombocytopenia, hemolytic anemia, three pregnancies, and death. A supplementary case report. Am. J. Clin. Path., 51:780, 1969.

LEVI, A. J., GATMAITAN, Z., and ARIAS, I.: Deficiency of hepatic organic anion-binding protein, impaired organic anion uptake by liver and "physiologic" jaundice in newborn monkeys. New Eng. J. Med., 283:1136, 1970.

LEVIN, S. E.: Shigella septicemia in the newborn infant. J. Pediat., 71:917, 1967.

LEVINE, P.: Serological factors as possible causes of spontaneous abortion. J. Hered., 34:71, 1943.

LEVINE, P., BURNHAM, L., KATZIN, E. M., and VOGEL, P.: The role of iso-immuniza-tion in the pathogenesis of erythroblastosis fetalis. Am. J. Obst. Gynec., 42:925, 1941.

LEVINE, P., KATZIN, E. M., and BURNHAM, L.: Iso-immunization in pregnancy, its possible bearing on the etiology of erythroblastosis fetalis. J.A.M.A., 116:825, 1941.

LICHTENSTEIN, A.: Hämatologeska studier å for tidigt födda barn under de första levnadsåren med särskild hansyn til anämiska tillstånd. Svenska Läk.-Sällsk. Handl., 43:1533, 1917.

LIE-INJO, L. E.: Haemoglobin of newborn infants in Indonesia. Nature, 183:1125, 1959.

LIE-INJO, L. E.: Alpha-chain thalassaemia and hydrops fetalis in Malaya: report of 5 cases. Blood, 20:581, 1962.

LIGGINS, G. C.: Fetal transfusion by the impaling technic. Obstet. Gynec., 27:617, 1966.

LILEY, A. W.: Diagnosis and treatment of erythroblastosis in the fetus. Adv. Ped., 15:29, 1968. (Yearbook Medical Publishers, Chicago, Ill.)

LILEY, A. W.: Liquor amnii analysis in the management of the pregnancy complicated by Rhesus sensitization. Am. J. Obst. Gynec., 82:1359, 1961.

LILEY, A. W.: Errors in the assessment of hemolytic disease from amniotic fluid. Am. J. Obst. Gynec., 86:485, 1963.

LILEY, A. W.: Intrauterine transfusion of foetus in haemolytic disease. Brit. Med. J., 2:1107, 1963.

LILEY, A. W.: Amniocentesis. New Eng. J. Med., 272:731, 1965.

LILEY, A. W.: The use of amniocentesis and fetal transfusion in erythroblastosis fetalis. Pediatrics, 35:836, 1965.

LINTZEL, W., RECHENBERGER, J., and SCHAIRER, E.: Über den Eisenstoffwechsel des Neugeboren und des Säughlings. Z. Ges. Exp. Med., 113:591, 1944.

LIPPMAN, H. S.: Morphologic and quantitative study of blood corpuscles in newborn period. Am. J. Dis. Child., 27:473, 1924.

LIPSITZ, P. J., and CORNET, J. M.: Blood cultures from the umbilical vein in the new-born infant. Pediatrics, 26:657, 1960.

LIPTON, E. L.: Elliptocytosis with hemolytic anemia: the effects of splenectomy. Pedi-atrics, 15:67, 1955.

LITWAK, O., TASWELL, H. F., BANNER, E. A., and KEITH, L.: Fetal erythrocytes in maternal circulation after spontaneous abortion. J.A.M.A., 214:513, 1970.

LO, S. S., HITZIG, W. H., and MARTI, H. R.: Hereditary methemoglobinemia due to diaphorase deficiency. Acta Haemat., 43:177, 1970.

LOCK, S. P., SMITH, R. S., and HARDISTY, R. M.: Stomatocytosis: a hereditary red cell anomaly associated with haemolytic anaemia. Brit. J. Haemat., 7:303, 1961.

LOELIGER, A., and KOLLER, F.: Behavior of factor VII and prothrombin in late preg-nancy and in newborn. Acta Haemat., 7:157, 1952.

LÖHR, G. S., and WALLER, H. D.: Zur Biochemie einiger angeborener hämolytischer Anämien. Folia Haemat. (Frankfurt), 8:377, 1963.

LONDON, W. T., DiFIGLIA, M., and RODGERS, J.: Failure of transplacental transmission of Australia antigen. Lancet, 2:900, 1969.

LONGPRÉ, B., COUSINEAU, L., and LOSITO, R.: Association du syndrome d'Evans et de la grossesse. L'Union Méd. du Canada, 99:1825, 1970.

LOPEZ, R., and COOPERMAN, J. M.: Glucose-6-phosphate dehydrogenase deficiency and hyperbilirubinemia in the newborn. Amer. J. Dis. Child. 122:66, 1971.

LOUKOPOULOS, D., KALTSOYA, A., and FESSAS, P.: On the chemical abnormality of Hb "Alexandra," a fetal hemoglobin variant. Blood, 33:114, 1969.

LOW, J. A., KERR, N. D., and COCHON, A. R.: Plasma and blood volume of the normal newborn infant and patterns of adjustment in initial 24 hours of the neonatal period. Am. J. Obst. Gynec., 86:886, 1963.

LUBIN, B., and OSKI, F. A.: Irreversible oxidant injury in the erythrocytes of the newborn infant. Program, Society Ped. Research, 1971, p. 86.

LUBIN, B., OSKI, F. A., NATHAN, D., and SCHNEIDER, A.: Hereditary stomatocytosis: a disease or a syndrome. Soc. Pediatric Research, Atlantic City, April, 1966.

LUCAS, W. P.: Blood studies in new-born; morphological; chemical; coagulation; urobilin and bilirubin. Am. J. Dis. Child., 22:525, 1921.

LUCEY, J. F.: Symposium on bilirubin metabolism. Original Article Series, National Foundation, New York City, 1970.

LUCEY, J. F., in: Intrauterine transfusion and erythroblastosis fetalis, Report of the Fifty-third Ross Conference on Pediatric Research, Lucey, J. F., and Butterfield, L. J., eds. Columbus, Ross Laboratories, 1966, p. 10.

LUCEY, J. F., and DOLAN, R. G.: Hyperbilirubinemia of newborn infants associated with the parenteral administration of a vitamin K analogue to the mothers. Pediatrics, 23:553, 1959.

LUCEY, J. F., ARIAS, I. M., and McKAY, R. J.: Transient familial neonatal hyperbilirubinemia. Am. J. Dis. Child., 100:787, 1960.

LUCEY, J. F., FERREIRO, M., and HEWITT, J.: Prevention of hyperbilirubinemia of prematurity by phototherapy. Pediat. 41:1047, 1968.

LUCEY, J. F., VALAES, T., and DOXIADIS, S. A.: Serum albumin reserve PSP dye binding capacity in infants with kernicterus. Pediatrics, 39:876, 1967.

LUHBY, A. L., SPEER, F. D., LEE, R., and SHAPIRO, A. D.: Congenital genetic agranulocytosis. Am. J. Dis. Child., 94:552, 1957.

LUNDH, B., OSKI, F. A., and GARDNER, F. H.: Plasma hemopexin and haptoglobin in hemolytic diseases of the newborn. Acta Paediat. Scand., 59:121, 1970.

LUNDMARK, K. M.: Bone marrow cell proliferation in health and haematological disease during childhood. Acta Paed., Suppl. 162, 1966.

LUNDSTRÖM, R.: Rubella during pregnancy. Acta Paediat., 51:1, 1962.

LUSHER, J. M.: Hemophilia A in chromosomal female subjects. J. Pediatrics, 74:265, 1969.

LUTZNER, M. A., and HECHT, F.: Nuclear anomalies of the neutrophil in a chromosomal triplication: the D_1 (13–15) trisomy syndrome. Lab. Invest., 15:597, 1966.

LUZZATTO, L., ESAN, G. J. F., and OGIEMUDIA, S. E.: The osmotic fragility of red cells in newborns and infants. Acta Haemat., 43:248, 1970.

LYON, M. F.: Gene action in the X-chromosome of the mouse (Mus musculinus L.). Nature, 190:372, 1961.

LYONS, K. P. and GUZE, L. B.: Australia antigen associated hepatitis. Radioimmunoassay in mother and infant. J.A.M.A., 215:981, 1971.

MacKINNEY, A. A., JR., MORTON, N. E., KOSOWER, M. S., and SCHILLING, R. F.: Ascertaining genetic carriers of hereditary spherocytosis by statistical analyses of multiple laboratory tests. J. Clin. Invest., 41:554, 1962.

MACRES, N. T., HELLMAN, L. M., and WATSON, R. J.: The transmission of transfused sickle-trait cells from mother to fetus. Am. J. Obst. Gyn., 76:1214, 1958.

MAGGIONI, G.: Observations on haemoglobin F and A_2 in newborns with haemolytic disease before and after exchange transfusion. Minerva Pediat., 11:498, 1959.

MAISELS, M. J., LI, T.-K., PIECHOCKI, J. T., and WERTHMAN, M. W.: Effect of exchange transfusion on serum ionized calcium. Abstract, Soc. Pediat. Research, Atlantic City, April, 1971, p. 99.

MAIZELS, M.: Factors in the active transport of cations. J. Physiol., 112:59, 1951.

MANIOS, S. G., SCHENCK, W., and KÜNZER, W.: Congenital fibrinogen deficiency. Acta Paed. Scand., 57:151, 1968.

MANN, D. L., SITES, M. D., DONATI, R. M., and GALLAGHER, M. I.: Erythropoietic stimulating activity during the first ninety days of life. Proc. Soc. Exp. Biol. Med., 118:212, 1965.

MANN, J., and GRAVEN, S. N.: Erythrocyte morphology in hemolytic disease. Am. J. Dis. Child., 108:611, 1964.

MANSON, M. M., LOGAN, W. P. D., and LOY, R. M.: Rubella and other virus infections during pregnancy. Reports on Public Health and Medical Subjects No. 101, Ministry of Health. Her Majesty's Stationery Office, London, 1960.

MARCUS, A. J.: Platelet function. New Eng. J. Med., 280:1213, 1969.

MARKARIAN, M., GITHENS, J. H., JACKSON, J. J., BANNON, A. E., LINDLEY, A., ROSENBLÜT, E., MARTORELL, R., and LUBCHENCO, L. O.: Fibrinolytic activity in premature infants. Am. J. Dis. Child., 113:312, 1967.

MARKS, J., GAIRDNER, D., and ROSCOE, J. D.: Blood formation in infancy. III. Cord blood. Arch. Dis. Child., 30:117, 1955.

MARKS, P. A., and BANKS, J.: Drug induced hemolytic anemias associated with glucose-6-phosphate dehydrogenase deficiency: a genetically heterogenous trait. Ann. N. Y. Acad. Sci., 123:198, 1965.

MARKS, P. A., SZEINBERG, A., and BANKS, J.: Erythrocyte glucose-6-phosphate dehydrogenase of normal and mutant human subjects: properties of the purified enzymes. J. Biol. Chem., 236:10–17, 1961.

MARSH, G. W., STIRLING, Y., and MOLLISON, P. L.: Accidental injection of anti-D immunoglobulin to an infant. Vox Sang., 19:468, 1970.

MARTIN, H., and HUISMAN, T. H. J.: Formation of ferrihaemoglobin of isolated human haemoglobin types by sodium nitrite. Nature, 200:898, 1963.

MATOTH, Y.: Phagocytic and ameboid activities of the leukocytes in the newborn infant. Pediatrics, 9:748, 1952.

MATOTH, Y., ZAIZOV, R., and VARSANO, I.: Postnatal changes in some red cell parameters. Acta Paediat. Scand., 60:317, 1971.

MATSUDA, G., SCHROEDER, W. A., JONES, R. T., and WELIKY, N.: Is there an "embryonic" or "primitive" fetal hemoglobin? Blood, 16:984, 1960.

MATTELAER, P. M., and RILEY, H. D., JR.: Leukemia in the perinatal period. Ann. Paed., 203:124–136, 1964.

MAUER, A. M., DEVAUX, L. O., and LAHEY, M. E.: Neonatal and maternal thrombocytopenic purpura due to quinine. Pediatrics, 19:84, 1957.

MAUER, H. M., WOLFF, J. A., FINSTER, M., POPPERS, P. J., PANTUCK, E., KUNTZMAN, R., and CONNEY, A. H.: Reduction in concentration of total serum bilirubin in offspring of women treated with phenobarbitone during pregnancy. Lancet, 2:122, 1968.

MAURER, H. M., and CAUL, J.: Bilirubin-induced platelet staining, aggregation and adenine nucleotide release. Abstr., Soc. Pediat. Research, Atlantic City, May, 1970., p. 75.

MAXIMOV, A. A.: Relation of blood cells to connective tissue and endothelium. Physiol. Rev., 4:533, 1924.

McCORMICK, W. F., and WALKER, R. H.: Immunologically different "normal" fetal hemoglobins. Am. J. Clin. Path., 33:500, 1960.

McCRACKEN, G. H. and EICHENWALD, H. F.: Leukocyte function and the development of opsonic and complement activity in the neonate. Am. J. Dis. Child., 121:120, 1971.

McCUISTION, C. H., and SCHOCH, E. P.: Possible discoid lupus erythematosus in newborn infant. Arch. Dermat. Syph., 70:782, 1954.

McDONALD, C. D., and HUISMAN, T. H. J.: A comparative study of enzymic activities in normal adult and cord blood erythrocytes as related to the reduction of methemoglobin. Clin. Chim. Acta, 7:555, 1962.

McELFRESH, A. E.: Coagulation during the neonatal period. Am. J. Med. Sci., 240:771, 1961.

McGOVERN, J. J., DRISCOLL, R., DUTOIT, C. H., GROVE-RASMUSSEN, M., and BEDELL, R. F.: Iron deficiency anemia resulting from fetomaternal transfusion, New Eng. J. Med., 258:1149, 1958.

McKAY, R. J.: Current status of exchange transfusion in newborn infants. Pediatrics, 33:763, 1964.

McLAREY, D. C., and FISH, S. A.: Fetal erythrocytes in the maternal circulation. Am. J. Obstet. Gynec., 95:824, 1966.

MEADOW, S. R.: Stomatocytosis, Proc. Roy. Soc. Med., 60:13, 1967.

MEDEARIS, D. N., JR.: Cytomegalic inclusion disease: analysis of clinical features based on literature and six additional cases. Pediatrics, *19*:467, 1957.

MEDEARIS, D. N., JR.: Observations concerning human cytomegalovirus infection and disease. Bull. Johns Hopkins Hosp., *114*:181, 1964.

MEDOFF, H. S., and BARBERO, G. J.: Total blood eosinophil counts in the newborn period. Pediatrics, 6:737, 1950.

MEDOFF, H. S.: Platelet counts in premature infants. J. Pediat., *64*:287, 1964.

MELLMAN, W. J., WOLMAN, I. J., WURZEL, H. A., MOORHEAD, P. S., and QUALLS, D. H.: Chromosomal female with hemophilia A. Blood, *17*:719, 1961.

MENGERT, W. F., RIGHTS, C. S., BATES, C. R., JR., REID, A. F., WOLF, G. R., and NABORS, G. D.: Placental transmission of erythrocytes. Am. J. Obst. Gynec., 96: 678, 1955.

MENTZER, W. C., JR., BAEHNER, R. L., SCHMIDT-SCHÖNBEIN, H., ROBINSON, S. H., and NATHAN, D. G.: Selective reticulocyte destruction in erythrocyte pyruvate kinase deficiency. J. Clin. Invest., *50*:688, 1971.

MERENSTEIN, G. B., BLACKMON, L. R., and KUSHNER, J.: Nucleated red-cells in the newborn. Lancet, *1*:1293, 1970.

MERENSTEIN, G. B., O'LOUGHLIN, E. P., and PLUNKET, D. C.: Effects of maternal thiazides on platelet counts of newborn infants. J. Pediat., 76:766, 1970.

MERSKEY, C., LALEZARI, P., and JOHNSON, A. J.: A rapid, simple, sensitive method for measuring fibrinolytic split products in human serum. Proc. Soc. Exper. Biol. Med., *131*:871, 1969.

MICHAEL, A. F., JR., and MAUER, A. M.: Maternal-fetal transfusion as a cause of plethora in the neonatal period. Pediatrics, *28*:458, 1961.

MICHAELSSON, M., and SJÖLIN, S.: Haemolysis in blood samples from newborn infants. Acta Paediat. Scand., *54*:325, 1965.

MILES, R. M., MAURER, H. M., and VALDES, O. S.: Iron deficiency anemia at birth. Two examples secondary to chronic fetal-maternal hemorrhage. Clin. Pediat. *10*:223, 1971.

MILLER, A. A.: Congenital sulfhemoglobinemia. J. Pediat., *51*:233, 1957.

MILLER, D. F., and PETRIE, S. J.: Fatal erythroblastosis fetalis secondary to ABO incompatibility. Obst. Gynec., *22*:773, 1963.

MILLER, D. R., FREED, B. A., and LAPEY, J. D.: Congenital neutropenia. Am. J. Dis. Child., *115*:337, 1968.

MILLER, D. R., HANSHAW, J. B., O'LEARY, D. S., and HNILICKA, J. V.: Fatal disseminated herpes simplex virus infection and hemorrhage in the neonate. Coagulation studies in a case and a review. J. Pediatrics, 76:409, 1970.

MILLER, D. R., NEWSTEAD, G. J., and YOUNG, L. W.: Perinatal leukemia with possible variant of the Ellis-van Creveld syndrome. J. Pediat., *74*:300, 1969.

MILLER, D. R., RICKLES, F. R., LICHTMAN, M. A., LaCELLE, P. L., and WEED, R. I.: A new variant of hereditary stomatocytosis. Blood, 36:839, 1970.

MILLER, G., TOWNES, P. L., and MacWHINNEY, J. B.: A new congenital hemolytic anemia with deformed erythrocytes (? "stomatocytes") and remarkable susceptibility of erythrocytes to cold hemolysis in vitro. I. Clinical and hematologic studies. Pediatrics, 35:906, 1965.

MILLER, J. M., SHERRILL, J. G., and HATHAWAY, W. E.: Thrombocythemia in the myeloproliferative disorder of Down's syndrome. Pediatrics, *40*:847, 1967.

MILLER, M. E.: Chemotactic function in the human neonate: humoral and cellular aspects. Pediat. Res., 5:492, 1971.

MILLER, M. E.: Leukocytes of neonates. J. Pediat., 76:158, 1970.

MILLER, M. E.: Phagocytosis in the newborn infant: humoral and cellular factors. J. Pediat., 74:255, 1969.

MILLER, M. E., OSKI, F. A., and HARRIS, M. B.: Lazy-leukocyte syndrome. Lancet, *1*:665, 1971.

MILLER, M. E., SEALS, J., KAYE, R., and LEVITSKY, L. C.: A familial, plasma-associated defect in phagocytosis. Lancet, 2:60, 1968.

MILLS, D. C. B., ROBB, I. A., and ROBERTS, G. C. K.: Release of nucleotides, 5-hydroxytryptamine and enzymes from human blood platelets during aggregation. J. Physiol., *195*:715, 1968.

MINKOWSKI, A.: Acute cardiac failure in connection with neonatal polycythemia (in monovular and single newborn infants). Biol. Neonat., 4:61, 1962.

MINNICH, V., CORDONNIER, J. K., WILLIAMS, W. J., and MOORE, C. V.: Alpha, beta and gamma polypeptide chains during the neonatal period with description of a fetal form of hemoglobin Dα-St. Louis. Blood, 19:137, 1962.

MISENHIMER, H. R.: Fetal hemorrhage associated with amniocentesis. Am. J. Obstet. Gynec., 94:1133, 1966.

MITTWOCH, U.: Inclusions of mucopolysaccharide in the lymphocytes of patients with gargoylism. Nature, 191:1315, 1961.

MOE, P. J.: Umbilical cord blood and capillary blood in the evaluation of anemia in erythroblastosis fetalis. Acta Paediat. Scand., 56:391, 1967.

MOHLER, D. N.: Adenosine triphosphate metabolism in hereditary spherocytosis. J. Clin. Invest., 44:1417, 1965.

MOHLER, D. N., MAJERUS, P. W., MENNICH, V., HESS, C. E., and GARRICK, M. D.: Glutathione synthetase deficiency as a cause of hereditary hemolytic disease. New Eng. J. Med., 283:1253, 1970.

MOLLICA, F.: On the behavior of the level of foetal haemoglobin in infancy. Pediatria, 70:231, 1962.

MOLLISON, P. L.: The survival of transfused erythrocytes in haemolytic disease of the newborn. Arch. Dis. Child., 18:161, 1943.

MOLLISON, P. L.: *Blood Transfusion in Clinical Medicine.* 1st Ed., Oxford, Blackwell, 1951.

MOLLISON, P. L.: *Blood Transfusion in Clinical Medicine.* 3rd Ed., Oxford, Blackwell, 1961, p. 614.

MOLLISON, P. L.: *Blood Transfusion in Clinical Medicine.* 4th Ed., Oxford, Blackwell, 1967, p. 275.

MOLLISON, P. L.: Suppression of Rh-immunization by passively administered anti-Rh. Brit. J. Haemat., 14:1, 1968.

MOLLISON, P. L., and CUTBUSH, M.: Hemolytic disease of the newborn due to fetal-maternal ABO incompatibility. Prog. Hemat., 2:153, 1959.

MOLLISON, P. L., FRAME, M., and ROSS, M. E.: Differences between Rh (D) negative subjects in response to Rh (D) antigen. Brit. J. Haemat., 19:257, 1970.

MOLLISON, P. L., VEALL, N., and CUTBUSH, M.: Red cell and plasma volume in newborn infants. Arch. Dis. Child., 25:242, 1950.

MOLONEY, W. C.: Management of leukemia in pregnancy. Ann. N. Y. Acad. Sci., 114:587, 1964.

MOLTHAN, L.: Unpublished data. Personal communication, 1971.

MONNENS, L. A. H., and RETERA, R. J. M.: Thrombotic thrombocytopenic purpura in a neonatal infant. J. Pediat., 71:118, 1967.

MONTAGUE, A. C. W., and KREVANS, J. R.: Transplacental hemorrhage in cesarean section. Am. J. Obs. Gynec., 95:1115, 1968.

MOORE, C. M., MCADAMS, A. J., and SUTHERLAND, J. M.: Intrauterine disseminated intravascular coagulation: A syndrome of multiple pregnancy with a dead twin fetus. J. Pediat., 74:523, 1969.

MOORE, T. J., and HALL, N.: Kinetics of glucose transfer in adult and fetal human erythrocytes. Pediat. Res. 5:356, 1971.

MORROW, G., III, BARNESS, L. A., AUERBACH, V. H., DIGEORGE, A. M., ANDO, T., and NYHAN W. L.: Observations on the coexistence of methylmalonic acidemia and glycinemia. J. Pediat., 74:680, 1969.

MOSES, S. W., CHAYOTH, R., LEVIN, S., LAZAROVITZ, E., and RUBENSTEIN, D.: Glucose and glycogen metabolism in erythrocytes from normal and glycogen storage type III subjects. J. Clin. Invest., 47:1343, 1968.

MOSS, A. J., DUFFIE, E. R., JR., and FAGAN, L.: Respiratory distress syndrome in the newborn. J.A.M.A., 184:48, 1963.

MOTULSKY, A. G.: Pharmacogenetics. *In Progress in Medical Genetics* (Steinberg, A. G., and Bearn, A. G., eds.). New York, Grune & Stratton, 1964, Vol. III, p. 49.

MOTULSKY, A. G., and CAMPBELL-KRAUT, J. M.: Population genetics of glucose-6-phosphate dehydrogenase deficiency of the red cell. In *Proceedings of the Conference on Genetic and Geographic Variations in Disease* (Blumberg, B. S., ed.). New York, Grune & Stratton, 1961, p. 159.

MOUNTAIN, K. R., HIRSH, J., and GALLUS, A. S.: Neonatal coagulation defect due to anticonvulsant drug treatment in pregnancy. Lancet, *1*:265, 1970,

MUGRAGE, E. R., and ANDRESEN, M. I.: Values for red blood cells of average infants and children. Am. J. Dis. Child., *51*:775, 1936.

MULL, M. M., and HATHAWAY, W. E.: Altered platelet function in newborns. Pediat. Res., *4*:229, 1970.

MULLER-EBERHARD, U., and BASHORE, R.: Assessment of Rh disease by ratios of bilirubin to albumin and hemopexin to albumin in amniotic fluid. New. Eng. J. Med., *282*:1163, 1970.

MURPHY, J. R.: Erythrocyte metabolism. II.Glucose metabolism and pathways. J. Lab. Clin. Med., *55*:286, 1960.

MURPHY, S., OSKI, F. A., and GARDNER, F. H.: Hereditary thrombocytopenia with an intrinsic platelet defect. New Eng. J. Med., *281*:857, 1969.

MURPHY, S., OSKI, F. A., NAIMAN, J. L., LUSCH, C. J., SMALLEY, R. V., GOLDBERG, S., and GARDNER, F. H.: Platelet volume measurements in hereditary and acquired thrombocytopenia. Blood, *36*:856, 1970.

NADER, P. R., and MARGOLIN, F.: Hemangioma causing gastrointestinal bleeding. Case report and review of the literature. Am. J. Dis. Child., *111*:215, 1966.

NAESLUND, J.: Studies on placental permeability with radioactive isotopes of phosphorus and iron. Acta Obst. Gynec. Scand., *30*:231, 1951.

NAEYE, R. L.: Human intrauterine parabiotic syndrome and its complications. New Eng. J. Med., *268*:804, 1963.

NAGAO, T., LAMPKIN, B. C., and HUG, G.: A neonate with Down's syndrome and transient abnormal myelopoiesis: serial blood and bone marrow studies. Blood, *36*: 443, 1970.

NAIMAN, J. L., and GERALD, P. S.: Fetal hemoglobin: improved separation by a modified agar gel electrophoresis. J. Lab. Clin. Med., *61*:508, 1963.

NAIMAN, J. L., and KOSOY, M. H.: Red cell glucose-6-phosphate dehydrogenase deficiency—a newly recognized cause of neonatal jaundice and kernicterus in Canada. Canad. M. A. J., *91*:1243, 1964.

NAIMAN, J. L., PUNNETT, H. H., LISCHNER, H. W., DESTINÉ, M. L., and AREY, J. B.: Possible graft-versus-host reaction after intrauterine transfusion for Rh erythroblastosis fetalis. New Eng. J. Med., *281*:697, 1969.

NAIMAN, J. L., and SCHLACKMAN, N.: Transient thrombocytopenia in the neonatal polycythemia syndrome. Prog. Soc. Pediat. Res., 1971, p. 241.

NAKAO, M., NAKAO, T., YAMAZOE, S., and YOSHIKAWA, H.: Adenosine triphosphate and shape of erythrocytes. J. Biochem., *49*:487, 1961.

NA-NAKORN, S., and WASI, P.: Alpha-thalassemia in northern Thailand. Amer. J. Human Genet., *22*:645, 1970.

NA-NAKORN, S., WASI, P., PORNPATKUL, M., and POOTRAKUL, S.: Further evidence for a genetic basis of haemoglobin H disease from newborn offspring of parents. Nature, *223*:59, 1969.

NATHAN, D. G., GERALD, P. S., DRISCOLL, S., and CRAIG, J. M.: Hydrops fetalis and erythroblastosis in homozygous alpha thalassemia. Abstract, Society for Pediatric Research, Atlantic City, 1966.

NATHAN, D. G., OSKI, F. A., MILLER, D. R., and GARDNER, F. H.: Life span and organ sequestration of the red cells in pyruvate kinase deficiency. New Eng. J. Med., *278*:73, 1968.

NATHAN, D. J., and SNAPPER, I.: Simultaneous placental transfer of factors responsible for L. E. cell formation and thrombocytopenia. Am. J. Med., *25*:647, 1958.

NATHAN, E.: Severe hydrops foetalis treated with peritoneal dialysis and positive-pressure ventilation. Lancet, *1*:1393, 1968.

NAVEH, D., SCHWART, J. M., PANG, K. W., FELDMAN, F., BUNN, H. F., GIDARI, A. S., ZANJANI, E. D., and GORDON, A. S.: Neonatal polycythemia and elevated plasma erythropoietin (ESF) in Down's syndrome. Prog. Amer. Soc. Hemat., p. 142, 1971.

NEBESKY, O.: Beitrag zur Nabelschurzerreissung intra partum. Arch. Gynäk., *100*: 601, 1913.

NECHELES, T. F., and ALLEN, D. M.: Heinz-body anemias. New Eng. J. Med., *280*:203, 1969.

NECHELES, T. F., BOLES, T. A., and ALLEN, D. M.: Erythrocyte glutathione peroxidase deficiency and hemolytic disease of the newborn infant. J. Pediat., *72*:319, 1968.

NECHELES, T. F., RAI, V. S., and CAMERON, D.: Congenital nonspherocytic hemolytic anemia associated with an unusual erythrocyte hexokinase abnormality. J. Lab. Clin. Med., *76*:593, 1970.

NEERHOUT, R. C.: Erythrocyte lipids in the neonate. Pediat. Res., *2*:172, 1968.

NELIGAN, G. A., and RUSSELL, J. K.: Blood loss from the foetal circulation, a hazard of lower segment caesarean section in cases of placenta praevia. J. Obst. Gynaec. Brit. Emp., 61:2, 1954.

NELSON, J. D., RICHARDSON, J., and SHELTON, S.: The significance of bacteremia with exchange transfusions. J. Pediat., 66:291, 1965.

NELSON, N. A., and STRUVE, V. R.: Prevention of congenital syphilis by treatment of syphilis in pregnancy. J.A.M.A., 161:869, 1956.

NELSON, T. C.: The relationship between melena and hyperbilirubinemia in mature neonates. Biol. Neonat., 8:267, 1965.

NEUMAYER, E.: Der fetale Hb-Gehalt im Nabelvenenblut bei Neugeborenen von müttern mit einer Spätgestose. Zbl. Gynaek, 88:1348, 1966.

NEWMAN, A. J., and GROSS, S.: Hyperbilirubinemia in breast-fed infants. Pediatrics, 32:995, 1963.

NEWTON, W. A., JR., and BASS, J. C.: Glutathione-sensitive chronic nonspherocytic hemolytic anemia. A.M.A. Am. J. Dis. Child., 96:501, 1958.

NG, W. G., DONNELL, G. N., and BERGREN, W. R.: Galactokinase activity in human erythrocytes of individuals at different ages. J. Lab. Clin. Med., 66:115, 1965.

NIEDERHOFF, H., SCHNEIDER, J., STACHOW, P., and KÜNZER, W.: The effect of anti-D immunoglobulin in Rh-positive persons. German. Med. Monthly. 14:501, 1969.

NIELSEN, J. A., and STRUNK, K. W.: Homozygous hereditary elliptocytosis as the cause of haemolytic anemia in infancy. Scand. J. Haem., 5:454, 1968.

NILSSON, L. R., and LUNDHOLM, G.: Congenital thrombocytopenia with aplasia of the radius. Acta Paediat., 49:291, 1960.

NITSCHKE, E.: Blutbefunde bei angeborener Syphilis. Arch. Kinderh., 72:136, 1924.

NOLDEKE, H.: Geburtskomplikationen bei insertio velamentosa. Zbl. Gynäk., 58:351, 1934.

NORDLUND, J. J., DeVITA, V. T., and CARBONE, P. P.: Severe vinblastine-induced leukopenia during late pregnancy with delivery of a normal infant. Ann. Int. Med., 69:581, 1968.

NOVAK, F.: Posthemorrhagic shock in newborns during labor and after delivery. Acta Med. Iugosl., 7:280, 1953.

NOWELL, R.: Personal communication (1965).

NURSE, D. S.: Congenital methaemoglobinaemia. Med. J. Austr., 47:692, 1960.

NYGAARD, K. K.: Prophylactic and curative effect of vitamin K in hemorrhagic disease of the newborn. Acta Obst. Gynec. Scand., 19:361, 1939.

NYHAN, W. L., and FOUSEK, M. D.: Septicemia of the newborn. Pediatrics, 22:268, 1958.

OBERHOLZER, V. G., LEVIN, B., BURGESS, E. A., and YOUNG, W. F.: Methylmalonic acidemia—an inborn error of metabolism leading to chronic metabolic acidosis. Arch. Dis. Childh., 42:492, 1967.

OBES-POLLARI, J., and HILL, W. S.: La fototerapia en las ictericias del recien nacido. Rev. Chile Ped., 25:638, 1964.

O'CONNOR, R. E., McKAY, R. N., and SMITH, J.: Congenital leukemia with septicemia as a terminal event. A.M.A. Am. J. Dis. Child., 88:740, 1954.

O'CONNOR, W. J., SHIELDS, G., KOHL, S., and SUSSMAN, M.: The occurrence of anemia of the newborn in association with the appearance of fetal hemoglobin in the maternal circulation. Am. J. Obst. Gynec., 73:768, 1957.

ODELL, G. B.: "Physiologic" hyperbilirubinemia in the neonatal period. New Eng. J. Med., 277:193, 1967.

ODELL, G. B.: The dissociation of bilirubin from albumin and its clinical implications. J. Pediat., 55:268, 1959.

ODELL, G. B.: The distribution and toxicity of bilirubin. Pediatrics, 46:16, 1970.

ODELL, G. B.: Discussion of paper by Waters and Odell (Amer. Pediat. Soc., 1965). J. Pediat., 67:1043, 1965.

ODELL, G. B., BRYAN, W. B., and RICHMOND, M. D.: Exchange transfusion. Ped. Clin. North Am., 9:605, 1962.

ODELL, G. B., COHEN, S. N., and GORDES, E. H.: Administration of albumin in the management of hyperbilirubinemia by exchange transfusions. Pediatrics, 30:613, 1962.

ODELL, G. B., COHEN, S. N., and KELLY, P. C.: Studies in kernicterus. II. The determination of the saturation of serum albumin with bilirubin. J. Pediat., 74:214, 1969.

ODELL, G. B., STOREY, G. N. B., and ROSENBERG, L. A.: Studies in kernicterus. III. The saturation of serum proteins with bilirubin during neonatal life and its relationship to brain damage at five years. J. Pediat., 76:12, 1970.

OETTINGER, L., JR., and MILLS, W. B.: Simultaneous capillary and venous hemoglobin determinations in newborn infant. J. Pediat., 35:362, 1949.

O'FLYNN, M. E. D., and HSIA, D. Y.: Serum bilirubin levels and glucose-6-phosphate dehydrogenase deficiency in newborn American Negroes. J. Pediat., 63:160, 1963.

O'GORMAN HUGHES, D. W.: Neonatal thrombocytopenia: assessment of aetiology and prognosis. Aust. Paediat., J., 3:226, 1967.

OH, W., and LIND, J.: Venous and capillary hematocrit in newborn infants and placental transfusion. Acta Paediat. Scand., 55:38, 1966.

OH, W., BLANKENSHIP, W., and LIND, J.: Further study of neonatal blood volume in relation to placental transfusion. Ann. Paed., 207:147, 1966.

OH, W., OH, M. A., and LIND, J.: Renal function and blood volume in newborn infant related to placental transfusion. Acta Paediat. Scand., 55:197, 1966.

OH, W., LIND, J., and GESSNER, I. H.: The circulatory and respiratory adaptation to early and late cord clamping in newborn infants. Acta Paediat. Scand., 55:17, 1966.

O'KELL, R. T.: Leukocyte alkaline phosphatase in the infant. Ann. N. Y. Acad. Sci., 155:980, 1968.

OLIVEIRA, M. M., and VAUGHAN, M.: Incorporation of fatty acids into phospholipids of erythrocyte membranes. J. Lipid Res., 5:156, 1964.

OORT, M., LOOS, J. A., and PRINS, H. K.: Hereditary absence of reduced glutathione in erythrocytes—a new clinical and biochemical entity. Vox Sang., 6:370, 1961.

OPPE, T. E., and FRASER, I. D.: Foetal haemoglobin in haemolytic disease of the newborn. Arch. Dis. Child., 36:507, 1961.

ORZALESI, M. M., and HAY, W. W.: The regulation of oxygen affinity of fetal blood. 1: In vivo experiments and results in normal infants. Pediatrics, 48:857, 1971.

OSGOOD, E. E.: Development and growth of hematopoietic tissues. Pediatrics, 15:733, 1955.

OSKI, F. A.: Red cell metabolism in the newborn infant. V. Glycolytic intermediates and glycolytic enzymes. Pediatrics, 44:84, 1969.

OSKI, F. A.: (Unpublished observations, 1971).

OSKI, F. A., ALLEN, D. M., and DIAMOND, L. K.: Portal hypertension—a complication of umbilical vein catheterization. Pediatrics, 31:297, 1963.

OSKI, F. A., and ALTMAN, A. A.: Carboxyhemoglobin levels in hemolytic disease of the newborn. J. Pediat., 61:709, 1962.

OSKI, F. A., and BOWMAN, H.: A low K_m phosphoenolpyruvate mutant in the Amish with red cell pyruvate kinase deficiency. Brit. J. Haemat., 17:289, 1969.

OSKI, F. A., and DIAMOND, L. K.: Erythrocyte pyruvate kinase deficiency: report of three cases. New Eng. J. Med., 269:763, 1963.

OSKI, F. A., ESHAGHPOUR, E., and WILLIAMS, M. L.: Red cell glucose-6-phosphate dehydrogenase (G-6-PO) deficiency as a cause of hyperbilirubinemia in the premature infant. American Pediatric Society, Atlantic City, April, 1966.

OSKI, F. A., and FULLER, E.: Glucose-phosphate isomerase (GPI) deficiency associated with abnormal osmotic fragility and spherocytes. Clin. Res., 19:427, 1971.

OSKI, F. A., and NAIMAN, J. L.: Red cell binding of bilirubin. J. Pediat., 63:1034, 1963.

OSKI, F. A., and NAIMAN, J. L.: Red cell metabolism in the premature infant. I. Adenosine triphosphate levels, adenosine triphosphate stability, and glucose consumption. Pediatrics, 36:104, 1965.

OSKI, F. A., NAIMAN, J. L., ALLEN, D. M., and DIAMOND, L. K.: Leukocytic inclusions— Döhle bodies—associated with platelet abnormality (the May-Hegglin anomaly). Report of a family and review of the literature. Blood, 20:657, 1962.

OSKI, F. A., NAIMAN, J. L., BLUM, S. F., ZARKOWSKY, H. S., WHAUN, J., SHOHET, S. B., GREEN, A., and NATHAN, D. G.: Congenital hemolytic anemia with high sodium, low potassium red cells. Studies of three generations of a family with a new variant. New Eng. J. Med., 280:909, 1969.

OSKI, F. A., NAIMAN, J. L., and DIAMOND, L. K.: Use of the plasma acid phosphatase value in the differentiation of thrombocytopenic states. New Eng. J. Med., 268: 1423, 1963.

OSKI, F. A., NATHAN, D. G., SIDEL, V. W., and DIAMOND, L. K.: The common metabolic pathway to red cell death in hemolytic anemias (abstract). J. Pediat., 65:1074, 1964.

OSKI, F. A., NATHAN, D. G., SIDEL, V. W., and DIAMOND, L. K.: Extreme hemolysis and red-cell distortion in erythrocyte pyruvate kinase deficiency. I. Morphology, erythrokinetics and family enzyme studies. New Eng. J. Med., 270:1023, 1964.

OSKI, F. A., and SMITH, C.: Red cell metabolism in the premature infant. III. Apparent inappropriate glucose consumption for cell age. Pediatrics, 41:473, 1968.

OSKI, F., and WHAUN, J.: Hemolytic anemia and red cell glyceraldehyde-3-phosphate dehydrogenase (G-3-PD) deficiency. Clin. Res., 17:601, 1969.

OUDART, J.-L., DIADHIOU, F., SARRAT, H., and SATGE, P.: L'hémoglobine du nouveau-né Africain. Ann. Pediat. (Paris), 15:773, 1968.

OXORN, H.: Rubella and pregnancy, a study of 47 cases. Am. J. Obst. Gynec., 77:628, 1959.

OZER, L., and MILLS, G. C.: Elliptocytosis with haemolytic anemia. Brit. J. Haemat., 10:468, 1964.

PACHMAN, D. J.: Massive hemorrhage in the scalp of the newborn infant. Hemorrhagic caput succedaneum. Pediatrics, 29:907, 1962.

PAGE, A. R.: Neutropenia in infancy and childhood. J. Lancet, 82:439, 1962.

PAGE, A. R., BERENDES, H., WARNER, J., and GOOD, R. A.: The Chediak-Higashi syndrome. Blood, 20:330, 1962.

PAGLIA, D. E., HOLLAND, P., BAUGHAN, M. A., and VALENTINE, W. N.: Occurrence of defective hexosephosphate isomerization in human erythrocytes and leukocytes. New Eng. J. Med., 280:66, 1969.

PAGLIA, D. E., VALENTINE, W. N., BAUGHAN, M. A., MILLER, D. R., REED, C. F., and McINTYRE, O. R.: An inherited molecular lesion of erythrocyte pyruvate kinase. J. Clin. Invest., 47:1929, 1968.

PANIZON, I.: L'ictère grave du nouveau-né associé à une deficience en glucose-6-phosphate dehydrogénase. Biol. Neonat., 2:167, 1960.

PANTAROTTO, M. F.: Un caso di aplasia midollare transitoria in neonato da farmaci anticonvulsivanti somministrati alla madre durante tutta la gravidanza. Clinica Ostet. Ginec., 67:343, 1965.

PARK, B. H., FIKRIG, S. M., and SMITHWICK, E. M.: Infection and nitroblue tetrazolium reduction by neutrophils. Lancet, 2:532, 1968.

PARK, B. H., HOLMES, B., and GOOD, R. A.: Metabolic activities in leukocytes of newborn infants. J. Pediat., 76:237, 1970.

PARKIN, J. M. and WALKER, W.: Peritoneal dialysis in severe hydrops foetalis. Lancet, 2:283, 1968.

PASTERNAK, A., FURUHJELM, V., VON KNORING, J., SKREFVARS, B., and KUHLBÄCK, B.: Acute renal failure after haemolysis, probably due to foeto-maternal transfusion. Acta Med., Scand., 180:13, 1966.

PATEL, D. A., PILDES, R. S., and BEHRMAN, R. E.: Failure of phototherapy to reduce serum bilirubin in newborn infants. J. Pediat., 77:1048, 1970.

PAYNE, R.: The development and persistence of leukoagglutinins in parous women. Blood, 19:411, 1962.

PAYNE, R., ROLFS, M. R., TRIPP, M., and WEIGLE, J.: Neonatal neutropenia and leukoagglutinins. Pediatrics, 33:194, 1964.

PEARSON, H. A.: The binding of Cr^{51} to hemoglobin. I. In vitro studies. Blood, 22:218, 1963.

PEARSON, H. A.: Life span of the fetal red blood cell. J. Pediat., 70:166, 1967.

PEARSON, H. A.: The binding of Cr^{51} to hemoglobin. II. In vivo elution of Cr^{51} from Hb CC, Hb CS and placental red cells. Blood, 28:563, 1966.

PEARSON, H. A., and DIAMOND, L. K.: Fetomaternal transfusion. Am. J. Dis. Child., 97:267, 1959.

PEARSON, H. A., and LORINCZ, A. E.: A characteristic bone marrow finding in the Hurler syndrome. Pediatrics, 34:280, 1964.

PEARSON, H. A., SHANKLIN, D. R., and BRODINE, C. R.: Alpha-thalassemia as cause of nonimmunological hydrops. Am. J. Dis. Child., 109:168, 1965.

PEARSON, H. A., SHULMAN, N. R., MARDER, V. J., and CONE, T. E., JR.: Isoimmune neonatal thrombocytopenic purpura. Clinical and therapeutic considerations. Blood, 23:154, 1964.

PEARSON, H. A., SHULMAN, N. R., OSKI, F. A., and EITZMAN, D. V.: Platelet survival in Wiskott-Aldrich syndrome. J. Pediat., 68:754, 1966.

PEARSON, H. A., and VERTREES, K. M.: Site of binding to chromium-51 by haemoglobin. Nature, *189*:1019, 1961.

PEDDLE, L. J.: Increase of antibody titer following amniocentesis. Am. J. Obst. and Gynec., *100*:567, 1968.

PENFOLD, J. B., and LIPSCOMB, J. M.: Elliptocytosis in man, associated with hereditary hemorrhagic telangiectasia. Quart. J. Med., *12*:157, 1943.

PERLSTEIN, M. A.: The late clinical syndrome of posticteric encephalopathy. Ped. Clin. North Am., *7*:665, 1960.

PERONA, G. P., and SARTORELLI, C.: The plasmatic haemoglobin in the newborn: its behaviour in the first four days of life. Biol. Neonat., *10*:1, 1966.

PERUTZ, M. F.: The hemoglobin molecule. Sci. Am., *211*:64, 1964.

PHIBBS, R., and TOOLEY, W.: Circulatory changes in newborns with erythroblastosis fetalis. Unpublished manuscript. Cited by Lucey, J. F., Pediatrics, *41*:139, 1968.

PHIBBS, R. H., HARVIN, D., JONES, G., TALBOT, C., COHEN, M., CROWTHER, D., and TOOLEY, W. H.: Development of children who had received intra-uterine transfusions. Pediatrics, *47*:689, 1971.

PHILIPSBORN, H. F., JR., TRAISMAN, H. S., and GREER, D., JR.: Rupture of the spleen: a complication of erythroblastosis fetalis. New Eng. J. Med., *252*:159, 1955.

PHILLIPS, G. B., and ROOME, N. S.: Quantitative chromatographic analysis of the phospholipids of abnormal human red blood cells. Proc. Soc. Exp. Biol., *109*:360, 1962.

PIERCE, M.: Leukemia in the newborn infant. J. Pediat., *54*:691, 1959.

PIERSON, W. E., BARRETT, C. T., and OLIVER, T. K., JR.: The effect of buffered and non-buffered ACD blood on electrolyte and acid-base homeostasis during exchange transfusion. Pediatrics, *41*:802, 1968.

PIHLAJA, T., VÄLIMÄKI, I., and YRJÄNÄ, T.: Effect of peroral ascorbic acid on blood methemoglobin of newborn infants. Biol. neonat., *13*:62, 1968.

PINKERTON, P. H., and COHEN, M. M.: Persistence of hemoglobin F in D/D translocation with trisomy 13–15 (D$_1$). J.A.M.A., *200*:647, 1967.

PIOMELLI, S., CORASH, L. M., DAVENPORT, D. D., MIRAGLIA, J., and AMOROSI, E. L.: In vivo lability of glucose-6-phosphate dehydrogenase in Gd^{A-} and Gd^{Mediterranean} deficiency. J. Clin. Invest., *47*:940, 1968.

PLAYFAIR, J. H. L., WOLFENDALE, M. R., and KAY, H. E. M.: The leucocytes of peripheral blood in the human foetus. Brit. J. Haemat., *9*:336, 1963.

PLOTKIN, S. A., OSKI, F. A., HARTNETT, E. M., HERVADA, A. R., FRIEDMAN, S., and GOWIG, J.: Some recently recognized manifestations of the rubella syndrome. J. Pediat., *67*:182, 1965.

POBLETE, E., THIBEAULT, D. W., and AULD, P. A. M.: Carbonic anhydrase in the premature. Pediatrics, *42*:429, 1968.

POCHEDLY, G.: Thrombocytopenic purpura of the newborn. Obst. Gynec. Survey, *26*:63, 1971.

POCHEDLY, C., and MUSIKER, S.: Twin-to-twin transfusion syndrome. Postgrad. Med., *47*:172, 1970.

POLAND, R. L., and ODELL, G. B.: Physiologic jaundice: the enterohepatic circulation of bilirubin. New Eng. J. Med., *284*:1, 1971.

POLEY, J. R., and STICKLER, G. B.: Petechiae in the newborn infant. Am. J. Dis. Child., *102*:365, 1961.

POLLACK, A.: Transplacental hemorrhage after external cephalic version. Lancet, *1*:612, 1968.

POLLACK, M., and MONTAGUE, A. C. W.: Transplacental hemorrhage in postterm pregnancies. Am. J. Obst. Gynec., *102*:383, 1968.

POLLACK, W. J., GORMAN, J. G., and FREDA, V. J.: Prevention of Rh-hemolytic disease. Progr. Hematol., *6*:121, 1969.

POLLEY, M. J., MOLLISON, P. L., ROSE, J., and WALKER, W.: A simple serological test for antibodies causing ABO-haemolytic disease of the newborn. Lancet, *1*:291, 1965.

POOL, J. G., and ROBINSON, J.: In vitro synthesis of coagulation factors by rat liver slices. Am. J. Physiol., *196*:423, 1959.

POOTRAKUL, S., WASI, P., and NA-NAKORN, S.: Haemoglobin Bart's hydrops foetalis in Thailand. Ann. Hum. Genet., *30*:293, 1967.

POOTRAKUL, S., WASI, P., and NA-NAKORN, S.: Studies on haemoglobin Bart's (Hb $-\gamma_4$) in Thailand: the incidence and the mechanism of occurrence in cord blood. Ann. Hum, Genet., *31*:49, 1967.

PORTER, E., and WATERS, W. J.: A rapid micromethod for measuring the reserve albumin binding capacity (abstract). Philadelphia, Soc. Ped. Res., May, 1965.

PORTER, E. G., and WATERS, W. J.: A rapid micromethod for measuring the reserve albumin binding capacity in serum from newborn infants with hyperbilirubinemia. J. Lab. Clin. Med., *67*:660, 1966.

PORTER, F. S., and THURMAN, W. G.: Studies of sickle cell disease. Am. J. Dis. Child., *106*:35, 1963.

POTTER, E. L.: Fetal and neonatal deaths: a statistical analysis of 2000 autopsies. J.A.M.A., *115*:996, 1940.

POTTER, E. L.: The effect on infant mortality of vitamin K administered during labor. Am. J. Obst. Gynec., *50*:235, 1945.

POVEY, M. J. C.: pH changes during exchange transfusion. Lancet, *2*:339, 1964.

POWARS, D., ROHDE, R., and GRAVES, D.: Foetal haemoglobin and neutrophil anomaly in the D_1-trisomy syndrome. Lancet, *1*:1363, 1964.

PRENDERGAST, J. J.: Congenital cataract and other anomalies following rubella in the mother during pregnancy. Arch. Ophthal., *92*:39, 1946.

PRIBILLA, W., BATHWELL, T., and FINCH, C. A.: Iron transport to the fetus in man. In *Iron in Clinical Medicine* (Wallerstein, R. O., and Mettier, S. R., eds.). Los Angeles, University of California Press, 1958, p. 58.

PRIDIE, G., and DUMITRESCU-PIRVU, D.: Laucemie acută sindrom Bonnevie-Ullrich la un nou născut. Pediatria, *10*:345, 1961.

PRINDULL, G.: Cellular inflammatory reactions in newborns and older infants. Zeistschrift für die Gesamte Blutforschung, *17*:279, 1968.

PRITCHARD, J. A., WHALLEY, P. J., and SCOTT, D. E.: The influence of maternal folate and iron deficiencies on intrauterine life. Am. J. Obst. and Gynec., *104*:388, 1969.

PROPP, R. P., and SCHARFMAN, W. B.: Hemangioma-thrombocytopenia syndrome associated with microangiopathic hemolytic anemia. Blood, *28*:623, 1966.

PROPP, S., BROWN, C., and TARTAGLIA, A. P.: Down syndrome and congenital leukemia. New York State J. Med., *66*:3067, 1966.

QUEENAN, J. T.: MODERN MANAGEMENT OF THE RH PROBLEM. New York, 1967, Hoeber Medical Division, Harper and Row, Publishers, p. 152.

QUEENAN, J. T., and ADAMS, D. W.: Amniocentesis: a possible immunizing hazard. Obst. Gynec., *24*:530, 1964.

QUEENAN, J. T., LANDESMAN, R., NAKAMOTO, M., and WILSON, K. H.: Postpartum immunization. Obst. Gynec., *20*:774, 1962.

QUEENAN, J. T., LANZKOWSKY, P., and GOLUBOW, J.: Significance of amniotic fluid volume in the interpretation of amniotic fluid-spectrophotometric analysis in antenatal management of erythroblastosis fetalis. Abstract, Soc. Pediat. Research, Atlantic City, May, 1968, p. 128.

QUEENAN, J. T., and NAKAMOTO, M.: Postpartum immunization: the hypothetical hazard of manual removal of the placenta. Obst. Gynec., *23*:392, 1964.

QUEENAN, J. T., SHAH, S., KUBARYCH, S. F., and HOLLAND, B.: Role of induced abortion in Rhesus immunization. Lancet, *1*:815, 1971.

QUIE, P. G., FISCH, R. O., and RAILE, R.: Methemoglobinemia and hemolytic anemia in normal newborns and normal prematures. Journal-Lancet, *82*:428, 1962.

QUIE, P. G., WHITE, J. G., WINDHORST, D. B., and GOOD, R. A.: In vitro bactericidal capacity of human polymorphonuclear leukocytes: diminished activity in chronic granulomatous disease of childhood. J. Clin. Invest., *46*:668, 1967.

RADDE, I. C., PARKINSON, D. K., HOFFKEN, B., FRIEDMAN, Z., and HANLEY, W. B.: Ionized calcium in infants treated with exchange transfusion. Abstract, Soc. Pediat. Research, Atlantic City, May, 1971, p. 99.

RÄDL, J., MASOPUST, J., JODL, J., and KITHIER, K.: Paraproteinemia in the pregnant woman and her child. II. Transient paraproteinemia in the child. Helv. Paediat. Acta, *23*:555, 1968.

RAMBOER, C., THOMPSON, R. P. H., and WILLIAMS, R.: Controlled trials of phenobarbitone therapy in neonatal jaundice. Lancet, *1*:966, 1969.

RANNEY, H. M.: Clinically important variants of human hemoglobin. New Eng. J. Med., 282:144, 1970.

RAPOPORT, S., and LUEBERING, J.: The 2,3-diphosphoglycerate cycle in human erythrocytes. J. Biol. Chem., 196:583, 1952.

RATTEN, G. J.: Spontaneous haematoma of the umbilical cord. Austral. New Zeal. J. Obstet. Gynec., 9:125, 1969.

RAUSEN, A. R., and DIAMOND, L. K.: Enclosed hemorrhage and neonatal jaundice. Am. J. Dis. Child., 101:164, 1961.

RAUSEN, A. R., GERALD, P. S., and DIAMOND, L. K.: Genetical evidence for synthesis of transferrin in the foetus. Nature, 192:182, 1961.

RAUSEN, A. R., LONDON, R. D., MIZRAHI, A., and COOPER, L. Q.: Generalized bone changes and thrombocytopenic purpura in association with intra-uterine rubella. Pediatrics, 36:264, 1965.

RAUSEN, A. R., RICHTER, P., TALLAL, L., and COOPER, L. Z.: Hematologic effects of intrauterine rubella. J.A.M.A., 199:75, 1967.

RAUSEN, A. R., SEKI, M., and STRAUSS, L.: Twin transfusion syndrome. A review of 19 cases studied at one institution. J. Pediat., 66:613, 1965.

RAYE, J. R., GUTBERLET, R. L., and STAHLMAN, M.: Symptomatic posthemorrhagic anemia in the newborn. Ped. Clin. N.A., 17:401, 1970.

REBUCK, J., and CROWLEY, J.: A method of studying leukocytic functions in vivo. Ann. N. Y. Acad. Sci., 59:757, 1955.

REDMOND, A., ISANA, S., and INGALL, D.: Relation of onset of respiration to placental transfusion. Lancet, 1:283, 1965.

REILLY, W. A.: The granules in the leukocytes in gargoylism. Am. J. Dis. Child., 62:489, 1941.

REIMAN, D. L., CLEMMENS, R. L., and PILLSBURY, W. A.: Congenital acute leukemia; skin nodules, first sign. J. Pediat., 46:415, 1955.

REIMANN, H. A., and DE BERNARDINIS, C. T.: Periodic (cyclic) neutropenia, an entity; a collection of sixteen cases. Blood, 4:1109, 1949.

REISS, J. S., and PRYLES, C. V.: Thrombocytopenia in congenital rubella. New Eng. J. Med., 275:264, 1966.

RIGBY, P. G., HANSON, T. A., and SMITH, R. S.: Passage of leukemic cells across the placenta. New Eng. J. Med., 271:124, 1964.

RISEL, H.: Blutbefunde bei angeborener syphilis. Arch. Kinderh., 72:136, 1924.

ROBERTS, J. T., GRAY, O. P., and BLOOM, A. L.: An abnormality of the thrombin-fibrinogen reaction in the newborn. Acta Paed. Scand., 55:148, 1966.

ROBINSON, A., and BARRIE, H.: The electrocardiogram during exchange transfusion. Arch. Dis. Child., 38:334, 1963.

ROBSON, H. N., and WALKER, C. H. M.: Congenital and neonatal thrombocytopenic purpura. Arch. Dis. Child., 26:175, 1951.

RODDY, R.: Clinical conferences at St. Christopher's Hospital for Children. J. Pediat., 44:213, 1954.

RODRIGUEZ, S., LEIKIN, S., and HILLER, M.: Neonatal thrombocytopenia associated with ante-partum administration of thiazide drugs. New Eng. J. Med., 270:881, 1964.

RODRÍGUEZ-ERDMANN, F.: Bleeding due to increased intravascular blood coagulation. New Eng. J. Med., 273:1370, 1965.

ROLANDI, L., and SIGNORELLI, I.: La reticolocitosi materna quale espressione di sofferenza fetale. Clin. Ginec., 4:351, 1962.

ROOTH, G., and SJÖSTEDT, S.: Haemoglobin in cord blood in normal and prolonged pregnancy. Arch. Dis. Child., 32:91, 1957.

ROSE, I. A., and WARMS, J. V. B.: Control of glycolysis in the human red blood cell. J. Biol. Chem., 241:4848, 1966.

ROSEN, F. S.: The lymphocyte and the thymus gland—congenital and hereditary abnormalities. New Eng. J. Med. 279:643, 1968.

ROZENSZAJN, L., KLAJMAN, A., YAFFE, D., and EFRATI, P.: Jordans' anomaly in white blood cells. Blood, 28:258, 1966.

ROSNER, F., and SUSSMAN, S. N.: Aplastic anemia in pregnancy. Report of a case. Obst. Gynec., 23:99, 1964.

Ross, J. D.: Deficient activity of DPNH-dependent methemoglobin diaphorase in cord blood erythrocytes. Blood, 21:51, 1963.

Ross, J. D., Maloney, W. C., and Desforges, J. F.: Ineffective regulation of granulopoiesis masquerading as congenital leukemia in a mongoloid child. J. Pediat., 63:1, 1963.

Rossi, J. P., and Brandt, I. K.: Transient granulocytopenia of the newborn associated with sepsis due to *Shigella* alkalescens and maternal leukocyte agglutinins. J. Pediat., 56:639, 1960.

Rubin, S. L.: A case of congenital amegakaryocytic thrombocytopenia with leukemoid blood picture and congenital deformities. Arch. Pediat., 76:251, 1959.

Rucker, M. P., and Tureman, G. R.: Vasa previa. Virginia Med. Month., 72:202, 1945.

Rudolph, A. J., Yow, M. D., Phillips, C. A., Desmond, M. M., Blattner, R. J., and Melnick, J. L.: Transplacental rubella infection in newly born infants. J.A.M.A., 191:843, 1965.

Rudolph, N.: Adenylate kinase activity in red cells of newborn infants. Program, Society Ped. Research, 1969, p. 160.

Rudolph, N., and Gross, R. T.: Studies on in-vitro autohaemolysis in blood from newborn infants. Brit. J. Haemat., 12:351, 1966.

Ruedda, cited by Baar, H. S., Baar, S., Rogers, K. B., and Stransky, E.: *Disorders of Blood and Blood-Forming Organs in Childhood.* New York, Hafner, 1963, p. 473.

Russell, S. J. M.: Blood volume studies in healthy children. Arch. Dis. Child., 24:88, 1949.

Sachtleben, V. P., Lehmann, H., Ruhenstroth-Bauer, G.: Zur Frage der Strukturspezifität der Membranen von Neugeborenen-Erythrozyten. Blut, 7:369, 1961.

Sachs, J. R., Wicker, D. J., Gilcher, R. D., Conrad, M. E., and Cohen, R. J.: Familial hemolytic anemia resulting from an abnormal red blood cell pyruvate kinase. J. Lab. Clin. Med., 72:359, 1968.

Sacker, L. S., Beale, D., Black, A. J., Huntsman, R. G., Lehmann, H., and Lorkin, P. A.: Haemoglobin F Hull, homozygous with haemoglobins O Arab and O Indonesia. Brit. Med. J., 2:531, 1967.

Sacks, J. J., and Labate, J. S.: Dicumarol in the treatment of antenatal thromboembolic disease. Report of a case with hemorrhagic manifestations in the fetus. Am. J. Obst. Gynec., 57:965, 1949.

Sacks, M. O.: Occurrence of anemia and polycythemia in plenotypically dissimilar single ovum human twins. Pediatrics, 24:604, 1959.

Salazar de Sousa, C.: Alterations de la coagulation sanguigne chez le nouveau-né. Pediatrics, 9:787, 1954.

Salzberger, M.: Foetal and adult hemoglobin fractions in dizygotic twins. Exp. Med. Surg., 14:130, 1956.

Salzman, E. W.: Measurement of platelet adhesiveness. J. Lab. Clin. Med., 62:724, 1963.

Sanford, H. N., Gesteyer, T. H., and Wyat, L.: The substances involved in the coagulation of blood of the newborn. Am. J. Dis. Child., 43:58, 1932.

Sansone, G., and Veneziano, G.: Erroneous administration of anti-D gamma-globulin to newborn children. Lancet, 1:952, 1970.

Saragea, T.: Le diamètre des hématies de l'homme aux différents âges de la vie. Compt. Rend. Soc. Biol., 86:312, 1922.

Sass, M. D., and Caruso, C. J.: cited by Spear, P. W., and Sass, M. D.: Some current concepts of red cell metabolism. I. Metabolic processes in red cell. Metabolism, 13:911, 1964.

Sato, T.: The phagocytosis of India ink by leukocytes in premature infants. Nigata Med. J., 73:24, 1959.

Schaar, F. E.: Familial idiopathic thrombocytopenic purpura. J. Pediat., 62:546, 1963.

Schade, H., Schoeller, L., and Schultze, K. W.: D-trisomie (Patau-syndrom) mit kongenitaler myeloescher Leukämie. Med. Welt., 50:2690, 1962.

Schafer, E. L.: Non-lipid reticuloendotheliosis: Letterer-Siwe disease. A report of 3 cases. Am. J. Path., 25:49, 1949.

Schaffer, A. J.: *Diseases of the Newborn.* 1st Ed., Philadelphia, W. B. Saunders, 1960.

SCHÄRER, K., HERZKA, H., and MARTI, H. R.: Kernicterus bei Mangei an Glukose-6-phosphat-Dehydrogenase der Erythrocytes. Helv. Paediat. Acta, *18*:148, 1963.

SCHENKER, J. G., and POLISHUK, W. Z.: Idiopathic thrombocytopenia and pregnancy. Gynaecologia, *165*:271, 1968.

SCHETTINI, F., BRATTA, A., MAUTONE, A., and ZIZZADORO, P.: Acid lysis of red blood cells in normal children. Acta Paediat. Scand., *60*:17, 1971.

SCHEUCH, D., KAHRIG, C., OCKEL, E., WAGENKNECHT, C., and RAPOPORT, S. M.: Role of glutathione and of a self stabilizing chain of SH enzymes and substrates in the metabolic regulation of erythrocytes. Nature, *190*:631, 1961.

SCHIFF, D., ARANDA, J. V., CHAN, G., COLLE, E., and STERN, L.: Metabolic effects of exchange transfusions. I. Effect of citrated and of heparinized blood or glucose, nonesterified fatty acids, 2 -(4 hydroxybenzeneazo) benzoic acid binding, and insulin. J. Pediat., 78:603, 1971.

SCHIFF, D., ARANDA, J. V., COLLE, E., and STERN, L.: Metabolic effects of exchange transfusion. II. Delayed hypoglycemia following exchange transfusion with citrated blood. J. Pediat., 79:589, 1971a.

SCHIFF, D., ARANDA, J. V., and STERN, L.: Neonatal thrombocytopenia and congenital malformations associated with administration of tolbutamide to the mother. J. Pediat., 77:457, 1970.

SCHMID, R., BRECHER, G., and CLEMENS, T.: Familial hemolytic anemia with erythrocyte inclusion bodies and a defect in pigment metabolism. Blood, *14*:991, 1959.

SCHNEIDER, A. S., VALENTINE, W. N., BAUGHAN, M. A., PAGLIA, D. E., SHORE, N. A., and HEINS, H. F., JR.: Triosephosphate isomerase deficiency. A. A multisystem inherited enzyme disorder. Clinical and genetic aspects. In Beutler, E. (ed.): *Hereditary Disorders of Erythrocyte Metabolism.* New York, Grune & Stratton, 1968, p. 265.

SCHNEIDER, A. S., VALENTINE, W. N., HATTORE, M., and HEINS, H. L., JR.: A new erythrocyte enzyme defect with hemolytic anemia-triose phosphate isomerase (TPI) deficiency. New Eng. J. Med., 272:229, 1965.

SCHNEIDER, H. J., and LASCARI, A. D.: Consumption coagulopathy in an infant with Kasabach-Merrit syndrome. Helvet. Paed. Acta, 23:674, 1968.

SCHNEIDER, K. M., BECKER, J. M., and KRASNA, I. H.: Neonatal neuroblastoma. Pediatrics, 36:359, 1965.

SCHNEIDER, R. G., and ARAT, F.: Immunological relationships of various types of haemoglobin. I. Reactions of antisera A, F and Bart's to haemoglobins with various polypeptide chains. Brit. J. Haemat., *10*:15, 1964.

SCHNEIDER, R. G., ARAT, F., and HAGGARD, M. E.: An inhomogeneous foetal haemoglobin variant (Texas type). Nature, 202:1346, 1964.

SCHNEIDER, R. G., and HAGGARD, M. E.: Sickling, a quantitatively delayed genetic character. Proc. Soc. Exp. Biol. Med., 89:196, 1955.

SCHNEIDER, R. G., HAGGARD, M. E., and GUSTAVSON, L. P.: Hemoglobin Bart's in newborns with adult genotypes AA, AS and AC. Blood, 38:796, 1971.

SCHNEIDER, R. G., JONES, R. T., and SUZUKI, K.: Hemoglobin F$_{Houston}$: a fetal variant. Blood, 27:670, 1966.

SCHRIER, S. L., MOORE, L. D., and CHIAPELLA, A. P.: Inhibition of human erythrocyte membrane mediated ATP synthesis by anti-D antibody. Am. J. Med. Sci., 256:340, 1968.

SCHROEDER, W. A., CUA, J. T., MATSUDA, G., and FENNINGER, W. D.: Hemoglobin F$_I$, an acetyl-containing hemoglobin. Biochim. Biophys. Acta, 63:532, 1962.

SCHROEDER, W. A., HUISMAN, T. H. J., BROWN, A. K., UY, R., BOUVER, N. G., LERCH, P. O., SHELTON, J. R., SHELTON, J. B., and APELL, G.: Postnatal changes in the chemical heterogeneity of human fetal hemoglobin. Pediat. Res., 5:493, 1971.

SCHROEDER, W. A., JONES, R. T., SHELTON, J. R., SHELTON, J. B., CORMICK, J., and McCALLA, K.: A partial sequence of the amino acid residues in the γ-chain of human hemoglobin F. Proc. Nat. Acad. Sci., 47:811, 1961.

SCHRÖTER, W.: Kongenitale nicht-sphärocytarocytäre hämolytische Anämie bei 2,3-Diphosphoglyceratmutase-Mangel der Erythrocyten im frühen Säuglingsalter. Klin. Wschr., 43:1147, 1965.

SCHRÖTER, W., and VON HEYDEN, H.: Kinetik des 2,3-diphosphoglyceratumsatzes in menschlichen erythrocyten. Biochem. Ztschr., 341:387, 1965.

SCHRÖTER, W., and WINTER, P.: Der 2,3-diphosphoglyceratsloff-wechsel in den erythrocyten neugeborener und erwachsener. Klin. Wschr., 45:255, 1967.

SCHULER, D., KISS, S., and SIEGLER, J.: About the glycolysis of lymphocytes and granulocytes in infancy and childhood. Ann. Paediat., *198*:279, 1962.

SCHULMAN, I.: Characteristics of the blood in foetal life. In *Oxygen Supply to the Human Fetus*. J. Walker and A. C. Turnbull, eds. Charles C Thomas, Springfield, Ill., 1959, p. 43.

SCHULMAN, I.: Pediatric aspects of the mild hemophilias. Med. Clin. North Am., *46*:93, 1962.

SCHULMAN, I., PIERCE, M., LUKENS, A., and CURRIMBHOY, Z.: Studies on thrombopoiesis. I. A factor in normal human plasma required for platelet production; chronic thrombocytopenia due to its deficiency. Blood, *16*:943, 1960.

SCHULMAN, I., and SMITH, C. H.: Fetal and adult hemoglobins in hemolytic disease of the newborn. Am. J. Dis. Child., 87:167, 1954.

SCHULMAN, I., SMITH, C. H., and ANDO, R. E.: Congenital thrombocytopenic purpura: observations on three infants born of a nonaffected mother; demonstration of platelet agglutinins and evidence for platelet isoimmunization. Am. J. Dis. Child., 88:785, 1954.

SCHULMAN, I., SMITH, C. H., and STERN, G. S.: Studies on the anemia of prematurity. I. Fetal and adult hemoglobin in premature infants. Am. J. Dis. Child., 88:567, 1954.

SCHUMACHER, G. F. B., and SCHNEIDER, J.: Current problems in prophylactic treatment of Rh-erythroblastosis. J. Reprod. Med., 6:67, 1971.

SCHUNK, G. J., and LEHMAN, L. W.: Mongolism and congenital leukemia. J.A.M.A., *155*:250, 1954.

SCHWARTZ, H., and OTTENBERG, R.: The hemorrhagic disease of the newborn, with special reference to blood coagulation and serum treatment. Am. J. Med. Sci., *140*:17, 1910.

SCHWARTZ, S. O., and KOSOVA, L.: Multiple myeloma and normal pregnancy. Blood, *28*:102, 1966.

SCHWARTZ, S. O., and MOTTO, S. A.: The diagnostic significance of "burr" red blood cells. Am. J. Med. Sci., *218*:563, 1949.

SCHWARTZ, J., SURCHIN, H., LUPU, H., and COOPERBERG, A. A.: Severe hypochromic anemia in a newborn due to fetal-maternal transfusion. Can. Med. Assn. Jour., 95:369, 1966.

SCHWEITZER, I. L., and SPEARS, R. L.: Hepatitis-associated antigen (Australia antigen) in mother and infant. New Eng. J. Med., *283*:570, 1970.

SCIALOM, C., NAJEAN, Y., and BERNARD, J.: Anémie hémolytique congénitale non sphérocytaire avec déficit incomplet en 6-phosphogluconate deshydrogénase. Nouv. Rev. Française d'Hémat., 6:452, 1966.

SCOTT, E. M.: The relation of diaphorase of human erythrocytes to inheritance of methemoglobinemia. J. Clin. Invest., *39*:1176, 1960.

SCOTT, J. L., HAUT, A., CARTWRIGHT, G. E., and WINTROBE, M. M.: Congenital hemolytic anemia associated with red cell inclusion bodies, abnormal pigment metabolism and an electrophoretic hemoglobin abnormality. Blood, *16*:1239–52, 1960.

SCOTT, R. B., CRAWFORD, R. P., and JENKINS, M.: Incidence of sicklemia in the newborn Negro infant. Am. J. Dis. Child., 75:842, 1948.

SEELEMANN, K.: Untersuchungen über die Erythropoese beim Neugeborenen und jungen Säugling. Ztschr. Kinderh., 75:189, 1954.

SEIP, M.: The reticulocyte level and the erythrocyte production judged from reticulocyte studies, in newborn infants during the first week of life. Acta Paediat., *44*:355, 1955.

SEIP, M.: Systemic lupus erythematosus in pregnancy with haemolytic anaemia, leucopenia and thrombocytopenia in the mother and her newborn infant. Arch. Dis. Child., *35*:364, 1960.

SELLS, R. L., WALKER, S. A., and OWEN, C. A.: Vitamin K requirement of the newborn infant. Proc. Soc. Exp. Biol. Med., *47*:441, 1941.

SEYFARTH, C., and JURGENS, R.: Untersuchungen über das Verhalten der vitalgranulärten roten Blutzellen (Reticulocyten) bei Embroyonen und Neugeborenen. Arch. Path. Anat., *266*:676, 1928.

SHAHIDI, N. T., and DIAMOND, L. K.: Enzyme deficiency in erythrocytes in congenital non-spherocytic hemolytic anemia. Pediatrics, 24:245, 1959.

SHAPIRO, L. M., and BASSEN, F. A.: Sternal marrow changes during first week of life. Am. J. Med. Sci., 202:341, 1941.

SHAW, S., and OLIVER, R. A.: Congenital hypoplastic thrombocytopenia with skeletal deformities in siblings. Blood, 14:374, 1959.

SHELDON, W. H., and CALDWELL, J. B. H.: The mononuclear cell phase of inflammation in the newborn. Bull. Johns Hopkins Hosp., 113:258, 1963.

SHENKER, S., DAWBER, N. H., and SCHMID, R.: Bilirubin metabolism in the fetus. J. Clin. Invest., 43:32, 1964.

SHEPHERD, M. K., WEATHERALL, D. J., and CONLEY, C. L.: Semi-quantitative estimation of distribution of fetal hemoglobin in red cell populations. Bull. Johns Hopkins, Hosp., 110:293, 1962.

SHERSHOW, L. W., EKERT, H., SWANSON, V. L., WRIGHT, H. T., JR., and GILCHRIST, G. S.: Intravascular coagulation in generalized herpes simplex infection of the newborn. Acta Pediat. Scand., 58:535, 1969.

SHIELDS, G. S., LICHTMAN, H. C., MASSITE, J., and WATSON, R. J.: Studies in sickle cell disease. I. Quantitative aspects of sickling in the newborn period. Pediatrics, 22:309, 1958.

SHOJANIA, A. M., and GROSS, S.: Folic acid deficiency and prematurity. J. Pediat., 64:323, 1964.

SHORLAND, J.: Management of the twin transfusion syndrome. Clin. Pediat., 10:160, 1971.

SHORE, N. A., SCHNEIDER, A. S., and VALENTINE, W. N.: Erythrocyte triosephosphate isomerase deficiency. Prog. Soc. Ped. Res., p. 23, 1965.

SHOWN, T. E., and DURFEE, M. F.: Blueberry muffin baby: neonatal neuroblastoma with subcutaneous metastases. J. Urol., 104:193, 1970.

SHOTT, R. J., ANDREWS, B. F., and THOMAS, P. T.: Maternal and infant serum iron, and total iron binding capacity (TIBC) at birth in a high risk population. Clin. Res. 20:100, 1972.

SHULMAN, N. R.: Immunoreactions involving platelets. I. A steric and kinetic model for formation of a complex from a human antibody, quinidine as a haptene, and platelets; and for fixation of complement by the complex. J. Exp. Med., 107:665, 1958.

SHULMAN, N. R., ASTER, R. H., PEARSON, H. A., and HILLER, M. C.: Immunoreactions involving platelets. VI. Reactions of maternal isoantibodies responsible for neonatal purpura. Differentiation of a second platelet antigen system. J. Clin. Invest., 41:1059, 1962.

SHULMAN, N. R., MARDER, V. J., HILLER, M. C., and COLLIER, E. M.: Platelet and leukocyte isoantigens and their antibodies: serologic, physiologic and clinical studies. Prog. Hemat. 4:222, 1964.

SHWACHMAN, H., DIAMOND, L. K., OSKI, F. A., and KHAW, K. T.: The syndrome of pancreatic insufficiency and bone marrow dysfunction. J. Pediat., 65:645, 1964.

SIDDALL, R. S., and WEST, R. H.: Incision of placenta at caesarean section: cause of fetal anemia. Am. J. Obst. Gynec., 63:425, 1952.

SILVERMAN, W. A., and HOMAN, W. E.: Sepsis of obscure origin in the newborn. Pediatrics, 3:157, 1949.

SILVERSTEIN, M. N., AARO, L. A., and KEMPERS, R. D.: Evans' syndrome and pregnancy. Am. J. Med. Sci., 252:206, 1966.

SILVESTRONI, E., and BIANCO, I.: Haemoglobin Bart's in Italy. Nature, 195:394, 1962.

SILVESTRONI, E., and BIANCO, I.: A new variant of human fetal hemoglobin: Hb F$_{Roma}$. Blood, 22:545, 1963.

SINGER, K., CHERNOFF, A. I., and SINGER, L.: Studies on abnormal hemoglobins. I. Their demonstration in sickle cell anemia and other hematologic disorders by means of alkali denaturation. Blood, 6:413, 1951.

SINISCALCO, M., BERNINI, L., LATTE, B., and MOTULSKY, A. G.: Favism and thalassemia in Sardinia and their relationship to malaria. Nature, 190:1179, 1961.

SIRCHIA, G., FERRONE, S., MERCURIALI, F., and ZANELLA, A.: Red cell acetylcholinesterase activity in autoimmune hemolytic anemias. Brit. J. Haemat., 19:411, 1970.

SISSON, T. R. C.: Blood hemoglobin levels in the neonatal period. Quart. Rev. Pediat., 13:124–30, 1958.

SISSON, T. R. C., and LUND, C. J.: The influence of maternal iron deficiency on the newborn. Am. J. Dis. Child., 94:525, 1957.

SISSON, T. R. C., KENDALL, N., GLAUSER, S. C., KNUTSON, S., and BUNYAVIROCH, E.: Phototherapy of jaundice in newborn infants. I. ABO blood group incompatibility. J. Pediat., 79:904, 1971.

SISSON, T. R. C., LUND, C. J., WHALEN, L. E., and TELEK, A.: The blood volume of infants. I. The full-term infant in the first year of life. J. Pediat., 55:163–179, 1959.

SJÖLIN, S.: The resistance of red cells in vitro. A study of the osmotic properties, the mechanical resistance and the storage behavior of red cells of fetuses, children and adults. Acta Paediat., 43:1, 1954.

SKYBERG, D., and JACOBSEN, C. D.: Defibrination syndrome in a newborn, and its treatment with exchange transfusion. Acta Paediat. Scand., 58:83, 1969.

SMITH, C. A.: The Physiology of the Newborn Infant. 3rd Ed., Springfield, Ill., Charles C Thomas, 1959.

SMITH, C. H.: Blood Diseases of Infancy and Childhood. St. Louis, C. V. Mosby, 1960, p. 478.

SMITH, C. H., SCHULMAN, I., and MORGENTHAU, J. E.: Iron metabolism in infants and children: serum iron and iron-binding protein. Adv. Pediat., 5:195, 1952.

SMITH, D. M.: The No. 18 trisomy and D trisomy syndromes. Ped. Clin. North Am., 10:389, 1963.

SMITH, G. D., and VELLA, F.: Erythrocyte enzyme deficiency in unexplained kernicterus. Lancet, 1:1133, 1960.

SMITH, M. G.: Propagation of a cytopathogenic virus from salivary gland virus disease of infants in tissue cultures. Am. J. Path., 32:641, 1956.

SMITH, R. T., PLATOU, E. S., and GOOD, R. A.: Septicemia of the newborn; current status of the problem. Pediatrics, 17:549, 1956.

SMITHWICK, E. M., and GO, S. C.: Hepatitis-associated antigen in cord and maternal sera. Lancet, 2:1080, 1970.

SOLOMONSON, L., and NYGAARD, K. K.: The prothrombin content in relation to early and late feeding in the newborn. Acta Paediat., 188:207, 1957.

SPENNATI, G. F., ORZALESI, M., and BOTTINI, E.: Stability of acid phosphatase of fetal red blood cells during incubation with acetylphenylhydrazine. Acta Paediat. Scand., 60:192, 1971.

SPIESC, H., and WOLF, H.: Die osmotische Erythrocytenresistenz bei icterus gravis des Neugeborenen und anderen Hyperbilirubinämien. Klin. Wschr., 41:30, 1963.

STAHLIE, T. O. V.: Chronic benign neutropenia in infancy and early childhood. J. Pediat., 48:710, 1956.

STAMATOYANNOPOULOS, G.: Gamma-thalassemia. Lancet, 2:192, 1971.

STAMEY, C. C., and DIAMOND, L. K.: Congenital hemolytic anemia in the newborn. Am. J. Dis. Child., 94:616, 1957.

STAVE, U., and CARA, J.: Adenosinophosphate in Blut Frühgeborener Biol. Neonat., 3:160, 1961.

STAVE, U., and POHL, J.: Altersabhängige Veränderungen von Enzymen der Glykolyse in Erythrocyten. Ztsch. Kinderh., 83:618, 1960.

STEBEL, L., and ODELL, G. B.: UDP glucuronyl transferase in rat liver: genetic variation and maturation. Pediat. Res., 3:351, 1969.

STEFANINI, M., MELE, R. H., and SKINNER, D.: Transitory congenital neutropenia: a new syndrome. Am. J. Med., 25:749, 1958.

STEINBERG, M., BRAUER, M. J., and NECHELES, T. F.: Acute hemolytic anemia associated with erythrocyte glutathione-peroxidase deficiency. Arch. Int. Med., 125:302, 1970.

STEINER, M. L., and PEARSON, H. A.: Bone marrow plasmocyte values in childhood. J. Pediat., 68:562, 1966.

STEINKE, J., GRIES, F. A., and DRISCOLL, S. G.: In vitro studies of insulin inactivation with reference to erythroblastosis fetalis. Blood, 30:359, 1967.

STEVENSON, S. S.: Carbonic anhydrase in newborn infants. J. Clin. Invest., 22:403, 1943.

STEWART, A. G., and BIRKBECK, J. A.: The activities of LDH, transaminase, and G-6-PD in the erythrocytes and plasma of newborn infants. J. Pediat., 61:395–404, 1962.

STOCKER, F., TAMINELLI, F., and deMURALT, G.: Die erythrozyten-azetylcholinesterase als gutes kriterium für die indikation zur austauschtransfusion bei der ABO-hämolyse der neugeborenen. Helvet. Paediat. Acta, 24:448, 1969.

STONE, H. O., THOMPSON, H. K., JR., and SCHMIDT-NIELSEN, K.: Influence of erythrocytes on blood viscosity. Am. J. Physiol., 214:913, 1968.

STORMORKEN, H., and OWREN, P. A.: Physiopathology of hemostasis. Sem. Hemat., 8:3, 1971.

STORMORKEN, H., SVENKERUD, R., SLAGSVOLD, P., LIE, H., and LUNDEVALL, J.: Thrombocytopenic bleedings in young pigs due to maternal isoimmunization. Nature, 198:1116, 1963.

STOUTENBOROUGH, K. A., SUTHERLAND, J. M., MEINEKE, H. A., and LIGHT, I. J.: Erythropoietin levels in cord blood of control infants and infants with respiratory distress syndrome. Acta Paediat. Scand., 58:121, 1969.

STRANSKY, E.: Beiträge zur klinischen Hämatologie en Säuglingsalter. Monataschr. Kinderh., 29:654, 1925.

STRANSKY, E., and SARCIA, S. R.: On neonatal leukemia. Ann. Paediat., 203:68, 1964.

STRAUSS, H.: Clinical pathological conference. J. Pediat., 66:443, 1965.

STRAUSS, H., and OLSON, S. L.: Hemophilia B (Christmas Disease) in a female. Pediatrics, 44:268, 1969.

STRAUSS, L., and DRISCOLL, S. G.: Congenital neuroblastoma involving the placenta. Pediatrics, 34:23, 1964.

STRAUSS, M. B.: Anemia of infancy from maternal iron deficiency in pregnancy. J. Clin. Invest., 12:345, 1933.

STRICKLAND, M., and HU, S. C.: Erythrocyte glucose-6-phosphate dehydrogenase deficiency associated with acute haemolytic anaemia in three Chinese children. Bull. Hong Kong Med. A., 14:81, 1963.

STRÖDER, J.: Über den fibrinstabilisierender Faktor (FSF) in den verschiedenen Lebensabschnitten und bei bestimmten Krankheitendes Kindes. Ann. Paediat., 203:393, 1964.

STUART, R. K., and MICHEL, A.: Monitoring heparin therapy with activated partial thromboplastin time. Canad. Med. Assn. J., 104:385, 1971.

STURGEON, P.: Studies of iron requirements in infants and children. I. Normal values for serum iron, copper and free erythrocyte protoporphyrin. Pediatrics, 13:107, 1954.

STURGEON, P.: Iron metabolism. A review with special consideration of iron requirements during normal infancy. Pediatrics, 18:267, 1956.

STURGEON, P.: Studies of iron requirements in infants. III. Influence of supplemental iron during pregnancy on mother and infant. Brit. J. Haemat., 5:31, 1959.

SUDERMAN, H. J., WHITE, F. D., and ISRAELS, L. G.: Elution of chromium-51 from labelled hemoglobins of human adults and cord blood. Science, 126:650, 1957.

SULLIVAN, J. F., PECKHAM, N. H., and JENNINGS, E. R.: Rh isoimmunization. Its incidence, timing and relationship to fetal-maternal hemorrhage. Am. J. Obs. Gynec., 98:877, 1967.

SUMMERELL, J. M.: Cholelithiasis in the newborn infant in association with congenital toxoplasmosis and hereditary elliptocytosis. J. Pediat., 69:292, 1966.

SUTHERLAND, J. M.: Observations on the relationships between drug therapy and neonatal jaundice. Ann. N. Y. Acad. Sci., 111:461, 1963.

SUTHERLAND, J. M., GLUECK, H. I., and GLESER, G.: Hemorrhagic disease of the newborn. Breast feeding as a necessary factor in the pathogenesis. Am. J. Dis. Child., 113:524, 1967.

SUTTON, R. L.: Periadenitis mucosa necrotica recurrens. J. Cut. Dis., 29:65–71, 1911.

SUVANSRI, U., CHEUNG, W. H., and SAWITSKY, A.: The effect of bilirubin on the human platelet. J. Pediat., 74:240, 1969.

SVANE, S.: Foetal exsanguination from hemangioendothelioma of the skin. Acta Paed. Scand., 55:536, 1966.

SZEINBERG, A., GAVENDO, S., and CAHANE, D.: Erythrocyte adenylate-kinase deficiency. Lancet, 1:315, 1969.

SWIERCZEWSKI, P. E., GIBELIN, C., and MINKOWSKI, A.: Glutathion dans les globules rouges de la veine Vombilecale: comparaison avec le glutathion dans les globules rouges de la femme enceinte. Biol. Neonat., 3:321, 1961.

SZEINBERG, A., and MARKS, P. A.: Substances stimulating glucose catabolism by the oxidative reactions of the pentose phosphate pathway in human erythrocytes. J. Clin. Invest., 40:914, 1961.

SZEINBERG, A., OLIVER, M., SCHMIDT, R., ADAM, A., and SHEBA, C.: Glucose-6-phosphate dehydrogenase deficiency and hemolytic disease of the newborn in Israel. Arch. Dis. Child., 38:23, 1963.

SZEINBERG, A., RAMOT, B., SHEBA, C., ADAM, A., HALBRECHT, I., RIKOVER, M., WISH-NIEVSKY, S., and RABAU, E.: Glutathione metabolism in cord and newborn infant blood. J. Clin. Invest., 37:1436, 1958.

TADA, K. R., and WATANABE, Y.: Anemia of premature infant: the glucose-6-phosphate dehydrogenase activity in erythrocytes of cord blood from premature and full term infants. Tohoku J. Exp. Med., 76:307–12, 1962.

TAJ-ELDIN, S.: Favism in breast-fed infants. Arch. Dis. Childh. 46:121, 1971.

TANAKA, K. R., and VALENTINE, W. N.: Pyruvate kinase deficiency. In Beutler, E. (ed.): *Hereditary Disorders of Erythrocyte Metabolism.* New York, Grune & Stratton, 1968, p. 229.

TANAKA, K. R., VALENTINE, W. N., and MIWA, S.: Pyruvate kinase (PK) deficiency hereditary non-spherocytic hemolytic anemia. Blood, 19:267, 1962.

TARLOV, A. R., BREWER, G. J., CARSON, P. E., and ALVING, A. S.: Primaquine sensitivity. Arch. Int. Med., 109:137, 1962.

TARUI, S., KONO, N., NASU, T., and NISHIKAWA, M.: Enzymatic basis for the coexistence of myopathy and hemolytic disease in inherited muscle phosphofructokinase deficiency. Biochem. Biophys. Res. Commun., 34:77, 1969.

TAYLOR, A. I.: 13-15 Trisomy in arrhinencephaly. Lancet, 1:149, 1966.

TAYLOR, F. M., and GEPPERT, L. J.: Congenital myelogenous leukemia. A.M.A. Am. J. Dis. Child., 80:417, 1950.

TAYLOR, P. M., BRIGHT, N. H., and BIRCHARD, E. L.: Effect of early versus delayed clamping of the umbilical cord on the clinical condition of the newborn infant. Am. J. Obst. Gynec., 86:893, 1963.

THATCHER, L. G., CLATANOFF, D. V., and THIEM, E. R.: Splenic hemangioma with thrombocytopenia and afibrinogenemia. J. Pediat., 73:345, 1968.

THOMAIDIS, T., AGATHOPOULOS, A., and MATSANIOTIS, N.: Natural isohemagglutin production by the fetus. J. Pediat., 74:39, 1969.

THOMAS, D. B., and YOFFEY, J. M.: Human foetal haematopoiesis. I. The cellular composition of foetal blood. Brit. J. Haemat., 8:290, 1962.

THOMAS, D. B., and YOFFEY, J. M.: Human foetal haematopoiesis. II. Hepatic haematopoiesis in the human foetus. Brit. J. Haemat., 10:193, 1964.

THOMAS, E. D., LOCHTE, H. L., JR., GREENOUGH, W. B., and WALES, M.: In vitro synthesis of foetal and adult haemoglobin by foetal haematopoietic tissues. Nature, 185:396, 1960.

THUMASATHIT, B., NONDASUTA, A., SILPISORNKOSOL, S., LOUSUEBSAKUL, B., UN-CHALIPONGSE, P., and MANGKORNKANOK, M.: Hydrops fetalis associated with Bart's hemoglobin in northern Thailand. J. Pediat., 73:132, 1968.

THOMPSON, E. N., and SHERLOCK, S.: The aetiology of portal vein thrombosis with particular reference to the role of infection and exchange transfusion. Quart. J. Med., 33:465, 1964.

THOMPSON, R. B., WARRINGTON, R. L., ODOM, J., and BELL, W. N.: A naturally occurring foetal haemoglobin hybrid. Nature, 209:721, 1966.

THOMPSON, W. P.: Observations on a possible relation between agranulocytosis and menstruation with further studies on case of cyclic neutropenia. New Eng. J. Med., 210:176, 1934.

TODD, D., LAI, M., and BRAGA, C. A.: Thalassaemia and hydrops fetalis—family studies. Brit. Med. J., 11:347, 1967.

TODD, D., LAI, M. C. S., BEAVEN, G. H., and HUEHNS, E. R.: The abnormal haemoglobins in homozygous α-thalassemia. Brit. J. Haemat., 19:27, 1970.

TODD, D., LAI, M. C. S., BRAGA, C. A., and SOO, H. N.: Alpha-thalassaemia in Chinese: cord blood studies. Brit. J. Haemat., 16:551, 1969.

TOIVANEN, P., and HIRVONEN, T.: Iso- and heteroagglutinins in human fetal and neonatal sera. Scand. J. Haemat., 6:42, 1969.

TOIVANEN. P., and HIRVONEN, T.: Fetal development of red cell antigens K, k, Lu^a, Lu^b, Fy^a, Fy^b, Vel and Xg^a. Scand. J. Haemat., 6:49, 1969.

TOLAND, O. J., MANN, H. J., and HELSEL, C. M.: Haematoma of the umbilical cord: a case report. Obstet. Gynec., 14:799, 1959.

TORREY, W. E.: Vasa previa. Am. J. Obst. Gynec., 63:146, 1952.

TOWNSEND, C. W.: The hemorrhagic disease of the newborn. Arch. Pediat., 11:559, 1894.

TRAVIS, S. F., MORRISON, A. D., CLEMENTS, R. S., JR., WINEGRAD, A. I., and OSKI, F. A.: Metabolic alterations in the human erythrocyte produced by increases in glucose concentration. The role of the polyol pathway. J. Clin. Invest., 50:2104, 1971.

TROLLE, D.: Decrease of total serum bilirubin concentration in newborn infants after phenobarbitone treatment. Lancet, 2:705, 1968b.

TROLLE, D.: Phenobarbitone and neonatal icterus. Lancet, 1:251, 1968a.

TRUCCO, J. T., and BROWN, A. K.: Neonatal manifestations of hereditary spherocytosis. Am. J. Dis. Child., 113:263, 1967.

TUCHINDA, S., VAREENIL, C., BHANCHIT, P., and MINNICH, V.: 'Fast' hemoglobin component found in umbilical cord blood of Thai babies. Pediatrics, 24:43, 1959.

TÜDÖS, E., and KISS, P.: Über den Einflub des Wismuts auf das Blutbild. Jb. Kinderh., 11:219, 1926.

TUFFY, P., BROWN, A. K., and ZUELZER, W. W.: Infantile pyknocytosis: common erythrocyte abnormality of the first trimester. Am. J. Dis. Child., 98:227, 1959.

TUNICLIFFE, R.: Observations on anti-infectious power of blood of infants. J. Infect. Dis., 7:698, 1910.

TURNER, G. C., FIELD, A. M., LASHEEN, R. M., TODD, R. M., WHITE, G. B. B., and PORTER, A. A.: SH (Australia) antigen in early life. Arch. Dis. Childh. 46:616, 1971.

UNDRITZ, E.: Das Pelger-Huetsche Blutbid beim Tier und seine Bedeutung fur die Entwicklungs Geschichte des Blutes. Schweiz. Med. Wschr., 69:1177, 1939.

USHER, R., and LIND, J.: Blood volume of the newborn premature infant. Acta Paediat. Scand., 54:419, 1965.

USHER, R., SHEPARD, M., and LIND, J.: The blood volume of the newborn infant and placental transfusion. Acta Paediat., 52:497–512, 1963.

VAHLQUIST, B.: Das Serumeisen. Eine pädiatrischklinische und experimentelle Studie. Acta Paediat., 28:1, 1941.

VAHLQUIST, B.: Cyclic agranulocytosis. Acta Med. Scand., 170:531, 1946.

VALAES, T.: Bilirubin and red cell metabolism in relation to neonatal jaundice. Postgrad. Med. J., 45:86, 1969.

VALAES, T., KARAKLIS, A., STRAVRAKAKIS, D., BAVELA-STRAVRAKAKIS, K., PERAKIS, A., and DOXIADIS, S. A.: Incidence and mechanism of neonatal jaundice related to glucose-6-phosphate dehydrogenase deficiency. Pediat. Res., 3:448, 1969.

VALENTINE, W. N., HSIEH, H. S., PAGLIA, D. E., ANDERSON, H. M., BAUGHAN, M. A., JAFFÉ, E. R., and GARSON, O. M.: Hereditary hemolytic anemia associated with phosphoglycerate kinase deficiency in erythrocytes and leukocytes. A probable x-chromosome-linked syndrome. New Eng. J. Med., 280:528, 1969.

VALENTINE, W. N., OSKI, F. A., PAGLIA, D. E., BAUGHAN, M. A., SCHNEIDER, A. S., and NAIMAN, J. L.: Hereditary hemolytic anemia with hexokinase deficiency. Role of hexokinase in erythrocyte aging. New Eng. J. Med., 276:1, 1967.

VALENTINE, W. N., TANAKA, K. R., and MIWA, S.: Specific erythrocyte glycolytic enzyme defect (pyruvate kinase) in three subjects with congenital non-spherocytic hemolytic anemia. Tr. Ass. Am. Phys., 74:100, 1961.

VAN BAELEN, H., VANDEPITTE, J., and EECKELS, R.: Observations on sickle-cell anaemia and haemoglobin Bart's in Congolese neonates. Ann. Soc. belge Méd. trop., 49:157, 1969.

VAN CREVELD, S.: Morbus haemorrhagicus neonatorum. Mederl. Tijdochr. Geneesk., 101:2109, 1957.

VAN CREVELD, S., BAKER, H., NIESSING, T., SIPKEMA, J. J., and SMITS, C. A. A. M.: Thromboplastin formation in the blood of the newborn infant. II. Étud. Néo-natal., 3:217, 1954.

VAN CREVELD, S., NAGEL, C. G. M., NIJINKIUS, J. H., MIRANDA, S. I., and KIE, T. S.: Thromboplastin formation in the blood of the newborn. I. Étud. Néo-natal., 3:135, 1954.

VAN CREVELD, S., PAULSSEN, M. M. P., ENS, J. C., MEIJ, C. A. M., VERSTEEG, P., and VERSTEGH, E. T. B.: Proconvertin content in blood of newborn full-term and premature infants. Étud. Néo-natal., 3:53, 1954.

VAN EYS, J., and FLEXNER, J. M.: Transient spontaneous remission in a case of untreated congenital leukemia. Am. J. Dis. Child., 118:507, 1969.

VAN PRAAGH, R.: Diagnosis of kernicterus in the neonatal period. Pediatrics, 28:870, 1961.

VARADI, S., and HURWORTH, E.: Heinz-body anemia in the newborn. Brit. Med. J., 1:315, 1957.

VAUGHAN, V. C. III, ALLEN, F. H., JR., and DIAMOND, L. K.: Erythroblastosis fetalis. IV. Further observations on kernicterus. Pediatrics, 6:706, 1950.

VEIGA, S., and VAITHIANATHAN, T.: Massive intravascular sickling after exchange transfusion with sickle cell trait blood. Transfusion, 3:387, 1963.

VELLA, F.: Fast foetal haemoglobin in Khartoum. E. Afr. Med. J., 40:9, 1963.

VELLA, F., AGER, J. A. M., and LEHMANN, H.: New variant of human foetal haemoglobin. Nature, 183:31, 1959.

VENTRUTO, V.: Electrophoretic study of incidence of Bart's haemoglobin in cord blood. Pediatria, 70:245, 1962.

VEST, M.: Physiologu v. Pathologie des neugeborinicterus. Bibl. Paediat., Fasc. 69, 1959.

VEST, M., and GRIEDER, H.: Erythrocyte survival in the newborn infant, as measured by chromium-51 and its relation to the postnatal serum bilirubin level. J. Pediat., 59:194, 1961.

VESTERMARK, B., and VESTERMARK, S.: Familial sex-linked thrombocytopenia. Acta Paediat., 53:365, 1964.

VIDYASAGAR, D.: Birthweight in haemolytic disease of newborn. Arch. Dis. Childh., 46:113, 1971.

VIGIL, J., WARBURTON, S., HAYNES, W. S., and KAISER, L. R.: Nitrates in municipal water supply cause methemoglobinemia in infant. Pub. Health Rep., 80:1119, 1965.

VOAK, D., and WILLIAMS, M. A.: An explanation of the failure of the direct antiglobulin test to detect erythrocyte sensitization in ABO hemolytic disease of the newborn and observations on pinocytosis of IgG anti-A antibodies by infant (cord) red cells. Brit. J. Haemat., 20:9, 1971.

VOIGHT, J. C., and BRITT, R. P.: Feto-maternal haemorrhage in therapeutic abortion. Brit. Med. J., 4:395, 1969.

VON FELTEN, A., and STRAUB, P. W.: Coagulation studies of cord blood, with special reference to "fetal fibrinogen". Thrombos. Diathes. Haemorrh., 22:274, 1969.

VON GILARDI, A., and MIESCHER, P.: Die Lebensdauer von autologen und homologen Erythrocyten bei frühgeborenen und ältersen Kindern. Schweiz. Med. Wschr., 87:1456, 1957.

VON SYDOW, G.: Hypoprotrombinemi och hjärnsda hos barn till dikumarinbehandlad moder. Nord. Med., 34:1171, 1947.

VOS, G. H.: The frequency of ABO-incompatible combinations in relation to maternal Rhesus antibody values in Rh immunized women. Am. J. Hum. Genet., 17:202, 1965.

VULLO, C., and TUNIOLI, A. M.: Ittero neonatale con defetto transitorio della glucoseo-6-fosfato deidrogenasi eritrocitaria. Pediatria, 69:327, 1961.

WACKSMAN, S. J., FLESSA, H. C., GLUECK, H. I., and WILL, J.: Coagulation defects and giant cavernous hemangioma. Am. J. Dis. Child., 111:71, 1966.

WAGNER, H. P., and SMITH, N. J.: A study of detoxification mechanisms in children with aplastic anemia. Blood, 19:676, 1962.

WAGNER, H. P., TONZ, O., and GREYERZ-GLOOR, R. D. V.: Congenital lymphoid leukaemia. Case report with chromosomal studies. Helv. Paediat. Acta, 23:591, 1968.

WAGNER, R.: The estimation of glycogen in whole blood and white blood cells. Arch. Biochem., 11:249, 1946.

WALKER, J. L., and TURNBULL, E. P. N.: Haemoglobin and red cells in the human fetus and their relation to the oxygen content of the blood in the vessels of the umbilical cord. Lancet, 2:312, 1953.

WALKER, J. L., and TURNBULL, E. P. N.: Haemoglobin and red cells in the human foetus. III. Foetal and adult haemoglobin. Arch. Dis. Child., 30:111, 1955.

WALKER, W.: Role of liquor examination in Rh haemolytic disease: recent advances in Rh isoimmunization prevention, ed. Finn, R. Brit. Med. J., 2:219, 1970.

WALKER, W., and ELLIS, M. I.: Intrauterine transfusion, in Rh haemolytic disease, recent advances in Rh isoimmunization prevention, ed. Finn, R. Brit. Med. J., 2:219, 1970.

WALLER, H. D.: Glutathione reductase deficiency. In Beutler, E. (ed.): Hereditary Disorders of Erythrocyte Metabolism. New York, Grune & Stratton, 1968, p. 185.

WALLERSTEIN, R. O.: Spontaneous involution of giant hemangioma. Simultaneous regression of tumor and thrombocytopenia in a newborn. Am. J. Dis. Child., 102:233, 1961.

WALSH, R. J., REYE, R. D. K., and STAPLETON, T.: Polycythaemia and hepatitis in a newborn. Arch. Dis. Child., 37:425, 1962.

WALTERS, T. R., and HOLDER, T. M.: Neonatal hyperbilirubinemia and renal vein thrombosis. Amer. J. Dis. Child., III: 433, 1966.

WALZER, S., GERALD, P. S., BREAU, G., O'NEILL, D., and DIAMOND, L. K.: Hematologic changes in the D_1 trisomy syndrome. Pediatrics, 38:419, 1966.

WANG, M. Y. F. W., and DESFORGES, J. F.: Complement in ABO-hemolytic disease of the newborn. Pediat., 48:650, 1971.

WASHBURN, A. H.: Blood cells in healthy young infants; study of 608 differential leukocyte counts, with final report on 908 total leukocyte counts. Am. J. Dis. Child., 50:413, 1935.

WASHBURN, A. H.: Plasma cells in the circulation in infants and children. Am. J. Dis. Child., 113:633, 1967.

WATERBURY, L., and FRENKEL, E. P.: Phosphofructokinase deficiency in congenital nonspherocytic hemolytic anemia. Clin. Res., 17:347, 1969.

WATERS, W. J.: The reserve albumin binding capacity as a criterion for exchange transfusion. J. Pediat., 70:185, 1967.

WATERS, W. J., and PORTER, E. G.: Dye-binding capacity of serum albumin in hemolytic disease of newborn. Am. J. Dis. Child., 102:807, 1961.

WATERS, W. J., and PORTER, E. G.: Indications for exchange transfusion based upon the role of albumin in the treatment of hemolytic disease of the newborn. Pediatrics, 33:749, 1964.

WATSON, D.: The absorption of bilirubin by erythrocytes. Clin. Chim. Acta, 7:733, 1962.

WATSON, R. J.: The significance of the paucity of sickle cells in newborn Negro infants. Am. J. Med. Sci., 215:419, 1948.

WAUGH, T. F., MERCHANT, F. T., and MAUGHAM, G. B.: Blood studies on newborn; determination of hemoglobin, volume of packed red cells, reticulocytes and fragility of erythrocytes over 9 day period. Am. J. Med. Sci., 198:646, 1939.

WEATHERALL, D. J.: Enzyme deficiency in haemolytic disease of the newborn. Lancet, 2:835, 1960.

WEATHERALL, D. J.: Abnormal haemoglobins in the neonatal period and their relationship to thalassemia. Brit. J. Haemat., 9:265, 1963.

WEED, R. I., LACELLE, P. L., and MERRILL, E. W.: Metabolic dependence of red cell deformability. J. Clin. Invest., 48:795, 1969.

WEGELIUS, R.: On changes in peripheral blood picture of newborn infant immediately after birth. Acta Paediat., 35:1, 1948.

WEGELIUS, R., VÄÄNÄNEN, I., and KOSKELA, S.: Down's syndrome and transient leukemia-like disease in a newborn. Acta Paediat. Scand., 56:301, 1967.

WEINBERGER, M. M., and OLEINICK, A.: Congenital marrow dysfunction in Down's syndrome. J. Pediat., 77:273, 1970.

WEINBERGER, M. M., and OLEINICK, A.: Neonatal polycythemia. Clin. Res., 29:209, 1971.

WEINER, A. S.: Diagnosis and treatment of anemia of the newborn caused by occult placental hemorrhage. Am. J. Obst. Gynec., 56:717, 1948.

WEINER, W., and WINGHAM, J.: Rhesus-immunized mothers and direct-Coombs-test-negative babies. Lancet, 2:85, 1966.

WEISERT, O., and MARSTRANDER, J.: Severe anaemia in a newborn caused by protracted feto-maternal "transfusion." Acta Paediat., 49:426, 1960.

WEISS, H. J.: Hereditary elliptocytosis with hemolytic anemia. Am. J. Med., 35:455, 1963.

WEISS, H. J., ALEDORT, L. M., and KOCHWA, S.: Effect of salicylates on hemostatic properties of platelets in man. J. Clin. Invest., 47:2169, 1968.

WELLER, S. D. V., APLEY, J., RAPER, A. B.: Malformations associated with precocious synthesis of adult hemoglobin—a new chromosomal anomaly syndrome. Lancet, 1:777, 1966.

WELLER, T. H., and HANSHAW, J. B.: Virologic and clinical observations on cytomegalic inclusion disease. New Eng. J. Med., 266:1233, 1962.

WELLER, T. H., MACAULEY, J. C., CRAIG, J. M., and WIRTH, P.: Isolation of intranuclear inclusion producing agents from infants with illness resembling cytomegalic inclusion disease. Proc. Soc. Exp. Biol. Med., 92:4, 1957.

WHAUN, J. M., and OSKI, F. A.: Characteristics of red cell phosphofructokinase (PFK). Studies of erythrocytes from newborn infants and adults. Clin. Res., 17:603, 1969.

WHAUN, J., and OSKI, F. A.: Red cell stromal adenosine triphosphatase (ATPase) of newborn infants. Pediat. Res., 3:105, 1969.

WHAUN, J. M., and OSKI, F. A.: Relation of red cell glutathione peroxidase to neonatal jaundice. J. Pediat., 76:555, 1970.

WHAUN, J. M., URMSON, J., and OSKI, F. A.: One year's experience with disseminated intravascular coagulation in a children's hospital. Program Am. Ped. Soc., p. 6, 1971.

WHIPPLE. G. H.: Hemorrhagic disease, antithrombin and prothrombin factors. Arch. Int. Med., 12:637, 1913.

WHISSELL, D. Y., HOAG, M. S., AGGELER, P. M., KROPATKIN, M., and GARNER. E.: Hemophilia in a woman. Am. J. Med., 38:119, 1965.

WHITAKER, J. A., SARTAIN, P., and SHAHEEDY, M.: Hematological aspects of congenital syphilis. J. Pediat., 66:629, 1965.

WHITTAM, R.: Transport and Diffusion in Red Blood Cells. London, Edward Arnold, 1964.

WIDDOWSON, E. M., and SPRAY, C. M.: Chemical development in utero. Arch. Dis. Child., 26:205, 1951.

WILSON, J. D., and NOSSAL, G. J. V.: Identification of human T and B lymphocytes in normal peripheral blood and in chronic lymphocytic leukemia. Lancet, 2:788, 1971.

WILSON, J. T.: Phenobarbital in the perinatal period. Pediatrics, 43:324, 1969.

WILSON, M. G., SCHROEDER, W. A., and GRAVES, D. A.: Postnatal change of hemoglobins F and A_2 in infants with Down's syndrome (G trisomy). Pediatrics, 42:349, 1968.

WILSON, M. G., SCHROEDER, W. A., GRAVES, D. A., and KACH, V. D.: Hemoglobin variations in D-trisomy syndrome. New Eng. J. Med., 277:953, 1967.

WINTROBE, M. M.: Clinical Hematology. 5th Ed., Philadelphia, Lea & Febiger, 1961, p. 32.

WINTROBE, M. M., and SHUMACKER, H. B., JR.: Comparison of hematopoiesis in the fetus and during recovery from pernicious anemia. J. Clin. Invest., 14:837, 1935.

WITT, I., MULLER, H., and KUNZER, W.: Vergleichende biochemische untersuchungen an erythrocyten aus neugeborenen und erwachsenen blut. Klin. Wschr., 45:262, 1967.

WITT. I., MÜLLER, H., and KÜNZER, W.: Evidence for the existence of foetal fibrinogen. Thrombos. Diathes. Haemorrh., 22:101, 1969.

WÖHLER, F.: Intermediary iron metabolism of the placenta, with special consideration of the transport of therapeutically administered iron through this organ. Curr. Ther. Res., 6:464, 1964.

WOLFF, J. A., GROSSMAN, B. H., and PAYA, K.: Neonatal serum bilirubin and glucose-6-phosphate dehydrogenase. Relationship of various perinatal factors to hyperbilirubinemia. Amer. J. Dis. Child., 113:255, 1967.

WOOD, B., COMLEY, A., and SHERWELL, J.: Effect of additional albumin administration during exchange transfusion on plasma albumin-binding capacity. Arch. Dis. Childh., 45:59, 1970.

WOOD, J. L.: Plethora in the newborn infant associated cyanosis and convulsions. J. Pediat., 54:143, 1959.

WOODROW, J. C., BOWLEY, C. C., GULLIVER, B. E., and STRONG, S. J.: Prevention of Rh immunization due to large volumes of Rh-positive blood. Brit. Med. J., 1:148, 1968.

WOODROW, J. C., and DONOHUE, W. T. A.: Rh-immunization by pregnancy: results of a survey and their relevance to prophylactic therapy. Brit. Med. J., 4:139, 1968.

WOODRUFF, C. W., and BRIDGEFORTH, E. B.: Relationship between the hemogram of the infant and that of the mother during pregnancy. Pediatrics, 12:681, 1953.

WOODRUFF, P.: Behavior of blood platelets in thyrotoxicosis. Med. J. Aust., 2:190, 1940.

WOO WANG, M. Y. F., McCUTCHEON, E., and DESFORGES, J. F.: Fetomaternal hemorrhage from diagnostic transabdominal amniocentesis. Am. J. Obst. Gynec., 97: 1123, 1967.

WRANNE, L.: Studies on erythrokinetics in infancy. Acta Paediat. Scand., 56:381, 1967.

WYANDT, H., BANCROFT, P. M., and WINSHIP, T. O.: Elliptic erythrocytes in man. Arch. Int. Med., 68:1043, 1941.

WYATT, J. P., SAXTON, J., LEE, R. S., and PINKERTON, H.: Generalized cytomegalic inclusion disease. J. Pediat., 36:271, 1950.

XANTHOU, M.: Leucocyte blood picture in healthy full-term and premature babies during neonatal period. Arch. Dis. Childh., 45:242, 1970.

YAO, A. C., MOINIAN, M., and LIND, J.: Distribution of blood between infant and placenta after birth. Lancet, 2:871, 1969.

YAO, A. C., LIND, J., TIISALA, R., and MICHELSSON, K.: Placental transfusion in the premature infant with observation on clinical course and outcome. Acta Paediat. Scand., 58:561, 1969.

YAO, A. C., HIRVENSALO, M., and LIND, J.: Placental transfusion rate and uterine contraction. Lancet, 1:380, 1968.

YAO, A. C., WIST, A., and LIND, J.: The blood volume of the newborn infant delivered by caesarean section. Acta Paediat. Scand., 56:585, 1967.

YOSHIDA, A.: Human glucose-6-phosphate dehydrogenase. Purification and characteristics of Negro type variant (A$^+$) and comparison with normal enzyme (B$^+$). Biochem. Genet., 1:81, 1967.

YOUNKIN, S., OSKI, F. A., and BARNESS, L. A.: Observations on the mechanism of the hydrogen peroxide hemolysis test and its reversal with phenols. Am. J. Clin. Nutr., 24:7, 1971.

YOUNG, L. E.: Hereditary spherocytosis. Am. J. Med., 18:486, 1955.

ZACHAU-CHRISTIANSEN, B., HOFF-JORGENSEN, E., and KRISTENSEN, H. P.: The relative haemoglobin, iron, vitamin B$_{12}$, and folic acid values in the blood of mothers and their newborn infants. Dan. Med. Bull., 9:157, 1962.

ZAIDI, Z. H., and MORTIMER, P. E.: Congenital thyrotoxicosis with hepatosplenomegaly and thrombocytopenia, associated with aniridia and dislocated lenses. Proc. Roy. Soc. Med., 58:390, 1965.

ZAIZOV, R., COHEN, I., and MATOTH, Y.: Thrombasthenia: A study of two siblings. Acta Paediat. Scand., 57:522, 1968.

ZANNOS-MARIOLEA, L., KATTAMIS, C., and PAIDOUCES, M.: Infantile pyknocytosis and glucose-6-phosphate dehydrogenase deficiency. Brit. J. Haemat., 8:258, 1962.

ZANNOS-MARIOLEA, L., THOMAIDES, T., GEORGIZAS, G., GAVRIELIDOU, E., and BENETOS, S.: Diagnostic problems in severe neonatal jaundice and G6PD deficiency in Greece. Arch. Dis. Childh., 43:36, 1968.

ZARKOWSKY, H. S., OSKI, F. A., SHÁAFI, R., SHOHET, S. B., and NATHAN, D. G.: Congenital hemolytic anemia with high sodium, low potassium red cells. I. Studies of membrane permeability. New Eng. J. Med., 278:593, 1968.

ZILLIACUS, H., and OTTELIN, A.-M.: Haemoglobins in the blood of human embryos. Biol. Neonat., 11:389, 1964.

ZINKHAM, W. H.: An in-vitro abnormality of glutathione metabolism in erythrocytes from normal newborns: mechanism and clinical significance. Pediatrics, 23:18, 1959.

ZINKHAM, W. H.: Peripheral blood and bilirubin values in normal full-term primaquine sensitive Negro infants: effects of vitamin K. Pediatrics, 31:983, 1963.

ZINKHAM, W. H., and CHILDS, B.: Effect of vitamin K and naphthalene metabolism on glutathione metabolism of erythrocytes from normal newborns and patients with naphthalene hemolytic anemia. Am. J. Dis. Child., 94:420, 1957.

ZINKHAM, W. H., and CHILDS, B.: A defect of glutathione metabolism in erythrocytes from patients with naphthalene-induced hemolytic anemia. Pediatrics, 22:461, 1958.

ZINKHAM, W. H., and MEDEARIS, D. N.: Blood and bone marrow picture in congenital rubella (abstract). J. Pediat., 67:985, 1965.

ZINKHAM, W. H., MEDEARIS, D. N., and OSBORN, J. E.: Blood and bone marrow findings in congenital rubella. J. Pediat., 71:512, 1967.

ZIPURSKY, A.: The erythrocytes of the newborn infant. Semin. Hematol., 2:167, 1965.

ZIPURSKY, A., HULL, A., WHITE, F. D., and ISRAELS, L. G.: Foetal erythrocytes in the maternal circulation. Lancet, 1:451, 1959.

ZIPURSKY, A., and ISRAELS, L. G.: The pathogenesis and prevention of Rh immunization. Canad. Med. Assoc. J., 97:1245, 1967.

ZIPURSKY, A., LaRUE, T., and ISRAELS, L. G.: The in vitro metabolism of erythrocytes from newborn infants. Canad. J. Biochem., 38:727, 1960.

ZIPURSKY, A., POLLOCK, J., CHOWN, B., and ISRAELS, L. G.: Transplacental foetal haemorrhage after placental injury during delivery or amniocentesis. Lancet, 2:493, 1963.

ZIPURSKY, A., POLLOCK, J., NEELANDS, P., CHOWN, B., and ISRAELS, L. G.: The transplacental passage of foetal red blood cells and the pathogenesis of Rh immunisation during pregnancy. Lancet, 2:489, 1963.

ZIPURSKY, A., ROWLAND, M., FORD, J. D., HAWORTH, J. C., and ISRAELS, L. G.: Erythrocyte metabolism in galactosemia. Pediatrics, 35:126, 1965.

ZUELZER, W. W.: Serological diagnosis and principles of management of ABO hemolytic disease. Sixth International Congress of the International Society of Hematology, Boston, 1956.

ZUELZER, W. W., and BAJOGHLI, M.: Chronic granulocytopenia in childhood. Blood, 23:359, 1964.

ZUELZER, W. W., and COHEN, F.: ABO hemolytic disease and heterospecific pregnancy. Ped. Clin. North Am., 4:405, 1957.

ZUELZER, W. W., and STULBERG, C. S.: Herpes simplex virus as the cause of fulminating visceral disease and hepatitis in infancy. Am. J. Dis. Child., 83:421, 1952.

ZUELZER, W. W., MASTRANGELO, R., STULBERG, C. S., POULIK, M. D., PAGE, R. H., and THOMPSON, R. I.: Autoimmune hemolytic anemia. Natural history and viral-immunologic interactions in childhood. Am. J. Med., 49:80, 1970.

ZUSSMAN, W. V., KHAN, A., and SHAYESTEH, P.: Congenital leukemia: Report of a case with chromosome abnormalities. Cancer, 20:1227, 1967.

Index